BIOLOGICAL BASIS OF GERIATRIC ONCOLOGY

edited by

LODOVICO BALDUCCI, MD
Professor of Oncology and Medicine
University of South Florida College of Medicine
Program Leader, Senior Adult Oncology Program
H. Lee Moffitt Cancer Center & Research Institute
Tampa, Florida, USA

MARTINE EXTERMANN, MD, PhD
Associate Professor of Oncology and Medicine
University of South Florida College of Medicine
Senior Adult Oncology Program
H. Lee Moffitt Cancer Center & Research Institute
Tampa, Florida, USA

Springer

Lodovico Balducci, MD
University of South Florida
College of Medicine
H. Lee Moffitt Cancer Center
and Research Institute
12902 Magnolia Drive
Tampa, FL 33612
USA
balducci@moffitt.usf.edu

Martine Extermann, MD, PhD
University of South Florida
College of Medicine
H. Lee Moffitt Cancer Center
and Research Institute
12902 Magnolia Drive
Tampa, FL 33612
USA
extermann@moffitt.usf.edu

Biological Basis of Geriatric Oncology

Library of Congress Cataloging-in-Publication Data

A C.I.P. Catalogue record for this book is available
from the Library of Congress.

ISBN 0-387-23961-8 e-ISBN 0-387-23962-6 Printed on acid-free paper.

Printed in the United States of America.

9 8 7 6 5 4 3 2 1 SPIN 11052470

springeronline.com

CONTENTS

FOREWORD

The population of Western countries is aging, and cancer in older aged persons is becoming increasingly common. The management of these neoplasms is a novel problem. Direct information on the outcome of cancer prevention and of cytotoxic chemotherapy in older individuals is scarce, especially for those aged 80 and over, and it is not clear whether the same process should direct medical decisions in younger and older persons. It is reasonable to assume that the benefits of cancer prevention and treatment diminish and the dangers increase with age. The expected gains from cancer treatment may be lessened by shorter life expectancy. The risk of therapeutic complications may be increased and the consequences of these complications may become more serious due to limited functional reserve of multiple organ-systems, and fading social support and economic resources. In addition, the biology of cancer may change with the age of the patient, due to a series of events that have been clarified only in part. For example, the prevalence of Multidrug Resistance in Acute Myelogenous Leukemia is much higher for patients over 60, which make the treatment less effective and the risk of treatment-related deaths higher. At the same time, the risk of local recurrence of breast cancer after partial mastectomy declines with age, indicating a more indolent disease.

Several publications, including books, review articles and original studies, related to cancer in the elderly have appeared during the last ten years and have highlighted important points that have become widely accepted:

- Age by itself is not and should never be a contraindication to cancer management, including prevention and treatment.
- The management of cancer in the older person should be individualized according to individual life expectancy, treatment tolerance, and risk of experiencing the complications of cancer including death, disability, and discomfort.

- A number of simple provisions may ameliorate the complications of cytotoxic chemotherapy and allow the administration of full doses of treatment. These provisions include prophylaxis of neutropenic infections, avoidance of severe anemia, timely management of mucositis, and provision of adequate home care giving.

The practical application of these directions remains somehow controversial however, as the methods to estimate life expectancy, functional reserve, and tumor behavior are poorly defined. The main goal of this book is to provide a simple blueprint enabling the practitioners of oncology, geriatrics, and primary care to decide when a patient may or may not benefit from cancer prevention and treatment. Based on the current knowledge of the biology of aging and cancer, the books examines several facets of patient assessment, including function, comorbidity, physical performance and laboratory tests, as well as the way these different forms of assessment may be integrated in medical decisions. At the meantime, the book explores future possibilities for understanding the interaction of aging and cancer biology and for predicting these interactions, and provides a rationale for clinical trials of chemoprevention of cancer in the older person by unraveling the mechanisms that associate aging and carcinogenesis. Some of these mechanisms, including the genomic changes of age, are predictable, while others, including proliferative senescence, are counter-intuitive, and open new, unsuspected opportunities for intervention. Aware of the rapid evolution of the field, we wanted for this book to become an expandable and adaptable frame of reference, able to accommodate new information and still able to direct the practitioner in the management of older individuals even when the current information will be outdated. The emphasis on current research directions in the biology of aging, of cancer, and of the hemopoietic system that is intimately connected to the management of cancer, should make the reader attuned to new developments and allow the reader to rapidly incorporate these developments into clinical thinking.

Another important goal of this book is to highlight the important lessons coming from the study of aging that may be collapsed into two points:

- To a large extent, the study of aging involves a movement from the bedside to the bench, which is directly opposed to the current trend of oncology. As underlined in the initial chapter, epidemiology is the main clue to the biological interactions of cancer and aging: epidemiology and clinical observation are still the main source for experimental hypothesis.
- Due to the scarcity of information, the study of geriatric oncology requires acceptance of some degree of uncertainty. In clinical practice this involves attention to unexpected and unpredictable occurrences; in clinical trials this involves readiness to accommodate a number of unknown parameters.

The best opportunity for real progresses in the field may come from the integration of these points in clinical practice and clinical research.

The third and final goal of this book is to provide an updated and practical research handbook for the increasingly large host of young investigators who want to become involved in the field. The need for such handbook is revealed by a number of recent initiatives aimed to promote research in geriatric oncology. Among them we would like to highlight the issuance of a RFA for program grants in geriatric oncology by a combined NCI/NIA effort, and the institution of a number of fellowships in geriatric oncology through a grant of the Hartford Foundation to the American Society of Clinical Oncology.

In addition to all excellent collaborators of the book, we would like to thank the numerous friends and colleagues who have been engaged with us in this adventure of geriatric oncology during the last ten years, and in particular, we would like to acknowledge the leadership of Rosemary Yancik, Ph.D., who single-handedly generated the field more than two decades ago, and the members of the Senior Adult Oncology Program at the H. Lee Moffitt Cancer Center, to whom this book is dedicated.

Lodovico Balducci M.D.

Martine Extermann M.D. Ph.D.

Chapter 1

EPIDEMIOLOGY OF CANCER AND AGING

Lodovico Balducci and Matti Aapro

Lodovico Balducci, Program Leader, Senior Adult Oncology Program, H. Lee Moffitt Cancer Center and Research Institute, Tampa, Florida, Professor of Oncology and Medicine, University of South Florida College of Medicine, Tampa, Florida. Matti Aapro, Director, Multidisciplinary Oncology Institute, Clinique de Genolier, Switzerland.

Epidemiology provides the initial clue to causes and mechanisms of diseases. It is well known that age is a risk factor for most common cancer and that incidence and prevalence of cancer increase with age[1]. In this chapter we explore the epidemiology of cancer and aging, in an attempt to understand the biologic interactions of these processes. In particular, we address the following questions:

1. Does aging enhance the susceptibility of older individuals to environmental carcinogens?
2. Is aging associated with increased risk of multiple malignancies?
3. Does the clinical behavior of cancer change with age?
4. Does cancer increase the risk of death of older individuals?

In conclusion we will examine the clinical implications of these questions and propose a research agenda aimed to improve the control of cancer in the older aged person.

1. AGE AND CARCINOGENESIS

The incidence of common cancers increases with age (Figure 1). This association is universal [2] and is observed with the aging of any population around the world. A clear explanation of this phenomenon is the time-length of carcinogenesis, a stepwise process involving the activation of cellular oncogenes, and the suppression of anti-proliferative genes (anti-oncogenes) [3]. It is reasonable to assume that the duration of carcinogenesis reflects the number of stages involved in the pathogenesis of different tumors, and that this number be highest for tumors whose incidence peaks late in life, such as adenocarcinoma of the prostate and of the large bowel, or non-melanomatous skin cancer [3]. In the era of chemoprevention and recognition and elimination of environmental carcinogens, an alternative possibility should be considered. These interventions may cause the prolongation of one or more carcinogenic steps and, in so doing; they may delay the development of cancer. For example, the incidence of lung cancer has decreased for individuals less than 60, while it has increased for older individuals [4]. As a result, the peak incidence of lung cancer has become more and more delayed. Interestingly, these changes have paralleled the incidence of smoking cessation in the Western population. In this case it is reasonable to assume that the length of carcinogenesis has increased as a result of a prolongation of the late carcinogenic stages, from reduced intensity of exposure to tobacco smoke [3]. If this hypothesis is correct, one may expect to see a progressive delay in the appearance of common cancer and an increased incidence of neoplasia in advanced ages.

Figure 1. The incidence of common cancers increases with age.

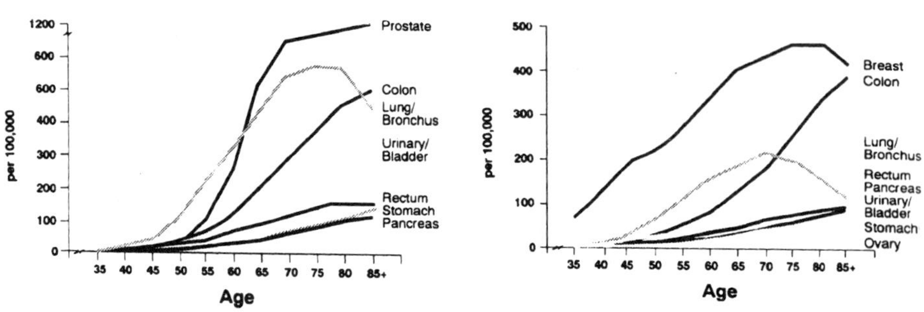

The duration of carcinogenesis may not account completely for association of cancer and aging. . The incidence of some neoplasms, such as prostate and non-melanomatous skin cancer increases more rapidly with age, than it would be expected from the time-length of carcinogenesis alone [3]. These findings suggest that the concentration of cells in advanced carcinogenic stages increases with the age of an organism, enhancing the susceptibility of older individuals to environmental carcinogens [3]. This possibility is supported by a host of studies of experimental carcinogenesis, summarized in another chapter of this book [3] and also by epidemiologic observations [5-9]. Barbone et al reported the risk of lung cancer after exposure to an environmental pollutant in the Italian city of Trieste increased with the age of the subject at the time of exposure [6]. Since 1970, the incidence of non-Hodgkin's lymphoma has increased 80% for individuals 60 and over, and that of malignant brain tumors seven fold (or 700%) for individuals 70 and older [8, 9]. It is tempting to infer that older individuals develop cancer after exposure to new environmental carcinogens earlier than the younger ones, because of increased susceptibility to these substances. In other words, older subjects may represent a natural monitoring system for new carcinogens. Unfortunately this hypothesis may have proven true, at least in the case of brain tumors, as the incidence of these neoplasms is now increasing also for individuals aged 50 and older [8].

For completeness, other biological changes of aging, beside advanced carcinogenesis, may favor the development of cancer. Immune-senescence may facilitate the growth of highly immunogenic tumors [10], while proliferative senescence may result in loss of cellular apoptosis, and the production of tumor growth factors and proteolytic enzymes that promote the growth and the spreading of cancer respectively [11].

Does the incidence of cancer increase indefinitely with age? The answer to these question as become highly relevant with the progressive aging of the Western population and with the expansion of the oldest segment of the population (those 85 and older), that is increasing more rapidly than any other segment. [12]. The observations of Stanta et al, who performed more than 350 autopsies of individuals aged 95 and older and in more than 100 aged 100 and older suggest that beyond a certain age the incidence of cancer might decrease [13]. These authors reported that not only the incidence of cancer as cause of death and the incidence of clinical cancer, but also the incidence of occult cancer decreased after age 95. Of interest, the decline in cancer was associated with increased incidence of sarcopenia, and atrophy of multiple tissues, which suggest that at the upper extreme of age the anabolic processes are reduced to an extent that they cannot support the rapid growth of neoplastic tissues. An alternative possibility is that genes involved in longevity may also be involved in protection from cancer.

2. AGE AND MULTIPLE NEOPLASMS

As aging is a risk factor for cancer, it is reasonable to ask whether the incidence of multiple primary malignancies is more common in older persons and in particular whether an aging phenotype of increased cancer risk may be defined. The recognition of such phenotype would have important practical consequences, which include the ability to target certain individuals for cancer prevention and new insight in the molecular pathogenesis of cancer. Luciani and Balducci have considered two alternative hypotheses (Figure 2) [14]. According to both hypotheses the incidence of multiple primary malignancies increases with age. In model A this increment reflects only the general risk of cancer associated with aging, whereas in model B previous history of cancer is itself a risk factor for new neoplasms. Model B implies an aging phenotype associated with increased risk of multiple malignancies. After review of the literature, the authors concluded that model A was more likely that model B. Absolute conclusions are not possible, however, due to the limitation of existing data (Table 1).
Universal consensus is wanted for the definition of multiple primary malignancies. In the majority of study series the definition of Warren and Gates has been utilized [15]. This implies the fulfillment of two conditions: each tumor must present an independent clinical and pathologic picture and the possibility that one neoplasm be a metastasis of the other should be excluded. A number of serious limitations related to this definition are self-evident. First, it fails to distinguish between clinically relevant and irrelevant neoplasms as it is based on autopsy studies. Second it fails to address the issues related to multifocal tumors occurring in the same organ, that are defined by two questions: how can it be established that multifocal tumors are distinct tumors; and should multifocal tumors be considered multiple primary malignancies.

The development of multifocal tumors is a consequence of "field carcinogenesis " implying that the same tissue may give origin to multiple neoplasms, as the whole tissue has been exposed to the same carcinogen for the same duration of time [16]. The development of multiple tumors in breast, large bowel, head and neck and bronchus support this theory [16]. The distinction of different tumors arising from the same organ may be problematic. The recognition of histologic differences (for example squamous cell carcinoma, adenocarcinoma or neuro-endocrine tumors) is by itself not a definitive proof of distinction, as it is well known that the same

Figure 2. Alternative hypotheses on the increased incidence of multiple primary malignancies with age [14]. Model A reflects only the general risk of cancer associated with aging. Model B implies an aging phenotype associated with increased risk of multiple malignancies.

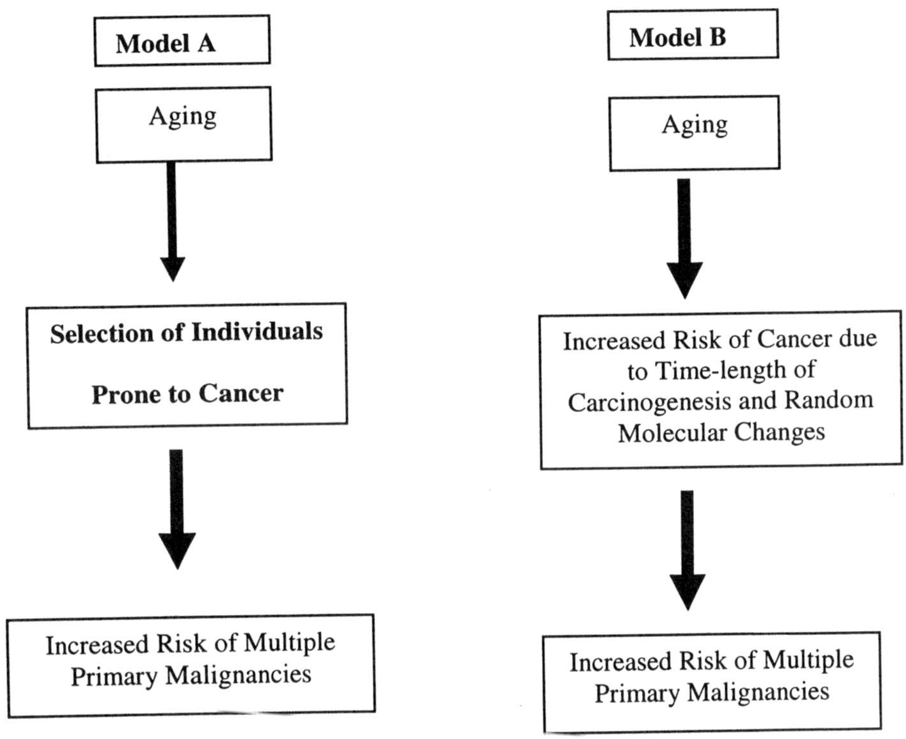

Table 1. Methodological difficulties related to the diagnosis of multiple primary malignancies

- Definition
- Clinical and pathologic recognition
- Influence of previous cancer treatment
- Selection bias
- Limitation of existing sources of data
- Tumor registries
- Autopsy series

epithelial stem cell can give origin to different neoplastic phenotypes [14]. Mortel proposed that two tumors arising in the same tissue be considered independent when the tissue separating the two neoplasms does not show neoplastic infiltration [17]. Though helpful, this criterion appears inadequate on two accounts: it relies on the correctness of individual observations, and it excludes the possibility of surface metastases.

Last but not least, there is an age-specific problem related to the association of age with multiple primary malignancies. This involves the decision whether one should consider that age at which the first or the subsequent tumors did occur. Conceptually, it appears reasonable to consider affected by age-related multiple primary malignancies only those patients whose first cancer was diagnosed during adulthood, but we recognize that this proposal only shifts the problem to the definition of adulthood.

One common problem in the definition of multiple primary malignancies is whether the subsequent neoplasms are metastases of the initial one. This difference can be established with absolute certainty only when the tissue of origin of the original and subsequent tumor is different (for example epithelial and mesenchymal neoplasms). Electron microscopy and immune-histochemistry have also helped to identify tumors of origin from different tissues [14]. In the case of some tumors, specific characteristics, such as the presence of hormone receptors in breast cancer allow establishing whether a tumor occurring in different organs is a metastasis of the original neoplasm.

The treatment of cancer may be itself a cause of new cancer, and enhance the risk of a second malignancy in patients who have received antineoplastic treatment. The association of acute myelogenous leukemia with cytotoxic chemotherapy [18] is well known. Cervical cancer has been associated with an increased risk of cancer of the bladder, small intestine, ovary, bones, and of multiple myeloma, but only in patients who had been treated with radiation therapy [19].

A number of selection biases may convey the impression that multiple primary malignancies after diagnosis of an initial cancer. Undoubtedly, patients with a diagnosis of cancer do receive more diagnostic tests, to stage the initial cancer and to establish the presence of recurrences. These tests may reveal concomitant occult malignancies. For example, staging of non-Hodgkin's lymphoma led to the diagnosis of a number of unsuspected renal cell carcinomas [14]. In addition to these diagnostic biases, there is a survival bias. That is the patients who survive the first cancer are more likely to carry the diagnosis of subsequent cancers as a consequence of the fact that they live longer [14]. Though not properly a "selection bias" another source of error may be the changing incidence of certain malignancies with time. For example, non-Hodgkin's lymphoma appeared more common in patients with previous diagnosis of renal cell carcinoma, before it was realized that this association reflected the increased incidence of lymphoma in the general population during that period of time [20].

The main source of information on multiple primary malignancies is tumor registries and autopsy studies. Tumor registry studies are cohort studies, whose value varies with the quality of the registry as well as with the quality of cancer care provided during the time covered by the registry. For example, studies performed during a time when women received routine mammographic screening are more likely to demonstrate the association of breast cancer with other malignancies, because breast cancer was diagnosed at an earlier stage and associated with a more prolonged survival. In general tumor registry studies showed that the risk of second malignancies increased with the duration of survival since the diagnosis of the initial neoplasm [14]. Autopsy studies are by there own nature selective, as they depend on the ability of physicians to obtain autopsy and on the willingness of patients' family to allow the procedure. These cross-sectional studies showed that the prevalence of multiple malignancies increased with the patient's age, but it was consistent with the general risk of cancer for that age [14]. In conclusion, both autopsy and registry studies demonstrated that the diagnosis of multiple primary malignancy was more likely in patients of advanced age, but age was not a risk factor for increased risk of multiple primary malignancies. These studies favored model B over model A in figure 1. It should be noticed that increased likelihood of association was found between certain types of cancer including smoking related cancer [16], papillary cancer of the kidney and cancer of the bladder and of the prostate [21], and breast and uterine cancer [22]. The latter was observed only in women aged 70 and older.

The increased possibility of multiple primary malignancies in older individuals has important clinical consequences:

- The development of a new lesion in patients with history of cancer should be investigated to rule out the possibility of a new and curable malignancy and should not be dismissed as a recurrence off the previous cancer. .
- Previous history of cancer should not prevent aggressive treatment of new cancer. It is not unusual for an older individual to carry a diagnosis of two or more primary malignancies, all of which have been curable.

3. AGE AND NATURAL HISTORY OF CANCER

It is well established that the biology of some malignancies may change with the age of the patient due to at least two underlying mechanisms (Table 2). One may think metaphorically of the tumor as a plant, whose growth is affected by changes in the seed (the neoplastic cell) and the soil (the aging tumor host). In the case of AML the seed is responsible for reduced responsiveness to chemotherapy and decreased likelihood of complete remission after chemotherapy-induced marrow aplasia [23]. A possible explanation for the worse prognosis of NHL in the aged [24] include the fact that aging is associated with increased circulating concentrations of IL-6 [25] one of the most powerful lymphatic growth factors [26]. Both seed and soil may conspire in making breast cancer a more indolent disease in older women: the prevalence of slowly proliferating [27], hormone-responsive tumors increase with the age of the patient, while endocrine senescence and, paradoxically, immune senescence may disfavor its growth. The role of immune senescence has been revealed in a couple of studies showing that the

Table 2. Age and behavior of common malignancies.

Tumor	Change in behavior
Acute myelogenous leukemia (AML)	Less responsive to chemotherapy after age 60 due to higher prevalence of Multi Drug Resistance (MDR). Less likely to yield remission after marrow aplasia, because the pluripotent hemopoietic stem cell may be involved by the disease The course of the disease may be more indolent than in older individuals due to higher prevalence of "smoldering acute leukemia" and "hypoplastic acute leukemia"
Non-Hodgkin's lymphoma, low and intermediate grade	Age may be associated with decreased response rate to chemotherapy and decreased remission duration. The worst prognosis may be due to increased circulating concentrations of Inteleukin-6 in older individuals
Breast Cancer	Diagnosed at more advanced stage in older women. Growth rate appears lower and may be due to a combination of factors, including higher prevalence of slow-growing, hormone-responsive tumors, endocrine senescence and immune senescence
Lung cancer, non small cell	More likely to be diagnosed at an early stage after age 70 Slower growth rate after age 70 Mechanism of change unknown
Ovarian cancer	Prognosis is worse with age, irrespective of stage and of treatment; mechanism unknown
Cancer of the large bowel	No clear relation between age and tumor behavior

growth of primary breast cancer was inversely related to the degree of mononuclear cell infiltration [10, 28], suggesting that these cells produce a cytokine promoting neoplastic growth. The statement that breast cancer becomes more indolent with age contrasts with some reports that age over 75 is associated with more advanced disease and reduced survival [29-31]. The contradiction may be only apparent, as the worst prognosis in women aged 75 and older may reflect lesser utilization of mammographic screening and of adjuvant treatment, and increased risk of mortality from comorbid conditions. Several lines of evidence suggest that breast cancer becomes more indolent with age including reduced risk of life-threatening hepatic and lymphangitic lung metastases, and reduced local recurrence rate after partial mastectomy [32-36].

In the case of non-small cell lung cancer a more indolent course is suggested by reports from different centers that lung cancer presented at an earlier stage in older than in younger individuals [37-39]. These reports may be fraught a referral bias, however, as only older patients with resectable tumors might have been referred to the centers for treatment. It is possible that lung cancer after age 70 involved preferentially ex-smokers, in whom reduced exposure to tobacco smoke resulted in more indolent tumors. While several studies have shown that age is associated with decreased treatment response and survival in women with ovarian cancer, the mechanism of this change has not been clarified [40].

The study of the natural history of cancer relies mainly on old reports, of questionable methodology, as in the last twenty years the majority of cancer patients have received some form of antinoplastic treatment. From a clinical standpoint the critical question is whether there are circumstances in which the management of cancer in older individuals may cause worse complications than the neoplasm itself. Clearly, the natural history of cancer is only one aspect of this decision that involves also the life expectancy and the functional reserve of individual patients [41, 42]. In addition is important to notice that major advances in cancer treatment may have minimized the risk of complications. These include more limited surgery, safer general anesthesia, laser surgery, cryosurgery, radiofrequency tumor ablation, radiosurgery, brachytherapy, conformal field radiation therapy, low dose weakly chemotherapy, and antidotes to chemotherapy-related toxicity, such as hemopoietic growth factors, and targeted therapy. In general, the same treatment of cancer that is beneficial to younger patients appears beneficial to the older ones, albeit to a lesser extent. Though the risk of local recurrence after partial mastectomy decreases with age, radiation therapy improves the chance of breast preservation even for older women [43]. Adjuvant hormonal therapy reduces the risk of breast cancer recurrence and death for women younger than 50 and older than 70 [44], while adjuvant chemotherapy may be beneficial to older post-menopausal women [45]. Likewise, age does not seem to reduce the benefits of adjuvant chemotherapy in patients with stage III cancer of the large bowel [46]. The only situations in which the natural history of cancer may suggest to forgo the use of antineoplastic treatment include smoldering AML and early stage prostate cancer in man aged 70 and older. Though smoldering acute leukemia is an obsolete term, this definition may still be helpful to encompass two conditions: hypoplastic acute leukemia, that is AML with a marrow cellularity lower than 10% and AML associated with Myelodysplasia, with a percentage of blasts in the bone marrow between 20 and 30%, that does not undergo any significant change over three months. In both cases the predominant clinical picture is pancytopenia, the incidence of leukostasis is negligible, cytotoxic chemotherapy is associated with low therapeutic response and high risk of early mortality, while supportive treatment with transfusion of blood products and possible erythropoietin may allow months of quality survival [47]. The value of local treatment of early prostate cancer in patients aged 70 and over has been debated [48]. A study in which patients aged 60 to 75 were randomized to observation and radical prostatectomy demonstrated that surgery was associated with decreased risk of prostate cancer-related deaths, but not overall survival benefits [49, 50].

4. PROFILE OF THE OLDER CANCER PATIENT

Aging is associated with reduced functional reserve of multiple organ systems, increased prevalence of comorbidity, memory disorders, depression, malnutrition, polypharmacy and functional dependence [51]. It is legitimate to ask whether these conditions may interfere with the treatment of cancer and may reduce the patient's life expectancy and tolerance of treatment to the point that treatment is futile or even harmful.

In three studies, cancer patients aged 70 and older had undergone a comprehensive geriatric assessment prior to the institution of treatment, with similar conclusions [52-54]. Some form of functional dependence was present in up to 70% of patients, some form of comorbidity in up to 90%, depression, malnutrition and memory disorders in approximately 20% and polypharmacy in 40%. . A review of the Surveillance, Epidemiology and End Results (SEER) data also revealed that some form of comorbidity was present in the majority of cancer patients aged 65 and older [55]. These studies show the benefits of a comprehensive evaluation of older individuals that allows an estimate of life expectancy and tolerance of treatment, recognition of conditions that should be reversed prior to treatment and the utilization of a common language in the definition of older individuals [56]. As a result of these studies should be highlighted the need to adjust the doses of chemotherapy to the renal function of older individuals, to investigate anemia, that is a risk factor for mortality, functional dependence, and chemotherapy related toxicity, the management of depression, and the provision of a home caregiver in patients at risk to develop functional dependence during cancer treatment.

Another series of study compared the survival and the general function of older cancer patients with that of individuals of same age without cancer. Diab et al review the SEER breast cancer experience and showed that for women aged 75 and older breast cancer was not associated with a change in survival. Unexpectedly, breast cancer was associated with a more prolonged survival in women aged 80 and older. This observation suggests that breast cancer may affect preferentially women in best general condition, who might have lived even longer if they had not developed breast cancer [57]. This hypothesis is supported by two other studies. Repetto et al compared functional dependence and comorbidity of patients 65 and older with and without cancer admitted to two general hospitals in Italy and found that cancer patients had lower prevalence of both conditions [58]. In a retrospective study of the population of Cusumano, Italy, Ferrucci demonstrated that patients who developed cancer had the highest degree of function and the lowest of comorbidity [59]. Similar conclusions were drawn by Stanta et al from autopsy studies of elderly persons with and without cancer [13].

It is reasonable to surmise that cancer is preferentially a disease of healthy elderly individuals and that the treatment of cancer in these individuals may result in prolongation of survival and quality of life improvement.

CONCLUSIONS

A review of the epidemiology of cancer and age allows concludes:

- Age is a risk factor both for cancer and carcinogenesis, at least up to age 95;
- Multiple primary malignancies are more common in older individuals. In many case each of these neoplasms is amenable to cure or life-prolonging treatment. Possible exceptions include localized low grade prostate cancer in men aged 70 plus and smoldering acute leukemia

- The biological behavior of cancer may be altered with age: in some cases the neoplasm may become more resistant to chemotherapy, in other cases more aggressive and in other cases more indolent;

- Cancer is prevalently a disease of healthy elderly individuals whose life expectancy and quality of life may be compromised by cancer.

REFERENCES

1. Yancik RM, Ries LAG: Aging and cancer in America. Demographic and epidemiologic perspectives. Hematol/Oncol Clin N Am 2000, 14, 17-23
2. LaVecchia C, Lucchini F, Negri E et al: Cancer mortality in the elderly, 1960-1998: a worldwide approach. Oncology Spectrums, 2001, 2, 386-394
3. Anisimov VN: Biological interactions of aging and carcinogenesis. In Balducci L, Extermann M: Biological Basis of Geriatric Oncology
4. Wingo PA; Cardinez CJ; Landis SH et al: Trends in cancer mortality in the United States, 1930-1998. Cancer, 2003, 97, 3133-3275
5. Glass AG, Hoover RH: The emerging epidemics of melanoma and squamous cell cancer. JAMA, 1989, 262, 2097-2100
6. Barbone S, Bovenzi M, Cavallieri F et al: Air pollution and lung cancer in Trieste, Italy. Am J Epidemiol, 1995, 141, 1161-1169
7. Halpern MT, Gillespie BW, Warner KE: Patterns of absolute risk of lung cancer mortality in former smokers. J Natl Cancer Inst, 1993,17, 457-464
8. Jukich PJ, McCarthy BJ, Surawicz TS et al: Trends in incidence of primary brain tumors in the United States, 1985-1994. Neuro-Oncology, 2001, 3, 141-151
9. O'Reilly SE, Connors JM, Klasa R, et al: Malignant lymphomas in the elderly. Clin Ger Med, 1997,13, 251-263
10. Kurtz JM; Jacquemier J, Amalric R, et al: Why are local recurrences after breast cancer conserving surgery more frequent in younger patients? J Clin Oncol, 1990, 10, 141-152
11. Hornsby PJ: Replicative senescence and cancer. In Balducci L, Extermann M: Biological Basis of Geriatric Oncology, 2004
12. Day JC. Population projections in the United States by age, sex, race, and Hispanic origin: 1995-2050. Washington DC, US Bureau of the Census, Current Population Reports, 1996, 25, 1130
13. Stanta G, Campagner L, Cavallieri F, et al: Cancer in the oldest old: what we have learned from autopsy studies. Clin Ger Med, 1997, 13, 55-68
14. Luciani A, Balducci L: Multiple primary malignancies. Sem Oncol, 2004, in press
15. Warren S, Gates O. Multiple primary malignant tumors: a survey of the literature and statistical study. Am J Cancer 1932, 16: 1358-1414
16. Begg CB, Zhanfg Z-F, Sun M, et al: Methodology for evaluating the incidence of second primary cancers with application of smoking-related cancers from the Surveillance, Epidemiology and End-Results (SEER) program. Am J Epidemiol, 1995, 142, 653-664
17. Moertel CG: Multiple primary malignant neoplasms: historical perspectives. Cancer, 1977, 40, 1786- 1792

18. Pedersen-Bjergaard J, Philip B, Olesen Larsen S, et al: Therapy-related myelodysplasia and acute myeloid leukemia. Cytogenetic characteristics of 115 consecutive cases and risk in seven cohorts of patients treated intensely for malignant diseases in the Copenhagen series. Leukemia, 1990, 7, 1975-1980
19. Boice TH, Day NE, Andersen A, et al: Second cancers following radiation treatment for cervical cancer: International Collaboration Among Cancer Registries. JNCI monograph, 1985, 74, 955- 975
20. Anderson CM; Pusztai L; Palmer JL, et al: Coincident renal cell carcinoma and non-Hodgkin's lymphoma: M.D. Anderson Experience and review of the literature. J Uro, 1998, 159, 714-717
21. Rabbani , Grimaldi G, Russo P: Multiple primary malignancies in renal cell carcinoma. J Urol, 1998, 160,1255-1259
22. Adami H-O, Bergkvist L, Krusemo UB, et al: Breast cancer as a risk factor of other primary malignant diseases. A nationwide cohort study. J Natl Cancer Inst, 1984,73, 1049-1055
23. Lancet JE, Willman CL, Bennett JM: Acute myelogenous leukemia and aging. Hematol Oncol Clin N Am, 2000, 14, 251-267
24. The International Non-Hodgkin's Lymphoma Prognostic Factors Project: A predictive model for aggressive non-Hodgkin's lymphoma. N Engl J med, 1993, 329, 987-994
25. Wilson CJ, Cohen HJ, Pieper CF: Cross-linked fibrin degradation products (D-Dimer), plasma cytokines, and cognitive decline in community dwelling elderly persons. J Am Ger Soc, 2003, 51, 1374-1381
26. Preti HA, Cabanillas F, Talpaz M, et al: Prognostic value of serum interleukin-6 in diffuse large-cell lymphoma. Ann Intern med, 1997, 127, 186-194
27. Balducci L, Silliman RA, Diaz N: Breast cancer in the older woman: the oncologist viewpoint. In Balducci L, Lyman GH, Ershler WB: Comprehensive Geriatric Oncology, Harwood Academic Publishers, Amsterdam, 2004
28. Nixon AJ, Neuberg D, Hayes DF, et al: Relationship of patients age to pathologic features of the tumor and prognosis for patients with stage I or II breast cancer. J Clin Oncol, 1994, 12, 888-894
29. Adami HO, Malker B, Holmberg L, et al: The relation between survival and age at diagnosis in breast cancer. N Engl J med, 1986, 315, 559-563
30. Greenfield S, Blanco DM, Elashoff RM, Ganz PA: Patterns of care related to age of breast cancer patients, JAMA, 1987, 257, 2766-2770
31. Yancik R, Ries LG, Yates JW: Breast cancer in aging women. A population based study of contrasts in stage, surgery, and survival. Cancer, 1989, 63, 976-981
32. Holmes FF: Clinical course of cancer in the elderly. Cancer Control, 1994, 1, 108-114
33. Ershler WB: Tumors and aging: the influence of age-associated immune changes upon tumor growth and spread. Adv Exp Med Biol, 1993,330, 77-92
34. Daidone MG, Luisi A, Silvestrini R, Di Fronzo G: Biologic characteristics of primary breast cancer in the elderly. Comprehensive Geriatric Oncology. L. Balducci, G.H. Lyman, W.B. Ershler. Harwood Academic Publishers, London, pp. 197-200, 1998
35. Veronesi U, Luini A, Del Vecchio M, et al : Radiotherapy after breast preserving surgery in women with localized cancer of the breast. N Engl J Med, 1993, 328, 1587-1591
36. Holmberg L, Lindgren A, Norden T, et al: Age as a determinant of axillary node involvement in invasive breast cancer. Acta Oncol, 1992, 31, 533-538
37. Goodwin JS, Samet JM, Key CR, et al: Stage at diagnosis of cancer varies with the age of the patient. J Am Ger Soc, 1986, 34, 20-26
38. DeMaria LC, Cohen HJ: Characteristics of lung cancer in elderly patients. J Gerontol, 1987, 42, 540-545

39. Guadagnoli E, Weitberg A, Mor V, et al: The influence of patient age on the diagnosis and treatment of lung and colorectal cancer. Arch Intern med, 1990, 150, 1485-1490
40. Thigpen T: Gynecological cancer in the elderly. In Balducci L, Lyman GH, Ershler WB: Comprehensive Geriatric Oncology, Harwood Academic Publishers, Amsterdam, 2004
41. Extermann M, Balducci L, Lyman G: What threshold for adjuvant tamoxifen in older breast cancer patients? A decision analysis. European Journal of Cancer 34(suppl 1):S40, 1998
42. Walter LC, Brand RJ, Counsell RS, et al: Development and validation of a prognostic index for one year mortality in older adults after hospitalization. JAMA 2001, 285,2987-2993
43. Morrow M, Harris JR, Schnitt SJ: Local control following breast cancer conserving surgery: results of clinical trials. J Natl Cancer Inst, 1995, 87, 1669-1673
44. Early Breast Cancer Trialists' Collaborative Group: Tamoxifen for early breast cancer: an overview of the randomized trials. Lancet 351:1451-1467, 1998
45. Early breast cancer Trialists' Collaborative Group: Polychemotherapy for early breast cancer; an overview of the randomised trials. Lancet, 1998, 352, 930-942
46. Sargent DJ, Goldberg RM, Jacobson SD, et al: A pooled analysis of adjuvant chemotherapy for resected colon cancer in elderly patients. N Engl J med, 2001, 345, 1091-1097
47. Vergilio JA, Bagg A: Myelodysplastic syndromes. Contemporary biologic concepts and emerging diagnostic approaches. Am J Clin Pathol, 2003, 119, s58-77
48. Chodak GW, Thisted RA, Gerber GS, et al: Results of conservative management of clinically localized prostate cancer. N Engl J med, 1994, 230, 242-248
49. Holmberg L, Bill-Axelson A, Hegelsen F, et al: A randomized trial comparing radical prostatectomy with watchful waiting in early prostate cancer. N Engl J med, 2002, 347, 781-789
50. Steineck G, Helgesen F, Adolfsson J, et al: Quality of life after radical prostatectomy or watchful waiting. N Engl J med, 2002, 347, 790-796
51. Ferrucci L: Clinical and Biological evaluation of aging. In Balducci L, Extermann M: Biological Basis of Geriatric Oncology, 2004
52. Extermann M, Overcash J, Lyman GH, et al: Comorbidity and functional status are independent in older cancer patients. J Clin Oncol, 1998, 16, 1582-1587
53. Repetto L, Fratino L, Audisio RA, et al: Comprehensive geriatric assessment adds information to the Eastern Cooperative Group performance status in elderly cancer patients. An Italian Group for Geriatric Oncology Study. J Clin Oncol, 2002, 20, 494-502
54. Ingram SS, Seo PH, Martell RE, et al: Comprehensive assessment of the elderly cancer patient: the feasibility of self-report methodology. J Clin Oncol, 2002, 20, 770-775
55. Yancik R, Ganz P, Varricchio CG, et al: Perspectives on comorbidity and cancer in older patients: approaches to expand the knowledge base. J Clin Oncol, 2001, 19, 1147-1151
56. Balducci L: Guidelines for the management of the older cancer patients. NCCN Journal, in press
57. Diab SG, Elledge RM, Clark GM: Tumor characteristics and clinical outcome of elderly women with breast cancer. J Natl Cancer Inst, 2000, 92, 550-556

58. Repetto L, Granetto C, Venturino A, et al: Prognostic evaluation of the older cancer patient. In Balducci L, Lyman GH, Ershler WB: Comprehensive Geriatric Oncology, Harwood Academic Publishers, Amsterdam, 1998, 281-286
59. Ferrrucci L: In Chianti. Invecchiare nel Chianti. Pacini Editore, Pisa, 2002

Chapter 2

BIOLOGICAL INTERACTIONS OF AGING AND CARCINOGENESIS

Vladimir N. Anisimov

Head, Department of Carcinogenesis and Oncogerontology,
N.N. Petrov Research Institute of Oncology, Pesochny-2, St. Petersburg, Russia

It is well documented that the incidence of malignant tumors increases progressively with age, both in animals and humans [1-3]. The relationship between aging and cancer is not clear. Considerable controversy surrounds the mechanisms that lead to increased incidence of cancer in the aged. Three major hypotheses have been proposed to explain the association of cancer and age.

The first hypothesis holds this association is a consequence of the duration of carcinogenesis. In other words, the high prevalence of cancer in older individuals simply reflects a more prolonged exposure to carcinogens [4]. The second hypothesis proposes that age-related progressive changes in the internal milieu of the organism may provide an increasingly favorable environment for the induction of new neoplasms and for the growth of already existent, but latent malignant cells [5-9]. These mechanisms may also include proliferative senescence, as the senescent cells loses their ability to undergo apoptosis and produce some factors which stimulate epithelial cells with oncogenic mutations [10]. The third hypothesis proposes that the cancer-prone phenotype of older humans might reflect the combined effects of cumulative mutational load, increased epigenetic gene silencing, telomere dysfunction and altered stromal milieu [11]. The elucidation of causes of an age-related increase in cancer incidence may be the key to a strategy for primary cancer prevention.

1. AGING AND MULTISTAGE MODEL OF CANCER

The homeostasis of most tissues is maintained thanks to a pool of stem cells able to reproduce themselves and to differentiate. Cell differentiation is followed by cell death and aging maybe construed as a progressive loss of stem cells to differentiation and death [12]. Another possibility involves the immortalization of the stem cell that is associated with a loss of differentiation and apoptosis. These immortalized stem cells may give origin to a clonal population with a survival advantage over the remaining tissues: this process is carcinogenesis [12,13]. (Figure 1). Both differentiation and death, and immortalization are multi-stage processes. Many steps of carcinogenesis are well-characterized [5,6,14,15] whereas the steps of aging need better recognition and definition [6,16]. Both models of cellular aging and immortalization involve delayed genomic instability that is a transmission of genomic aberrations to distant cellular progenies, accompanied by the occurrence of new aberrations. In one case this process results in cellular death; in the other, in cellular immortalization, and some steps may be shared by the two [16].

Carcinogenesis is a multistage process: neoplastic transformation implies the engagement of a cell through sequential stages, and different agents may affect the transition between contiguous stages [17,18]. Several lines of evidence support this conclusion [19]:

- Histopathology of tumors reveals multiple stages of tumor progression, such as dysplasia and carcinoma *in situ*
- The two-stage model of chemical carcinogenesis in mouse skin shows that different chemicals affect qualitatively different stages in the carcinogenic process
- The existence of individuals with genetic traits manifested by an early occurrence of cancer (e.g., familial retinoblastoma, colon and rectum adenomatosis) suggests that one of the carcinogenic steps is a germ-line mutation, but additional somatic effects are required for neoplastic development
- Mathematical models based on age-specific tumor incidence curves are consistent with the hypothesis that three to seven independent hits (effects of independent carcinogens) are required for tumor development
- Studies with chemical carcinogens in cell cultures reveal that different phenotypic properties of a tumor cell are required for tumor development
- Studies with viral and tumor-derived oncogenes in cell cultures show that neoplastic conversion of normal cells generally requires multiple cooperating oncogenes.

- Transgenic mice that carry activated proto-oncogenes in their germ-line develop focal tumors, which are apparently monoclonal in origin, suggesting that additional somatic events are required for full malignant progression.

Figure 1. Two strategies of stem cell

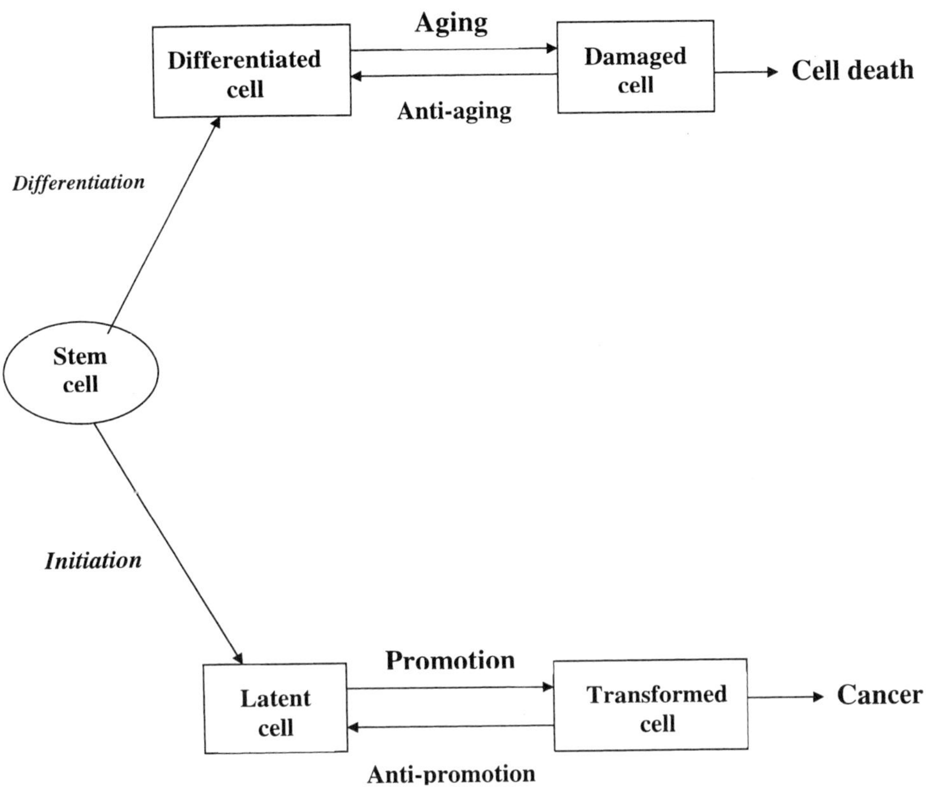

The process of neoplastic development is frequently divided into three operationally defined stages - initiation, promotion and progression. During the first stage of carcinogenesis (initiation) irreversible changes in the genotype of the normal target stem cell leading to its immortality take place. During the initiation the carcinogen or its active metabolite(s) (derived by simple degradation or by active enzymatic process) interacts with nucleic acids leading to mutations in oncogenes and in anti-oncogenes. During the second stage of carcinogenesis (promotion) initiated (latent, immortalized) cell acquires phenotypic features of transformed (malignant) cell, and under the exogenous influence, some of which at least are provided by the neoplastic stroma, tumor progression may occur. A carcinogen affects not only target cells but also influence a lot of factors in the microenvironment of the target cell creating the conditions for promotion of immortalized cell (growth factors, cytokines, immunodepression, biogenic amines, hormonal and metabolic imbalance). Some carcinogens, such as tobacco smoke may effect multiple carcinogenic steps.

Unlike initiation, promotion requires prolonged exposure to the carcinogen and may be reversible to a large extent. The dissection of carcinogenesis into initiation, promotion, and progression is useful as a frame of reference. It should not be assumed, however, that only three carcinogenic stages exist: each stage can be subdivided into multiple substages. Promotion may involve the activation of several enzymes, such as protein kinase C and ornithine decarboxylase; enhanced hexose transport; increased polyamine production, prevention of cell differentiation; and inhibition of cell-to-cell communication [20-21]. It was found that 12-O-tetradecanoylphorbol-13-acetate (TPA), a well-known skin tumor promoter, causes free radical-mediated DNA alterations, such as sister chromatid exchanges and expression of proviruses and retroviruses [22].

Discovery of oncogenes and of their function has provided new insight into the carcinogenic process. One may view carcinogenesis as a "cascade" phenomenon, resulting in serial activation of multiple cellular oncogenes and/or inactivation of tumor-suppressing genes (e.g., p53) [23].

To overcome the obvious limitations of two (three)-stage model, a multistage model of carcinogenesis has been conceived, in which the number of stages is not limited, the stages are envisioned as a continuum, and the influence of factors other than specific carcinogens may be properly accounted for in Figure 2 [24]. The principles of this model are as follows. First, neoplastic transformation involves the transition of target cells through multiple stages, the number of which varies for different neoplasms (with

Figure 2. Integral scheme of carcinogenesis

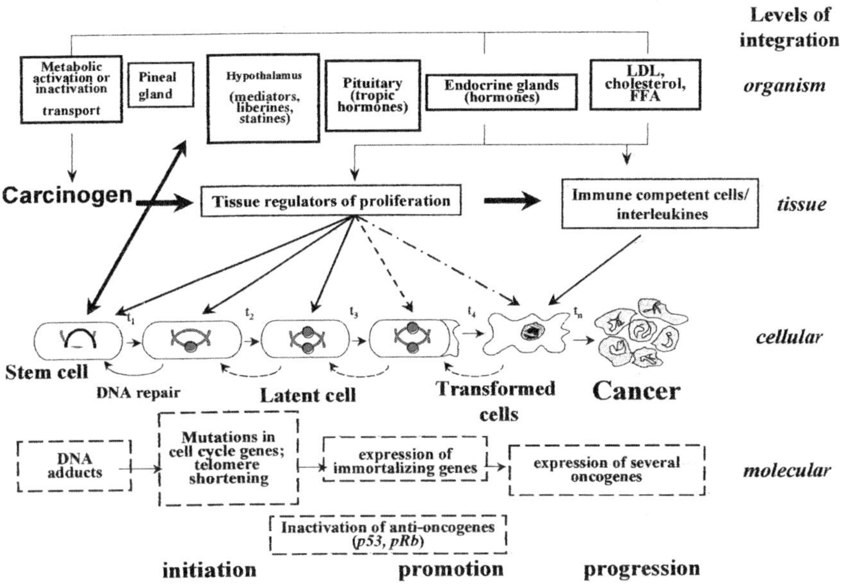

a minimum of one intermediate stage). Secondly, passage from one stage to another is a stochastic event, the rate of which depends on the dose of a carcinogen that affects the cell. Finally, all cells at any stage of carcinogenesis may enter the next stage independently of each other.

According to this model, the tumor develops only if at least one cell goes through all the necessary stages, and the clonal growth of this cell causes clinical cancer, as a critical volume of neoplastic cells accumulates. In this model, the exact origin of the various stages is ignored and the changes in cell function during the process of carcinogenesis are not assessed. The grade of malignancy is considered to increase with every stage. Various carcinogenic agents (exogenous as well as endogenous) may modulate the process. In addition, some agents act at early stages of carcinogenesis and others at later stages [24]. Epidemiological data, analyzed within the framework of a multi-stage model, have helped to estimate the contribution of various factors to the development of cancer. These factors include the time from the start of carcinogenic exposure, and the age of onset of exposure.

It is worthy to note that in every tissue the number of events occurring in the stem cell before its complete transformation is variable and depends on many factors, in particular the rate of aging of the target tissue and its regulatory system(s) [6,14]. This model is consistent with the analysis of age-related distribution of tumor incidence in different sites in humans and laboratory animals [1,3].

Important differences between early and late-stage carcinogens should be highlighted, to illustrate potential interactions of aging and carcinogenesis. Exposure to early stage carcinogens requires a latent period for the development of cancer. During the latent period the transformed cell goes through the subsequent carcinogenic stages. Clearly, elimination of early-stage carcinogens from the environment will not result in immediate cessation in the incidence of cancer. Carcinogens acting at late stages of carcinogenesis cause the tumor incidence rate to rise after a relatively short period of time. The increased rate of tumor incidence will be reversed almost immediately on cessation of exposure [24].

This risk of cancer after exposure to a carcinogen may be calculated as: $I = (age)^{k-1} - (t)^{k-1}$ where I is the risk of cancer, t is the time from initial exposure to the carcinogen, and k is the number of stages that the target cells have undergone before the exposure to the carcinogen. This formula is based on the assumption that with aging there is a progressive accumulation of partially transformed cells primed to the effect of late-stage carcinogens (Figure 3). Age is considered as a variable because older cells may already present in advanced carcinogenic stages, are primed to the effects of environmental carcinogens and consequently may develop cancer more rapidly and at higher rate when exposed to these substances. A number

Figure 3. The multistage carcinogenesis inducted by single exposure to a carcinogenicagent at different ages.

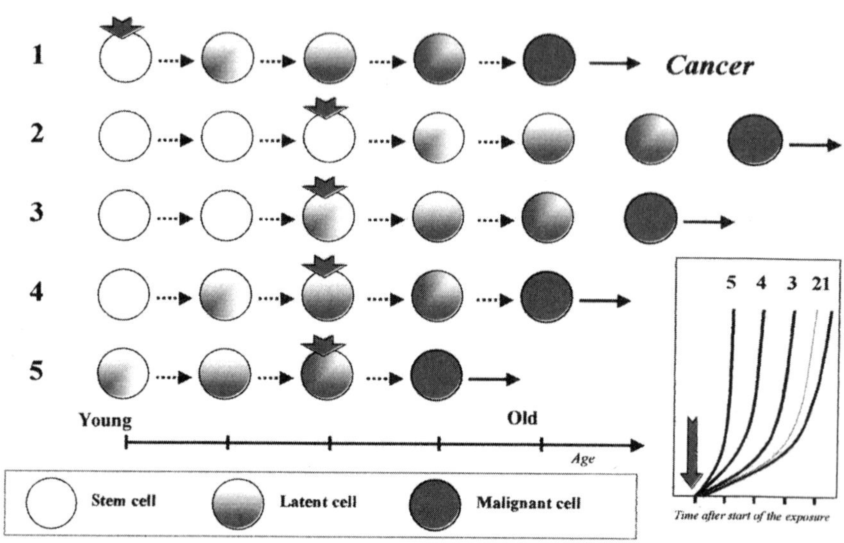

of factors, including genetic predisposition, oxidative stress, and previous exposure to carcinogens may be responsible of the molecular changes that prime aging cells to environmental carcinogens.

2. EFECT OF AGING ON THE SUSCEPTIBILITY TO CARCINOGENESIS IN VIVO

Animal experiments seem to confirm that there are age related differences in sensitivity to carcinogen in some tissues. Thus, with age, susceptibility to carcinogens in murine mammary gland, small intestine and colon, thyroid, ovarian follicular epithelium decreases, in subcutaneous tissue, cervix uteri and vagina increases and in others (lung, hemopoietic tissues) it remains stable (Table 1). For details see references 1,5-6). Age-related differences in cancer susceptibility have been observed after exposure to the same carcinogens in experimental systems. For example, in female rats exposed to N-nitrosomethylurea (NMU) in doses 10, 20 or 50 mg/kg at the age of 3 month developed mammary carcinomas, tumors of the kidney, ovaries and colon. In contrast to young animals, the rats exposed to the same doses of the carcinogen at the age of 15 months showed a higher frequency of tumors of the corpus and cervix uteri, and a lower frequency of mammary and intestinal adenocarcinomas and tumors of the ovary and kidney [25]. Comparison of the results with the data on DNA alkylation, synthesis and O^6-methylguanine repair obtained on the same model suggests a critical role of age-related proliferative activity changes occurring in the target tissues in the mechanism of age in modifying the effect on carcinogenesis. Obviously, there are no common patterns of age related changes in DNA synthesis and repair or in proliferative activity of different tissues with age [1,5,6].

There are several possible reasons for this wide variation in experimental results. These include factors related to the experimental model and factors related to the tumor-host. Model-related factors involve the characteristics of different carcinogens (direct or indirect action, chemical structure, mechanism of action), route of administration, exposure duration, presence of local and systemic activity, and time of observation. Host-related factors involve animal species, strain, sex, and age. The effective dose of an indirect carcinogen, requiring metabolic activation, may vary significantly in old and young animals, because the activity of the enzymes necessary for carcinogen activation in the liver and/or target tissue(s) may change with age [5,26,27]. Critical factors that determine the susceptibility of a tissue to carcinogenesis include DNA synthesis and proliferative activity of that tissue at the time of carcinogen exposure, and the efficacy of repair of damaged DNA. The

Table 1. Effect of aging on the susceptibility of laboratory rodents to carcinogenesis (Anisimov, 1987; 1998)

Target tissue	Carcinogenic agent	Effect of aging
Skin	DMBA, MCA, BP, TC, UV, β-irradiation	↑
	Fast neutrons, electrone-irradiation	↓
Subcutaneous soft tissues	BP, DMBA, MCA, NMU, polyurethane sponge, Moloney virus	↑
Bone	^{224}Ra, ^{227}Th, ^{239}Pu, radionuclides	=
Vascular vessel	DENA, DMH	=
	Vinylchloride	↑
Hematopoietic tissue	X-rays, γ-irradiation, estrogens	↓
	NMU, pristan	↑=
Mammary gland	DMBA, MCA, NMU, AAF, X-rays	↓
	Estrogens	↑
Uterus	DMH, NMU	↑
Vagina	DMBA	=
Ovary	X-rays, Biskind's operation	↓
Testis	Fast neutrons	↑
Thyroid gland	Fast neutrons, X-rays	↓
Lungs	DENA, DBA, urethane	↓
	NMU, fast neutrons, X-rays	↑
Pleura	Asbestos	↑
Liver	AAF, AFB_1, DMNA, DENA,	↓
	Phenobarbital, CCl_4	↑
Pancreas	NMU	↑
Esophagus	DENA	↓
Forestonach	DENA	↓
Stomach	MNNG	↓
Small intestine	MAMNA	↓
Colon	DMH, MAMNA	↓ (rat)
	DMH, NMU	↑ (mouse)
Kidney	AAF, NMU, DMNA	↓
Bladder	DMBA, BHBNA	↑

Abbreviations: AAF- 2-acetylaminofluorene; AFB_1 – aflatoxin B_1; BHBNA – N-butyl-N-(4-hydroxybutyl)nitrosamine; BP – benzo(a)pyrene; DBA – 1,2,5,6-dibenzanthracene; DENA – N-diethylnitrosamine; DMNA – N-dimethylnitrosamine; DMH- 1,2-dimethylhydrazine; MAMNA – N-methyl-(acethoxymethyl)nitrosamine; MCA – 20-methylcholanthrene; MNNG – N-methyl-N'-nitro-N-nitrosoguanidine; NMU – N-nitrosomethylurea; TC – tobacco smoke condensate; UV- ultra violet irradiation; CCl_4 – carbon tetrachloride; X-rays - Roentgen irradiation.

↑ - increase in incidence of tumors or decrease in tumor latency; ↓ - decrease in incidence of tumors or increase in tumor latency; = no effect.

available data concerning age related changes of these parameters have been discussed elsewhere [1-3,23,28]. Obviously, there are no common patterns of age related changes in DNA synthesis and repair or in proliferative activity of different tissues with age.

The homeostatic regulation of cell numbers in normal tissues reflects a precise balance between cell proliferation and cell death. Programmed cell death (apoptosis) provides a protective mechanism from cancer, by removing senescent, DNA damaged, or diseased cells that could potentially interfere with normal function or lead to neoplastic transformation [23, 29]. Apoptosis plays a substantial role in many other aspects of aging and cancer, including control of the life span of most members of transformed cells, and the rate of growth of tumors [30]. p53 mediated apoptosis was suggested as a safeguard mechanism to prevent cell proliferation induced by oncogene activation [31].

3. AGING AND SUSCEPTIBILITY TO CARCINOGENESIS IN VITRO

Some *in vitro* observations support the suggestion on accumulation in tissues of premalignant cells. Thus, transformed by 24-hours exposure to DMBA, foci in murine bladder epithelium have appeared earlier (on the 40th to the 60th day) and more often (25%) in explants of old (28-30 months) donors in comparison with 100 days and 0.9% in cultures received from five to seven month old mice. A spontaneous transformation of bladder epithelium occurred only in the explants received from old donors [32]. The aging of the tissue donor was associated with increased susceptibility of primary cultures of rat fibroblasts to transformation induced by SV-40 [33]. However rat embryonal fibroblasts were much susceptible to v-*scr* transformation than when they were isolated from an adult rat [34]. Nettesheim et al. [35] reported that the sensitivity of trachea epithelium explants of old animals to chemical carcinogens was lower in comparison to explants from young animals.

Susceptibility to transformation varies during the different stages of proliferative senescence depending on the carcinogen. Thus, young cells are more susceptible to transformation by chemical carcinogens and by low-dose ionizing radiation, susceptibility to ultraviolet radiation is identical throughout the life span of human fibroblasts, whereas susceptibility to a tumor promoter is identical through the cell life span with exception of the final stage, and susceptibility to SV40 is highest during the final stage [36,37].

Thus, experiments both *in vivo* and *in vitro* provide evidence that the age related factors limiting the susceptibility to carcinogens are tissue specific [1,6]. This conclusion may explain, at least in part, both age related changes in susceptibility to carcinogenesis in target tissues, and organ and tissue variability in age distribution of spontaneous tumor incidence. This conclusion generates a critical question: does the aging accompanied by the accumulation of premalignant lesions in target tissues?

4. EFFECT OF AGING ON THE SUSCEPTIBILITY TO TUMOR PROMOTERS IN VIVO

There is evidence of age-related accumulation of cells that are in the late stage of multi-stage process of carcinogenesis. Numerous experiments support this model. Thus, single skin application with 7,13-dimethylbenz[a]anthracene (DMBA) in mice aged 8 and 48 weeks at doses ranging from 10 to 300 μg caused increased skin papilloma incidence in older mice [38]. Also, the average diameter of the tumors was larger in the older animals. Of particular interest are the experiments using skin transplants. TPA failed to induce tumors in the skin of 2-month-old mice grafted to animals of different ages, but caused the same tumor incidence in the skin of 1-year-old donors irrespective of the recipient's age [39,40]. These results indicate that the age of the target tissue, more than the age of the host, determines susceptibility to late-stage agents. Delaying wounding 16 weeks after initiation with a carcinogen led to a more pronounced skin tumor response compared with delay of only 6 weeks in young mice [41]. Delaying promotion has also been reported to lead to an increased tumor response with the promoters chrysarobin [42] or mezerein [43]. These findings are in agreement with data on age-related decrease in cellular DNA repair capacity in skin [44,45] and increasing *p53* mutation frequency with advancing age in human normal skin [46] and in basal-cell skin carcinomas [47,48]. Post-ultraviolet DNA repair capacity was found to undergo an age-related decline to which corresponded age-related increase in post-ultraviolet mutability in cultured primary skin fibroblasts from normal donors from the first to the tenth decade of life [44]. It was suggested that there was the age-related increase in the number of telomerase positive basal cells in the skin [49]. However in some studies the papilloma response either decreased with age or was the same as the response in younger mice [50-52].

In Tg.AC transgenic (v-*Ha-ras*) mice, skin tumor incidence and multiplicity were strongly age-dependent, increasing with increasing age of the animal when first treated with TPA, or exposed to wounding, or UV-light [53]. The authors suggest that natural developmental changes in keratinocytes are co-opted by the molecular mechanisms that regulate the induction of transgene expression, thus stimulating tumor formation in older Tg.AC mice.

Age-related accumulation of cells in advanced carcinogenic stages may also be inferred by other types of experiments. The mouse model of hepatocarcinogenesis is very convenient for this purpose because of the availability of strains of animals with different susceptibility to hepatic carcinogenesis. In the liver of highly susceptible mice, the concentration of hepatocytes in advanced stages of carcinogenesis was increased early in life before the exposure to experimental carcinogens [54]. In the liver of F344 rats the number of spontaneous proliferative foci is proportional to the animal age [55,56]. The incidence of proliferative foci and hepatic tumors induced by phenobarbital, carbon tetrachloride or peroxisome proliferators in rodents is also a function of age [55-57].

Another pertinent model involves induction of lymphomas in mice receiving transplants of splenic, thymic and lymphoid cells from syngeneic donors [40]. The incidence of neoplasms was related to the age of the donor, but not to the age of the recipient. Geschickter [58] observed mammary tumor development in estrogen-treated one and 20 month-old rats with a latency period of 9.5 and 3.0 months, respectively. The data on age-related susceptibility to tumor promoters are given in Table 2.

Table 2. Effect of aging on susceptibility of different tissues to tumor promoters in rodents (Anisimov, 1998)

Target tissue	Species	Treatment, agent	Age groups, months	Effect of aging	References
Skin	Mouse	TPA*	4 and 14	↑	39
Liver	Mouse	Phenobarbital	1,5 and 12	↑	55
	Rat	Phenobarbital	1 and 26	↑	56
		Partial hepatectomy + phenobarbital	5 and 18	↑	154)
		CCl_4	1-6 and 12	↑	155
		Clofibrat, nafenopin	3 and 18	↑	57
		Clofibrat, Wy-14643	2,5 and 23	↑	156
Mammary gland	Rat	Estradiol	1 and 20	↑	58
Ovary	Rat	Biskinds' operation**	3 and 14	↑	157

*- 12-O-tetradecanoylphorbol-13-acetate
** Transplantation of the ovary into the spleen after ovaruectomy.

Single intravenous injection of NMU at doses of 10, 20 or 50 mg/kg was administered to female rats aged 3 or 15 months [25]. The NMU carcinogenic dose dependence in different age groups was considered in the context of a multi-stage model. It was calculated that the number of events necessary for complete malignant transformation in 15-month-old rats under the influence of NMU was lower than in three month-old. In this experiment as well as in another sets of experiments in rats and in mice it was shown that tumors developed earlier in older than in younger animals after exposure to the same doses of NMU [14,59-62]. The combined incidences of severe endometrial hyperplasia and adenocarcinomas tended to increase with the increase in intervals between a start of promoting estrasiol treatment after N-nitrosoethylurea initiation in mice [62].

5. EFFECT OF AGING ON TRANSPLANATABLE TUMOR GROWTH

An important question related to the integrated carcinogenic model (Figure 2) concerns age-related changes in tissue microenvironment as these changes may both favor or oppose carcinogenesis in different circumstances. Should aging alter the environment in which tumor develops, the growth rate of transplantable tumors may vary with the age of the tumor recipient [63]. These experiments bypass the effect of age on carcinogenesis itself and explore the role of age-related changes in the organism on the growth and progression of transformed cells. Evaluation criteria for such experiments should include: (a) tumor transplantability, (b) rate of tumor growth, and (c) survival time of tumor bearing animals. The natural history of spontaneous tumors in humans (the rate of tumor doubling, metastasizing potential) and on the survival of cancer patients newly diagnosed at different ages provide information on the effects of age on tumor growth in humans. Available data both in experimental animals and in humans are contradictory and support different effects of age on tumor development (Table 3) [1,6]. In general, an "age effect" may be recognized both in experimental and in human malignancies.

Tissue origin (histogenesis) and immunogenicity of tumor are the principal factors determining age-related differences in tumor growth. There is increasing evidence that age-related changes in tumor microenvironment might play also a significant role. In our experiments, lung-affine cells of rat rhabdomyosarcoma RA-2 were intravenously inoculated into rats of different ages [64]. It was observed that the number of lung tumor colonies was highest in one month-old and 15 month-old animals and lowest in 3 and 12 month-old animals. A positive correlation was found between the number of tumor lung colonies and somatomedine (IGF-1) activity in the lung.

Table 3. Effect of aging on growth of subcutaneously transplanted tumors in rodents (Anismov, 1987, 2003). ↑ - Increase in transplantability and/or the rate of growth and/or decrease in survival time; ↓ - Opposite effects; = No effect.

Tumor	Species	Age at the time of tumor transplantation, months	Effect of aging
Epidermoid carcinoma H.Ep.#3	Mouse	4-8 and 20-23	↑
Squamous-cell cervical carcinoma SCC	Mouse	3 and 12	=
		3 and 18	↑
Melanoma B16	Mouse	3 and 12	↓
		3 and 22	=
		3 and 24	↓
Mammary carcinoma: Spontanous	Mouse	3,5 and 16,5	↓
		10-11 and 21-22	↓
Ehrlich ascite carcinoma		3 and 16,5-18	↑
EMT6		3-4 and 20-28	↑
MAT-21		2 and 4- 5	↓
A-755		3 and 18	↑
64pT		3 and 24	↓
Walker-256	Крыса	2 and 24	↓
Lewis lung carcinoma	Mouse	3 and 18	=
		2 and 24	↑
		3 and 33	↓
Lung carcinoma-1	Mouse	3-8 and 18-23	↑
Hepatoma-22a	Mouse	3 and 14-16	↑
Novikoff's hepatoma	Крыса	4,5 and 27,5	↓
Teratocarcinoma OTT 6050	Mouse	2 and 16	↓
Methylchlanthrene sarcoma	Mouse	6 and 22	↑
		2-3 and 10-21	↑
	Крыса	1-10 and 12-15 8-20 and 29-32	↓ ↑
Fibrosarcoma 1023	Mouse	2 and 4-5	↑
Fibrosarcoma 1591	Mouse	2-6 and 10	↑
Sarcoma 180	Mouse	3 and 18	↑
Osteogenic sarcoma	Mouse	2-3 and 10-17	=
Uterine sarcoma	Mouse	3 and 12	=
Fibrosarcoma	Крыса	4 and 12	↓
Ascitic fibrosarcoma	Крыса	3-4 and 16-18	↑
Mastocytoma P815	Mouse	3 and 25 3-12 and 20-32	↑ ↑
Reticulocell tumor, type A	Mouse	8 and 11-17	↓
Leukemia L1210	Mouse	3 and 11	=
Hemocytoblastoma La	Mouse	3 and 18	=
Myeloma LCP-1	Mouse	2-3 and 19-20	↓

In another experiment, RA-2 cells from a 3-month-old donor were inoculated into 2-3 or 21-23- month-old recipients and 3 weeks later were separately taken from "young" and "old" hosts and transplanted into 3-month-old recipients. The number of lung colonies was significantly decreased in 3-month-old recipients injected with RA-2 cell passed via "old" host [60]. The results obtained suggest the critical role of host and donor microenvironment in lung colony forming potential of RA-2 cells.

McCullough *et al.* [65] have observed that transformed rat hepatocytic cells lines were only weakly tumorigenic following transplantation into the livers of young adult rats. The tumorigenicity of these cell lines increased progressively with the age of the tumor recipients. These results suggest strongly that the tissue microenvironment represents an important determinant in the age-related tumorigenic potential of transformed cells.

Krtolika and Campisi [66] have shown that senescent stromal fibroblasts can stimulate the hyperproliferation and malignant progression of preneoplastic and neoplastic cells in culture. They also tested the ability of senescent fibroblasts to stimulate epithelial cell growth in vivo by inoculation of preneoplastic epithelial cells with presenescent or senescent human fibroblasts into nude mice [67]. None of the tumors when injected alone. Both preneoplastic mouse mammary epithelial cells and preneoplastic human keratinocytes did not form tumors in the presence of presenescent fibroblasts but formed large lethal tumors in the presence of senescent fibroblasts. In the case of human breast cancer cells, senescent fibroblasts markedly stimulated the rate of tumor growth [67].

6. MECHANISMS OF INTERACTION OF AGING AND CARCINOGENESIS

Cancer is a common denomination given to a number of different diseases. Common features to all cancers include [23,68]

- potential immortality of cancer cells due to avoiding apoptosis
- ability to invade surrounding tissues due to reduced sensitivity to signals from neighboring cells aimed to offset proliferation
- cell de-differentiation with re-appearance of some embryonal proteins (e.g. α-fetoprotein) in cytoplasm
- growth signals autonomy, which allows cancer cells to proliferate in absence of outside signals due to only inner growth signals
- release of growth factors and promotion of angiogenesis in tissue, which favor tumor growth and metastasis
- increase in metabolism and number of mitochondria in cancer cells

Gene mutations, as well as changes in regulation of gene expression, which can produce these typical features, were suggested to be key genetic events leading to cancer development [23,68,69]. Down regulation of apoptosis gene, *p53*, as well as upregulation of *myc* and *ras* genes, which may favor excessive proliferation, could be examples of such events [69,70].

Both carcinogenesis and aging are associated with genomic alterations, which may act synergistically in causing cancer [23,68-71]. In particular, three age-related changes in DNA metabolism may favor cell transformation and cancer growth. These changes are genetic instability, DNA hypomethylation, and formation of DNA adducts.

Genetic instability involves activation of genes that are normally suppressed, such as the cellular proto-oncogenes, and/or inactivation of some tumor suppression genes (*p53, Rb*, etc.) [23,31]. DNA hypomethylation is characteristic of aging, as well as of transformed cells. Hypomethylation, a potential mechanism of oncogene activation, may result in spontaneous deamination of cytosine and consequent base transition, i.e., substitution of the pair thymine:adenine. Accumulation of inappropriate base pairs may cause cell transformation by activation of cellular proto-oncogenes [23]. Age-related abnormalities of DNA metabolism may be, to some extent, tissue- and gene-specific. For example, hypomethylation of the c-*myc* proto-oncogene has been found in the hepatocytes, but not in the neurons of old mice [72,73]. Within the same cell, different DNA segments express different degrees of age-related hypomethylation. The uneven distribution of hypomethylation may underlie selective overexpression of proto-oncogenes by senescent cells. For example, the transcription of c-*myc* is progressively increased in the liver but not in the brain of rats between the ages of 4-22 months, whereas the transcription of c-*sis* and c-*src* does not appear to be age-related in any tissues [72,73]. The different extent of DNA abnormalities among aging tissues may account in part for the different susceptibility of these tissues to carcinogens [74,75].

The damage caused by endogenous oxygen radicals has been proposed as a major contributor to both aging and cancer [76-78]. Endogenous oxidative damage to lipids and proteins increases with age [77,78]. It was shown that oxygen free radicals may induce active mutations of the human c-*Ha-ras* proto-oncogene [78]. The level of one oxidized nucleoside, 8-hydroxy-2'-deoxyguanosine (oh8dG) in the DNA increased with age in liver, kidney, and intestine but remained unchanged within brain and testes of rats, whereas the urinary excretion of the nucleoside decreased with age of rats [79]. A variety of cellular defense systems are involved in protecting cellular macromolecules against devastating action of oxygen-based radicals. These systems include antioxidant enzymes (Cu,Zn- superoxide dismutase (SOD), manganese-containing SOD, catalase, glutathione peroxidase, glutathione reductase, glucose-6-phosphate dehydrogenase), some vitamins (α-tocopherol, ascorbic acid), uric acid and the pineal indole hormone melatonin [80-83].

There is evidence of an age-related accumulation of spontaneous mutations in somatic and germ cells [71]. Accumulation with age of some spontaneous mutations or mutations evoked by endogenous mutagens can induce genome instability and, hence, increase the sensitivity to carcinogens and/or tumor promoters. It has been shown that clonally expanded mtDNA mutations accumulate with age in normal human tissues as well as in human tumors [84,85]. The finding that deleted mtDNA accumulated in human muscle tissue as well as evidence for partially duplicated mtDNA in aged human tissues [85] suggests the important role of clonal expansion of mutant mtDNA in the age-related increase of systemic oxidative stress in the whole organism [86]. A significant trend toward increasing *p53* mutations frequency with advancing age was found in some normal and malignant tissues [46,47]. Simpson [9] suggested that the aging human body accumulates enough mutations to account for multistep carcinogenesis by selection of preexisting mutations. The evidence showed that both genetics of the selected cellular clone and the epigenetics of the selective environment contribute to tumor development [87].

Thus, the data available show that some changes in structure and function of DNA are evolving with natural aging. The character of these changes could vary in different tissues and might cause uneven tissue aging. Dolle et al. [88] using a *lacZ* plasmid transgenic mouse model, determined spectra of spontaneous point mutations in different organs in young and old mice. While similar at a young age, the mutation spectra among these organs were significantly different in old age. The authors stressed that the replicative history *per se* is not the underlying causal factor of age-related organ-specific differences in mutations spectra. Rather, differences in organ function, possibly with association with replicative history, may explain the divergence in mutation spectra during aging. In turn, this may explain both age-related increase in spontaneous tumor incidence and age-related changes in susceptibility to carcinogens in various organs.

Multistage carcinogenesis is accompanied by disturbances in tissue homeostasis and perturbations in nervous, hormonal, and metabolic factors that may favor tumor growth and lessen natural antitumor defenses. The development of these changes depends on the susceptibility of various systems to a carcinogen and on the dose of the carcinogen. Changes in the microenvironment may condition key carcinogenic events and determine the duration of each carcinogenic stage, and sometimes they may even reverse the process of carcinogenesis. These microenvironmental changes influence the proliferation rate of transformed cells together, the total duration of carcinogenesis and, consequently, the latent period of tumor development (Figure 2).

Crosstalk between mesenchyme and epithelium has been described as a known driver of differentiation and development [89,90]. It was shown that changes in stromal behavior can promote epithelial transformation [66,89].

Thus, the data available show that some changes in structure and function of DNA are evolving with natural aging. The character of these changes could vary in different tissues and might cause uneven tissue aging. In turn, this may lead to both age-related increases in spontaneous tumor incidence and age-related changes in susceptibility to carcinogens in various organs. Table 4 summarizes the data available in literature and obtained in our experiments on some hormonal metabolic shifts in the organism and disturbances at tissue and cellular levels observed in natural aging and in different types of carcinogenesis in vivo. Despite incomplete data, it can be seen that there is a similarity between the shifts in aging and carcinogenesis. Carcinogens could be supposed to initiate a normal cell, interacting with its elements on the molecular level, on the one hand, and to produce diverse changes in the organism facilitating promotion and progression of tumor growth, on the other hand.

7. THE ROLE OF THE INSULIN/IGF-1 SIGNALING PATHWAY IN AGING AND CANCER

The potential link between aging and insulin/IGF-1 signaling has attracted substantial attention during last years, on the basis of evidence including age-related increase in incidence of insulin resistance and type 2 diabetes in accelerated aging syndromes and life span extension by caloric restriction in rodents. Concomitant reduction in plasma insulin and plasma glucose levels, which implies increased sensitivity to insulin, emerged as a hallmark of increased longevity [91,92]. Hyperglycemia is an important aging factor involved in generation of advanced glycosylation endproducts (AGEs) [93,94]. There are evidence that hyperinsulinemia favors accumulation of oxidized protein by reducing its degradation as well as facilitates protein oxidation by increasing steady-state level of oxidative stress [95]. Untreated diabetics with elevated glucose levels suffer many manifestations of accelerated aging, such as impaired wound healing, obesity, cataracts, vascular and microvascular damage [8]. It was shown that centenarians have a preserved glucose tolerance and sensitivity to insulin as well as lower degree of oxidative stress as compared to aged persons [96]. It is worthy to note that hyperinsulinemia is an important factor not only in aging but also in the development of cancer [8, 97,98].

The intensive investigations in *C. elegans* since 1990's, which have identified insulin signaling components including *daf-2, age-1* and *daf-16* as the genes whose mutations lead to life span extension shed new light on

Table 4. Similarity of changes developing in an organism during natural aging and carcinogenesis (Anisimov, 1997, 2003, with modifications)

Parameters	Aging	Carcinogenesis
	Molecular level	
Free radical generation	Increases	Increases
DNA adducts formation	Increases	Increases
DNA repair efficacy	Decreases	Decreases
DNA hypomethylation	Increases	Increases
Genomic instability	Increases	Increases
Telomere length	Decreases	Increases *
Error protein synthesis	Increases	Increases
Mutation rate	Increases	Increases
Oncogene expression	Increases	Increases
p53 mutations	Increases	Increases
	Cell/tissue level	
Oxidative stress	Increases	Increases
Chromosome aberrations	Increases	Increases
Growth factor production	Deceases	Increases *
Proliferative activity	Decreases	Clonal proliferation*
Focal hyperplasia	Increases	Increases
Apoptosis	Increases	Decreases *
Angiogenesis	Decreases	Increases *
Bioenergetics	Decreases	Anaerobic glycosis *
Cell-to-cell communication	Decreases	Decreases
Latent (dormant) cells number	Increases	Increases
	Systemic/ organism level	
Melatonin circadian rhythm	Damaged	Damaged
Serum melatonin level	Decreases	Decreases
Hypothalamic biogenic amines level	Decreases	Decreases
Hypothalamic threshold of senisitivity to homeostatic inhibition by steroids	Increases	Increases
Tolerance to glucose	Decreases	Decreases
Serum insulin level	Increases	Increases
Susceptibility to insulin	Decreases	Decreases
LDL and cholesterol level	Increases	Increases
Serum glucocorticoid level	Increases	Increases
Fertility	Decreases	Decreases
T-cell immunity	Decreases	Decreases
Cancer risk	Increases	Increases
	Population level	
Cancer incidence	Exponential pattern	Exponential pattern
Progeria	Acceleration	Increases
Exposure to 5-bromodeoxyguanine	Acceleration	Increases
Exposure to ionizing radiation	Acceleration	Increases
Treatment with geroprotectors	Postponement	Decreases or latency increases
Rate at the oldest age	Decreases in mortality	Decrease in incidence

* Related to clonally proliferating malignant cells

molecular mechanisms underlying aging [91,92,99]. In *D. melanogaster*, the mutation of genes operating in the signal transduction from insulin receptor to transcription factor *daf-16* (*age-1, daf-2, CHICO, InR* и др.) are strongly associated with longevity [99,100]. It was demonstrated that FKHR, FKHRL1 and AFX, which are mammalian homologues of *daf-16* forkhead transcription factor, function downstream of insulin signaling and akt/PKB under cellular conditions [101,102].

Daf-2 and InR are structural homologues of tyrosine kinase receptors in vertebrates that include the insulin receptor and the insulin-like growth factor type 1 receptor (IGF-1R). It was shown that in vertebrates the insulin receptor regulates energy metabolism whereas IGF-1R promotes growth. At least three genes ($Pit1^{dw}$, $Prop1^{dw}$, *Ghr*) whose knockout leads to dwarfism have been identified. The expression of these genes is associated with reduced levels of IGF-1 and insulin and increased longevity [103,104]. In Snell and Ames dwarf mice, sexual maturation is delayed, and only few males are fertile, while females are invariably sterile. These mice as well as $Ghr^{-/-}$ knockout mice have significantly reduced glucose levels and fasting insulin levels, decreased tolerance to glucose and increased sensitivity to insulin which appears to be combined with reduced ability to release glucose in response to acute challenge [91].

Recently, strong support for the role of insulin/IGF-1 signaling pathway in the control of mammalian aging and for the involvement of this pathway in longevity of IGF-1 deficient mice was provided by Hsieh et al [105,106]. It was shown that in the Snell dwarf mice, GH deficiency would lead to reduced insulin secretion and alterations in insulin signaling via InRβ, IRS-1 or IRS-2 and P13K affects genes involved in the control of longevity. The authors concluded that the *Pit1* mutation may result in physiological homeostasis that favors longevity.

Reduction in both glucose and insulin levels as well as an increase in the sensitivity to insulin are a well-documented response to caloric restriction in rodents and monkey [107,108]. It is worthy to note that $Ghr^{-/-}$ mice have a major increase in the level of insulin receptors [109], while Ames dwarf mice have a smaller increase in insulin receptor and substantially increased amount of insulin receptor substrates IRS-1 and IRS-2 [110]. The development of tumors in Ames dwarf mice was postponed and the incidence was reduced as compared to the control [108].

The crucial event of the effect of caloric restriction is low levels of insulin and IGF-1 and also the increase of insulin sensitivity in rodents [111] as well as in monkeys [112]. Many characteristics of these long-lived mutants and GH-receptor knockout mice resemble those of normal animals exposed to caloric restriction. These characteristics include reduced plasma levels of IGF-1, insulin and glucose, with the consequent reductions in growth and body size, delayed puberty, and significantly increased sensitivity to insulin action.

Holzenberger et al [113] inactivated the *Igf1r* gene by homologous recombination in mice. It was shown that *Igf1r*$^{-/-}$ mice dead early in life, whereas heterozygous *Igf1r*$^{+/-}$ mice live on average 26% longer than wild-type littermates. These mice did not develop dwarfism; their energy metabolism was normal. Food intake physical activity, fertility and reproduction were also unaffected in *Igf1r*$^{+/-}$ mice. These mice and embryonal fibroblasts derived from them were more resistant to oxidative stress than controls. The spontaneous tumor incidence in the aging cohort of *Igf1r*$^{+/-}$ mice was similar to that in wild-type controls. At the molecular level, insulin receptor substrate and the *p52* and *p66* isoforms of *Shc*, both main substrates of IGF-1 receptor, showed decreased tyrosine phosphorylation. *p66*^{Shc} mediated cellular responses to oxidative stress. Two main pathways - the extracellular-signal related kinase (ERK)/mitogen-activated protein kinase (MAPK) pathway and the phosphatidylinositol 3-kinase (PI3K)-Akt pathway – were downregulated in *Igf1r*$^{+/-}$ mice.

The extension of longevity was observed in fat-specific insulin receptor knockout (FIRKO) mice [114,115]. These animals have reduced fat mass and were protected against age-related obesity and its subsequent metabolic abnormalities including deterioration in glucose tolerance, although their food intake was normal. Both male and female FIRKO mice had increased mean life span (by 18%) with parallel increases in maximum life span. Extended longevity in FIRKO mice was associated with a higher age threshold beyond which age-dependent increase in mortality risk became appreciable and a decreased age-adjusted mortality rate, especially after 36 months of age. In FIRKO mice, the resistance to obesity, despite normal food intake, suggested that metabolic rate is increased, rather than decreased [115]. The authors believe that decreased fat mass could lead to a decrease in oxidative stress. Another possibility is that the increased longevity in these mice is the direct result of altered insulin signaling.

Shimokawa et al. [116] designed a transgenic strain of rats whose GH gene was suppressed by an anti-sense GH transgene. Male rats homozygous for the transgene (*tg/tg*) had a reduced number of pituitary GH cells, a lower plasma concentration of IGF-1, and a dwarf phenotype. Heterozygous rats (*tg/-*) had an intermediate phenotype in plasma IGF-1, food intake, and body weight between *tg/tg* and control (-/-) rats. The life span of *tg/tg* rats was 5 to 10% shorter than -/- rats. In contrast, the life span of *tg/-* rats was 7 to 10% longer than -/- rats. It was found that tumors caused earlier death in *tg/tg* rats; in contrast, *tg/-* rats had reduced nonneoplastic diseases and a prolonged life span. Immunological analysis revealed a smaller population and lower activity of splenic natural killer cells in homozygous *tg/tg* rats. These results provided evidence that an optimal level of the GH-IGF-1 axis function needs for longevity in mammals.

Recently it was shown that the incidence of mutations in insulin regulatory region (IRE) of APO C-III T-455 C directly correlates with longevity in humans. This is the first evidence showing that mutation located downstream to *daf-16* in insulin signal transduction system is associated with longevity [117]. It is worth noting that centenarians display lower degree of resistance to insulin and lower degree of oxidative stress as compared with elderly persons before 90 years [96]. The authors suggested that centenarians may have been selected for appropriate insulin regulation as well as for the appropriate regulation of tyrosine hydroxylase (TH) gene, whose product is rate limiting in the synthesis of catecholamines, stress-response mediators. It was shown that catecholamines may increase free radical production through induction of the metabolic rate and auto-oxidation in diabetic animals [118]. Recent study on aging parameters of young (up to 39 years) and old (over 70 years) individuals having similar IGF-1 serum levels provides evidence of important role of this peptide for life potential [119]. Roth et al. [120] analyzed data from the Baltimore Longitudinal Study of Aging and reported that survival was greater in men who maintained lower insulin level.

Several years ago, it was suggested to use biguanide antidiabetics as a potential anti-aging treatment [8]. The antidiabetic drugs, phenformin (1-phenylethylbiguanide), buformin (1-butylbiguanide hydrochloride) and metformin (N,N-dimethylbiguanide) were observed to reduce hyperglycemia, improve glucose utilization, reduce free fatty acid utilization, gluconeogenesis, serum lipids, insulin, somatomedin, reduce body weight and decrease metabolic immunodepression both in humans and rodents [8,121,122].

Buformin supplemented at the concentration of 0.1 mg/ml to nutrient medium during the larvae stage and over the life span of *C. elegans* increased the mean life span of the vorms by 23.4% and the maximum life span by 26.1% as compared to the controls [123]. The treatment with phenformin or buformin slightly decreased the body weight of rats, in comparison with the control slow down the age-related switching-off of the reproductive function in female rats prolonged the mean life span of female C3H/Sn mice and LIO rats [1,6,124-128]. Recently it was found that metformin significantly increases the life span of rats (G.S. Roth, personal communication).

Several other effects of treatment with antidiabetic biguanides related to reproduction and aging, are known from earlier studies. For example, it decreased hypothalamic threshold of the sensitivity to feedback inhibition by estrogens [125-128], which is one of the most important mechanisms regulating age-related decline and switch-off of the reproductive function [125-130]. Treatment with metformin may improve menstrual regularity, leading to spontaneous ovulation, and enhance the induction of ovulation with clomiphene citrate in women with polycystic ovary syndrome [131]. The treatment with phenformin also decreased hypothalamic threshold sensitivity to feedback regulation by glucocorticoids and by metabolic stimuli (glucose and insulin) [8]. It was recently shown that elements involved in the insulin/IGF-1 signaling pathway are regulated at the expression and/or functional level in the central nervous system. This regulation may play a role in the brain's insulin resistance [132], in the control of ovarian follicular development and ovulation [102], and brain's control of life span [111,133]. Antidiabetic biguanides also alleviated age-related metabolic immunodepression [8]. These mechanisms can be involved in geroprotective effect of biguanides. Treatment with chromium picolinate which elevated the insulin sensitivity in several tissues, including hypothalamus, significantly increased the mean life span and decreased the development of age-related pathology in rats [134]. We hypothesized that antidiabetic biguanides and possibly chromium picolinate regulate thyrosine hydroxylase and insulin/IGF-1 signaling pathway genes both associated with longevity [99,135]. It was shown that the polymorphism at TH-INS locus affects non-insulin dependent type 2 diabetes [136], and is associated with hypothalamic obesity [137], polycystosis ovary syndrome [138], hypertriglyceridemia and atherosclerosis [139].

The anticarcinogenic effect of antidiabetic biguanides has been demonstrated in several models of spontaneous and induced carcinogenesis. The treatment with phenformin normalized the tolerance to glucose and serum insulin and IGF-1 level in rats exposed to intravenous injections of N-nitrosomethylurea (NMU) and inhibited mammary carcinogenesis in these animals [124, 140]. Treatment of rats with 1,2-dimethylhydrazine (DMH) caused the decrease in the level of biogenic amines, particularly of in the hypothalamus, the decrease of glucose tolerance and the increase of the blood level of insulin and triglycerides. Administration of phenformin restored immunological indices and inhibited DMH-induced colon carcinogenesis [140, 141]. The colon 38 adenocarcinoma growth was significantly inhibited in liver-specific IGF-1-deficient mice, whereas injections with recombinant human IGF-1 displayed sufficiently promoted the tumor growth and metastasing [142].

A decrease of glucose utilization was found in the 3-month-old female progeny of rats exposed to NMU on the 21st day of pregnancy [124,140]. Postnatal treatment with biguanides started from the age of 2 months significantly inhibited the development of malignant neurogenic tumors in rats transplacentally exposed to NMU or NEU [143,144]. In high fat-fed hamsters, the treatment with N-nitrosobis-(2-oxopropyl)amine was followed by the development of pancreatic malignancies in 50% of cases, whereas no tumors were found in the hamsters treated with the carcinogen and metformin [145].

Figure 4. Proposed effects of metformin, calorie restriction and genetic modifications on insulin/IGF-1 signaling pathway in control of aging. The broken arrows on the figure show the targets for the genetic modifications, calorie restriction and for metformin in IGF-axis.

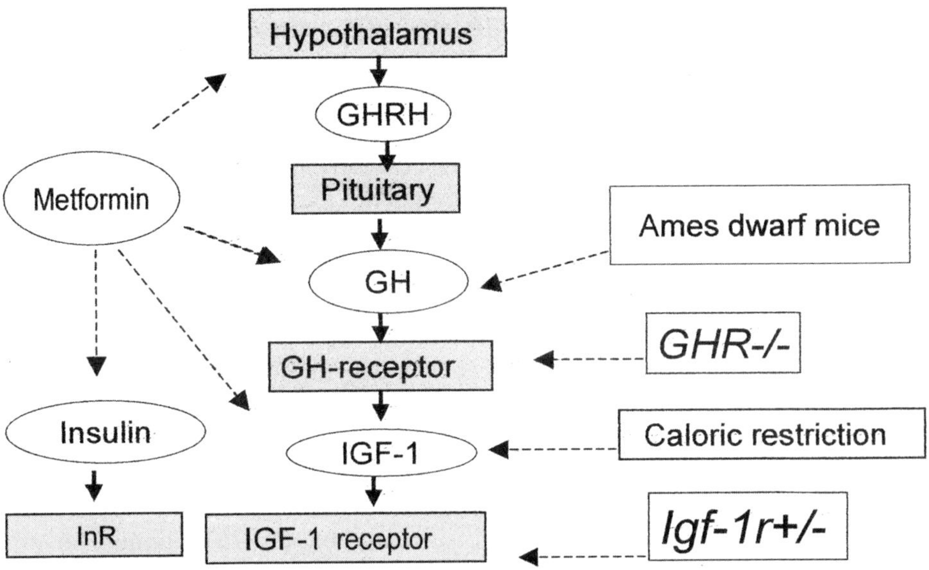

Thus, anticarcinogenic effect of antidiabetic biguanides has been demonstrated in relation to spontaneous carcinogenesis in mice and rats, in different models of chemical carcinogenesis in mice, rats and hamsters, and in radiation carcinogenesis model in rats. Phenformin administered orally to rodents potentiated the antitumor effect of cytostatic drugs on transplantable tumors [125-127].

The comparative study of 10-years results of metabolic rehabilitation (included fat and carbohydrate dietary restrictions and treatement with biguanides) of cancer patients had suggested increase in the survival of breast and colorectal cancer patients, increase in the length of cancer-free period, decrease in the incidence of metastasis as compared with control patients [122].

Although it is known that free radicals are produced during metabolic reactions, it is largely unknown which factor(s) modulate their production *in vivo*. It has been suggested that hyperinsulinemia may have increase free radicals and therefore promote aging, independent of glycemia [8,94,96]. Plasma levels of lipid hydroperoxides are higher, and antioxidant vitamins are lower in individuals who are resistant to insulin-stimulated glucose disposal but otherwise glucose tolerant, nonobese, and normotensive [93,95]. There is substantial evidence supporting the hypothesis that selective resistance to insulin-stimulated (muscle) glucose disposal consequent hyperinsulinemia triggers a variety of metabolic effects, likely resulting in accelerated oxidative stress and aging [8,93,95].

The anti-diabetics biguanides inhibit fatty acid oxidation, inhibit gluconeogenesis in the liver, increase the availability of insulin receptors, inhibit monoamine oxidase [121], increase sensitivity of hypothalamo-pituitary complex to negative feedback inhibition, reduce excretion of glucocorticoid metabolites and dehydroepiandrosterone-sulfate [8]. These drugs have been proposed for the prevention of the age-related increase of cancer and atherosclerosis, and for retardation of the aging process [8]. It has been shown that administration of antidiabetic biguanides into patients with hyperlipidemia lowers the level of blood cholesterol, triglycerides, and β-lipoproteins. It also inhibits the development of atherosclerosis, reduces hyperinsulinemia in men with coronary artery disease. It increases hypothalamo-pituitary sensitivity to inhibition by dexamethasone and estrogens, causes restoration of estrous cycle in persistent-estrous old rats, improves cellular immunity in atherosclerotic and cancer patients, lowers blood IGF-1 levels in cancer and atherosclerotic patients with Type IIb hyperlipoproteinemia, [8]. There are data on antioxidative effect of biguanides [133,146] and its neuroprotective activity [147]. It was shown that biguanides inhibits complex I of the respiratory chain in mitochondria that leads to an activation of physiological intracellular inhibition of mitochondrial respiration [148]. Biguanides stimulate a protein kinase cascade inhibiting an expression of transcription factor SREBP-1. An interaction of this factor with cholesterol leads to an increase in transcription of genes coding lipogenesis enzymes and to suppression of free fat acids oxidation. Thus, stimulation of uptake of glucose in tissues by biguanides inhibits lipogenesis and activates oxidation of FFA [149]. It was shown also that in vivo biguanides inhibits an appetite [150,151] and serum levels of leptin and IGF-1 [152]. It was suggested that biguanides regulate energy balance of the organism at the fat tissue level [153]. In general, results of bioguanides effects seem very similar to those of calorie restriction.

Table 5. Comparison of characteristics of rodents subjected to normal aging, caloric restriction, genetic modifications or treatment with antidiabetic biguanides.

Parameters	Aging	Calorie restriction	Dwarf mice	*GH R*$^{-/-}$	*Igf1r*$^{+/-}$	FIRKO	Biguanides
Life span extension	↓	+40-50%	+50%	+46 %	+33%	+18%	+20%
Tolerance to glucose	↓	↑	↓	↓	↑↓[a]	= or ↑	↑
Senstivity to insulin	↓	↑	↑	↑	↑	↑ in fat	↑
Serum level: Insulin	↑	↓	↓	↓	=	↓	↓
GH	↓	↓	Absent	↑	ND	↓	↓
IGF-1	↓	↓	↓	↓	↓	↓	↓
Body size	↑	↓	↓	↓	↓	↓	↓
Body fat content	↑	↓	↑	ND	↑↓	↓	↓
Reproductive function	↓	↓[b]	↓[b]	↓[b]	=[b]	ND	↑
Thyroid function	↓	↓	↓	↓	=	ND	↑
Serum cortico-sterone	↑	↑	=	=	ND	ND	↓
Immune function	↓	↓	= or ↓	ND	ND	ND	↑
Resistance to oxidatve stress	↓	↑	↓	↓	↑	↑	↑
Tumor incidence	↑	↓	= or ↓	=	=	ND	↓

Note: ↓ - decrease; ↑ - increase; = no effect; ND – no available data.

[a] The tolerance to glucose is increased in females but decreased in male.

[b] Reproductive function in relation to normal aging mice.

8. CONCLUSION

The incidence of cancer increases with age in humans and in laboratory animals alike, but patterns of age-related distribution of tumors is different for different tissues and different tumors. Aging may increase or decrease the susceptibility of individual tissues to early carcinogens and usually facilitates promotion and progression of carcinogenesis. Aging may predispose to cancer by two mechanisms: tissue accumulation of cells in late stages of carcinogenesis and alterations in internal homeostasis, in particular, alterations in immune and endocrine system. Increased susceptibility to the effect of late-stage carcinogens is found both in aged animals and elderly humans, as predicted by the multistage model of carcinogenesis. Studies in mammals have led to the suggestion that hyperglycemia and hyperinsulinemia are important factors both in aging and in the development of cancer. Insulin/insulin-like growth factor 1 (IGF-1) signaling molecules that have been linked to longevity include DAF-2 and InR and their homologues in mammals, and inactivation of the corresponding genes followed by the increase in life span in nematodes, fruit flies and mice. It is possible that the life-prolonging effects of caloric restriction are due to decreasing IGF-1 levels. A search of pharmacological modulators of insulin/IGF-1 signaling pathway mimetic effects of life span extending mutations or calorie restriction could be a perspective direction in regulation of longevity. Some old and new observations suggest that antidiabetic biguanides could be promising candidates for both the life span extension and the prevention of cancer.

REFERENCES

1. Anisimov VN: Carcinogenesis and Aging. Vols 1 and 2. Boca Raton, FL. CRC Press, 1987
2. Dix D; Cohen P: On the role of aging in carcinogenesis. Anticancer Res 1999;19:723-726
3. Parkin DM; Bray FI; Devesa SS: Cancer burden in the year 2000. The global picture. Eur J Cancer 2001; 37:S4-S66
4. Peto R; Parish SE; Gray RG: There is no such thing as aging, and cancer is not related to it. In Likhachev A; Anisimov V; Montesano R (eds): Age-related factors in carcinogenesis. IARC, Lyon. France. 1985; 58:43-53
5. Anisimov VN: Carcinogenesis and aging. Adv Cancer Res 1983; 40: 265-324
6. Anisimov V.N. The relationship between aging and carcinogenesis: a critical appraisal. Crit. Rev. Oncol. Hematol. 2003; 45:277-304
7. Miller RA: Gerontology as oncology. Cancer. 1991; 68:2496-2501
8. Dilman VM: Development, aging, and disease. A new rationale for and intervention strategy. Chur: Harwood Acad Publ Switzerland, 1994

9. Simpson AJG: A natural somatic mutation frequency and human carcinogenesis. Adv Cancer Res 1993;71:209-240
10. Campisi J: Cancer and ageing: rival demons? Nature Rev Cancer 2003;3:339-349
11. DePinho RA: The age of cancer. Nature 2000; 408:248-254
12. von Wangenheim KH; Peterson HP: Control of cell proliferation by progress in differentiation: clues to mechanisms of aging, cancer causation and therapy. J Theor Biol. 1998; 193:663-678
13. Reya T; Morrison SJ; Clarke MF; Weissman IL: Stem cells, cancer, and cancer stem cells. Nature 2001; 414:105-111
14. Anisimov VN: Age as a factor of risk in multistage carcinogenesis. In: Balducci L; Lyman GH; Ershler WB (eds): Comprehensive geriatric oncology. Amsterdam: Harwood Acad. Publ. 1998; 157-178
15. Moolgavkar S; Krewski D; Zeise L; Cardis E; Moller H (eds): Quantitative estimation and prediction of human cancer risk. IARC Sci Publ No 131. Lyon: IARC. 1999
16. Butov AA; Volkov MA; Anisimov VN: Mathematical and simulating model of accelerated aging induced by 5-bromodeoxyuridine. Adv Gerontol 2001; 8:70-76
17. Berenblum I: Sequential aspects of chemical carcinogenesis: skin. In Becker J (ed.): Cancer - A Comprehensive Treatise. Plenum Press. New York. 1975; 323-344
18. Consensus Report. In Vanio H, Magee PN, McGregor D, McMichael AJ (eds.): Mechanisms of Carcinogenesis in Risk Identification. IARC Scientific Publication No.116. IARC. Lyon. France. 1992; 9-56
19. Barrett JC: Mechanisms of action of known human carcinogens. In: Vainio H; Magee PN; McGregor DB; McMichael AJ (eds): Mechanisms of Carcinogenesis in Risk Identification. IARC. Lyon. France. 1992;116:115-134
20. Slaga TJ (ed.): Mechanisms of Tumor Promotion. Vols 1-4, CRC Press. Boca Raton, FL, 1983/84
21. Harris CC: Chemical and physical carcinogenesis: advances and perspectives for the 1990s. *Cancer Res.* 1991; 51:5023s-5044s
22. Slaga TJ: Can tumor Promotion be effectively inhibited? In Borzsonyi M, Day NE, Lapis K, Yamasaki H (eds): Models. Mechanisms and Etiology of Tumor Promotion. IARC Scientific Publication No. 56. IARC. Lyon, France. 1984; 497-506
23. Hanahan D; Weinberg RA: The hallmarks of cancer. Cell 2000;100:57-70
24. Kaldor JM; Day NE: Interpretation of epidemiological studies in the context of the multistage model of carcinogenesis. In: Barret JC (ed.): Mechanisms of Environmental carcinogenesis. Boca Raton. FL. CRC Press. 1987; 2:21-57
25. Anisimov VN; Zhukovskaya NV; Loktionov AS; et al: Influence of host age on lung colony forming capacity of injected rat rhabdomyosarcoma cells. Cancer Lett 1988; 40:77-82
26. Birnbaum LS: Pharmacokinetic basis of age-related changes in sensitivity to toxicants. Annu Rev Pharmacol Toxicol 1991; 31:101-128
27. Mayersohn M: Pharmacokinetics in the elderly. Environ Health Perspectives Suppl 11. 1994; 102:119-124
28. Preston-Martin S; Pike MC; Ross RK; Jones PA; Henderson BE: Increased cell division as a cause of human cancer. Cancer Res 1990; 50:7415-7421
29. Evan G; Littlewood T: A matter of life and cell death. Science 1998; 281:1317-1321
30. Zhang Y; Herman B: Ageing and apoptosis. Mech Aging Dev 2002; 123:245-260
31. Kinzler KW; Vogelstein B: Gatekeepers and caretakers. Nature 1997; 386:761-763
32. Summerhayes IC; Franks LM: Effect of donor age on neoplastic transformation of adult bladder epithelium in vitro. J Natl Cancer Inst 1979; 62:1017-1023
33. Kunisada T; Danner D; Friedman V; Schneider EL: Increased susceptibility to SV40 transformation with development and in vitro aging. Exp Cell Res 1990; 189:222-226
34. Tavoloni N; Inoue H: Cellular aging is a critical determinant of primary cell resistance to v-*src* transformation. J Virol 1997; 71: 237-247

35. Nettesheim P; Topping DC; Jamasbi R: Host and environmental factors enhancing carcinogenesis in the respiratory tract. Annu Rev Pharmacol Toxicol 1981; 21:133-163
36. Maciera-Coelho A: Neoplastic disease through the human life span. Biogerontology 2001; 2: 179-192
37. Maciera-Coelho A: Genome reorganization through cell division, implications for aging of the organism and cancer development. Ann NY Acad Sci 1994; 719: 108-128
38. Stenback F; Peto R; Shubik P: Initiation and promotion at different ages and doses in 2200 mice. III. Linear extrapolation from high doses may underestimate low-dose tumor risks. Br J Cancer 1981; 44:24-34
39. Ebbesen P: Papilloma development on TPA treated young and senescent mouse skin. In: Likhachev A; Anisimov V; Montesano R (eds): Age-related factors in carcinogenesis. IARC Sci Publ No 58. Lyon: IARC, 1985; 167-171
40. Ebbesen P: Reticulosarcoma and amyloid development in BALB/c mice inoculated with syngeneic cells from young and old donors. J Natl Cancer Inst 1971; 47:1241-1245
41. Hennings H; Boutwell RK: Studies on the mechanism of skin tumor promotion. Cancer Res 1970; 30:312-320
42. Kruszewski FH; Conti CJ; DiGiovanni J: Characterization of skin tumor promotion and progression by chrysarobin in SENCAR mice. Cancer Res 1987; 47:3783-3790
43. Hennings D; Yuspa SH: Two-stage tumor promotion in mouse skin: An alternative interpretation. J Natl Cancer Inst 1985; 74:735-740
44. Moriwaki S; Ray S; Tarone RE; Kraemer KH; Grossman L: The effect of donor age on the processing of UV-damaged DNA by cultured human cells: reduced DNA repair capacity and increased DNA mutability. Mutat Res 1996; 364:117-123
45. Wei Q: Effect of aging on DNA repair and skin carcinogenesis: a minireview of population-based studies. J Investig Dermatol Symp Proc 1998; 3(1):19-22
46. Ouhtit A; Ueda M; Nakazawa M; Dumaz N; Sarasin A; Yamasaki H: Quantitative detection of ultraviolet-specific p53 mutations in normal skin from Japanese patients. Cancer Epidemiol Biomarkers Prev 1997; 6:433-438
47. Liang S-B; Ohtsuki Y; Furihata M; Takeuchi T; Iwata J; Chen B-K;Sonobe H: Sun-exposure- and aging-dependent p53 protein accumulation results in growth advantage for tumour cells in carcinogenesis of nonmelanocytic skin cancer. Virchows Arch 2000; 434:193-199
48. D'Errico M; Calcagnile AS; Corona R, et al: p53 mutations and chromosome instability in basal cell carcinomas developed at an early or late age. Cancer Res 1997; 57:747-752
49. Ueda M: Telomerase in cutaneous carcinogenesis. J Dermatol Sci 2000; 23, Suppl 1:S37-S40
50. Boutwell RK: Some biological aspects of skin carcinogenesis. Prog Exp Tumor Res 1964; 4:207-250
51. Roe FJC; Carter RL; Mitchley R; Peto R; Hecker E: On the persistence of tumor initiation and the acceleration of tumor progression in mouse skin tumorigenesis. Int J Cancer 1972; 9:264-273
52. Van Duuren BL; Sivak A; Katz C; Steidman I; Melchionne S: The effect of aging and interval between primary and secondary treatment in two-stage carcinogenesis on mouse skin. Cancer Res 1975; 35:502-505
53. Battalora MStJ; Spadling JW; Szczesniak CJ et al: Age-dependent skin tumorigenesis and transgene expression in the Tg.AC (v-Ha-ras) transgenic mice. Carcinogenesis 2001; 22:651-659
54. Lee G-H; Sawada N; Mochizuki Y et al: Immortal epithelial cells of normal C3H mouse liver in culture: possible precursor populations for spontaneous hepatocellular carcinoma. Cancer Res 1989; 49:403-409

55. Ward JM; Lynch P; Riggs C: Rapid development of hepatocellular neoplasms in aging male C3H/HeNcr mice given phenobarbital. Cancer Lett 1988; 39:9-18
56. Ward JM: Increased susceptibility of liver of aged F.344/Ncr rats to the effects of phenobarbital on the incidence, morphology, and histochemistry of hepatocellular foci and neoplasms. J Natl Cancer Inst 1983; 71:815-823
57. Kraupp-Grasl B; Huber W; Taper H; Schulte-Hermann R: Increased susceptibility of aged rats to hepatocarcinogenesis by the peroxisome proliferator nafenopin and the possible involvement of altered liver foci occurring spontaneously. Cancer Res 1991; 51:666-671
58. Geschickter CF; Byrnes EW: Factor influencing the development and time of appearance of mammary cancer in the rat in response to estrogen. Arch Pathol 1942; 33:334-342
59. Anisimov VN: Age and dose-dependent carcinogenic effects of N-nitrosomethylurea administered intraperitoneally in a single dose to young and adult female mice. J Cancer Res Clin Oncol 1993; 119:657-664
60. Anisimov VN: Effect of aging and interval between primary and secondary treatment in carcinogenesis induced by neonatal exposure to 5-bromodeoxyuridine and subsequent administration of N-nitrosomethylurea in rats. Mutat Res 1995; 316:173-187
61. Anisimov VN; Birnbaum LS; Butenko GM et al: Principles for evaluating chemical effects on the aged population. Environmental Health Criteria 144. Geneva: WHO, 1993
62. Takahashi M; Nishimura S; Miyajima K; Sasahara K; Yoshida M; Ando J; Maekawa A: Time-dependent promotion activity of 17β-estradiol on uterine carcinogenesis in mice initiated with N-ethyl-N-nitrosourea. Cancer Lett 2001; 165: 123-130
63. Peto R; Roe FJC; Lee PN; Levy L; Clack J: Cancer and aging in mice and men. Br J Cancer 1975; 32:411-426
64. Anisimov VN: Effect of age on dose-response relationship in carcinogenesis induced by single administration of N-nitrosomethylurea in female rats. J Cancer Res Clin Oncol 1988; 114:628-635
65. McCullough KD; Coleman WB; Smith GJ; Grisham JW: Age-dependent regulation of the tumorigenic potential of neoplastically transformed rat liver epithelial cells by the liver micro- environment. Cancer Res 1994; 54:3668-3671
66. Krtolika A; Campisi J: Integrating epithelial cancer, aging stroma and cellular senescent. Adv. Gerontol 2003; 11:109-116
67. Krtolica A; Parinello S; Locckett S; Desprez P-Y; Campisi J: Senescent fibroblasts promote epithelial cell growth and tumorigenesis: a link between cancer and aging. Proc Natl Acad Sci USA 2001; 98:12072-12077
68. Pitot HC: The molecular biology of carcinogenesis. Cancer 1993; 72:962-970
69. Luzatto L: The mechanisms of neoplastic trasformation. Eur J Cancer 2001; 37:S114-S117
70. Ponten J: Cell biology of precancer. Eur J Cancer 2001; 37:S97-S113
71. Vijg J: Somatic mutations and aging: a re-evaluation. Mutat Res. 2000; 447:117-135
72. Matoha HF; Cosgrove JW; Atak JR; Rapoport SI: Selective elevation of c-myc transcript levels in the liver of the aging Fischer-344 rat. Biochem Biophys Res Commun 1987; 147:1-7
73. Ono T; Uehara Y; Kurishita A; Tawa R; Sakurai H: Biological significance of DNA methylation in the aging process. Age & Aging 1993; 22:534-543
74. Lindahl T: Instability and decay of the primary structure of DNA. Nature 1993; 362:709-715
75. Catania J; Fairweather DS: DNA methylation and cellular aging. Mutat Res 1991; 256: 283-293
76. Yu BP (ed): Free radicals in aging. Boca Raton: CRC Press, Inc, 1993
77. Barja G: Endogenous oxidative stress: relationship to aging, longevity and caloric restriction. Ageing Res Rev 2002; 1:397-411

78. Shigenaga MK; Hagen TV; Ames BN: Oxidative damage and mitochondrial decay in aging. Proc Natl Acad Sci USA. 1994; 91:10771-10778
79. Fraga CG; Shigenaga MK; Park J-W; Degan P; Ames BN: Oxidative damage to DNA during aging 8-hydroxy-2'deoxyganosine in rat organ DNA and urine. Proc Natl Acad Sci USA 1990; 87:4533-4537
80. Ames BN; Shigenaga MB; Hagen TM: Oxidants, antioxidants, and the degenerative diseases of aging. Proc Natl Acad Sci USA. 1993; 90:7915-7922
81. Anisimov VN; Semenchenko AV; Yashin AI: Insulin and longevity: antidiabetic biguanides as geroprotectors. Biogerontoloy 2003; 4: 303-313
82. Harman DH: Free-radical theory of aging: increasing the functional life span. Ann NY Acad Sci 1994; 717:257-266
83. Reiter RJ: Reactive oxygen species, DNA damage, and carcinogenesis: intervention with melatonin. In Bartsch C; Bartsch H; Blask DE; Cardinali DP; Hrushesky WJM; Mecke D (eds): The Pineal Gland and Cancer. Berlin: Springer-Verlag: 2001:442-455
84. Coller HA; Khrapko K; Bodyak ND et al: High frequency of homoplasmic mitochondrial DNA mutations in human tumors can be explained without selection. Nature Genet 2001; 28:147-150
85. Khrapko K; Nekhaeva E; Kraytsberg Y; Kunz W: Clonal expansion of mitochondrial genomes: implicatons for in vivo mutaton spectra. Mutat Res 2003; 522:13
86. de Grey AD: The reductive hotspot hypothesis: un update. Arch Biochem Biophys 2000; 373:295-301
87. Chow M; Rubin H: Clonal selection versus genetic instability as the driving force in neoplastic transformation. Cancer Res 2000; 60:6510-6518
88. Dolle ME; Snyder WK; Dunson DB; Vijg J: Mutational fingerprints of aging. Nucleic Acids Res 2002; 30:545-549
89. Aboseif S; El-Sakka A; Young P; Cunha G: Mesenchymal reprogramming of adult human epithelial differentiation. Differentiation 1999; 65: 113-118
90. Liotta LA; Kohn EC: The microenvironment of the tumor-host interface. Nature 2001; 411:375-379
91. Bartke A; Chandrashekar V; Dominici F et al: Insulin-like growth factor 1 (IGF01) and aging: controversies and new insights. Biogerontology 2003; 4:1-8
92. Tatar M; Bartke A; Antebi A: The endocrine regulation of aging by insulin-like signals. Science 2003; 299:1346-1351
93. Facchini FS; Hua N; Abbasi F; Reaven GM: Insulin resistance as a predictor of age-related diseases. J.Clin.Endocrinol Metab 2001; 86:3574-3578
94. Ulrich P; Cerami A: Protein glycation, diabetes, and aging. Recent Prog Horm Res 2001; 56:1-21
95. Facchini FS; Hua NW; Reaven GM; Stoohs RA: Hyperinsulinemia: the missing link among oxidative stress and age-related diseases? Free Radicals Biol. Med. 2000; 29:1302-1306
96. Barbieri M; Rizzo MR; Manzella D; Grella R; Ragno E; Carbonella M; Abbatecola AM; Paolisso G: Glucose regulation and oxidative stress in healthy centenarians. Exp. Gerontol 2003; 38:137-143
97. Colangelo LA; Gapstur SM; Gann PH; Dyer AR; Liu K: Colorectal cancer mortality and factors related to the insulin resistance syndrome. Cancer Epidemiol. Biomarkers Prev 2002; 11:385-391
98. Gupta K; Krishnaswamy G; Karnad A; Peiris AN: Insulin: a novel factor in carcinogenesis. Am. J. Med. Sci. 2002; 323:140-145
99. Kenyon C: A conserved regulatory system for aging. Cell 2001; 105:165-168
100. Dillin A; Crawford DK; Kenyon C: Timing requirements for insulin/IGF-1 signaling in *C. elegans.* Science 2002; 298:830-834

101. Ramaswamy S; Nakamura N; Sansal I; Bergeron L; Sellers WR: A novel mechanism of gene regulation and tumor suppression by the transcription factor FKHR. Cancer Cel 2002; 2:81-91
102. Richards JS; Sharma SC; Falender AE; Lo YH: Expression of FKHR, FKHRL1, and AFX genes in the rodent ovary: evidence for regulation by IGF-I, estrogen, and the gonadotropins. Mol Endocrinol 2002; 16: 590-599
103. Flurkey K; Papaconstantinou J; Miller RA; Harrison DE: Life-span extension and delayed immune and collagen aging in mutant mice with defects in growth hormone production. Proc Natl Acad Sci USA 2001; 98:6736-6741
104. Coschigano KT; Clemmons D; Bellush LL; Kopchick JJ: Assessment of growth parameters and life span of GHR/BP gene-disrupted mice. Endocrinology 2000; 141:2608-2613
105. Hsieh CC; Deord JH; Flurkey K; Harrison DE; Papaconstantinou J: Implications for the insulin signaling pathway in Snell dwarf mouse longevity: a similarity with the C. elegans longevity paradigm. Mech Aging Dev 2002; 123:1229-1244
106. Hsieh CC; DeFord JH; Flurkey K; Harrison DE; Papaconstantinou J: Effects of the Pit1 mutation on the insulin signaling pathway: implications on the longevity of the long-lived Snell dwarf mouse. Mech Aging Dev 2002; 123:1245-1255
107. Weindruch R; Sohal RS: Caloric intake and aging. The New Engl J Med 1997; 337: 986-994
108. Mattison JM; Wright C; Bronson RT; Roth GS; Ingram DK; Bartke A: Studies of aging in Ames dwarf mice: effects of caloric restriction. J Amer Aging Assoc 2000; 23:9-16
109. Dominici FP; Arosegui Diaz G; Bartke A; Kopchik JJ; Turyn D: Compensatory alterations of insulin signal transduction in liver of growth hormone receptor knockout mice. J Endocrinol 2000; 166:579-590
110. Dominici FP; Hauck S; Argention DP; Bartke A; Turyn D: Increased insulin sensitivity and upregulation of insulin receptor, insulin receptor substrate (ISR)-1 and IRS-2 in liver of Ames dwarf mice. J Endocrinol 2002; 173, 81-94
111. Chiba T; Yamaza H; Higami Y; Shimokawa I: Anti-aging effects of caloric restriction: Involvement of neuroendocrine adaptation by peripheral signaling. Microsc Res Tech 2002; 59: 317-324
112. Mattison JA; Lane MA; Roth GS; Ingram DK: Calorie restriction in rhesus monkeys. Exp. Gerontol 2003; 38: 35-46
113. Holzenberger M.; Dupond J; Ducos B; Leneuve P; Gefoen A.; Even PC; Cervera P; Le Bouc Y: IGF-1 receptor regulates lifespan and resistance to oxidative stress in mice. Nature 2003; 421:182-187
114. Bluher M; Kahn BB; Kahn CR.: Extended longevity in mice lacking the insulin receptor in adipose tissue. Science 2003; 299: 572-574
115. Bluher M; Michael M.D; Peroni OD; Ueki K; Carter N; Kahn BB; Kahn CR: Adipose tissue selective insulin receptor knockut protects against obesity and obesity-related glucose intolerance. Dev Cell 2002; 3: 25-38
116. Shimokawa I; Higami Y; Utsuyama M; Tuchiya T; Komatsu T; Chiba T; Yamaza H: Life span extension by reducing in growth hormone-insulin-growth factor-1 axis in a transgenic rat model. Am J Pathol 2002; 160, 2259-2265
117. Anisimov SV; Volkova MV; Lenskaya LV; Khavinson VKh; Solovieva DV; Schwartz EI: Age-associated accumulation of the Apolipoprotein C-III gene T-455C polymorphism C allele in a Russian population. J Gerontol Biol Sci 2001; 56A: B27-B32
118. Singal PK: Beamish RE; Dhalla NS: Potential oxidative pathways of catecholamine in the formation of lipid peroxides and genesis of heart disease. Adv Exp Biol Med 1983; 161: 391-401
119. Ruiz-Torres A; Soares de Melo Kirzner, M; Aging and longevity are related to growth hormone/insulin-like growth factor-1 secretion. Gerontology 2002; 48: 401-407

120. Roth GS; Lane MA; Ingram DK; Mattison JA; Elahi D; Tobin JD; Muller D; Metter EJ: Biomarkers of caloric restriction may predict longevity in humans. Science 2002; 297: 811
121. Muntoni, S., 1999. Metformin and fatty acids. Diabetes Care 22, 179-80
122. Berstein LM; Evtushenko TP; Tsyrlina EV; Bobrov YuF; Ostroumova MN; Kovalenko IG; Semiglazov VF; Simonov NN; Dilman VM: Comparative study of 5- and 10-year-long results of the metabolic rehabilitation of cancer patients. In: Hanson KP; Dilman VM (eds.): Neuroendocrine System, Metabolism, Immunity and Cancer (Clinical Aspects). N.N. Petrov Research Institute of Oncology Publ, St.Petersburg, 1992:102-112
123. Bakaev VV: Effect of 1-butylbiguanide hydrochloride on the longevity in the nematoda *Caenorhabditis elegans*. Biogerontology 3, 2002; Suppl. 1:23-24
124. Anisimov VN: Effect of buformin and diphenylhydantoin on life span, estrus function and spontaneous tumor incidence in female rats. Vopr Onkol 1980; 26 (6): 42-48
125. Anisimov VN; Semenchenko AV; Yashin AI: Insulin and longevity: antidiabetic biguanides as geroprotectors. Biogerontology 2003; 4: 297-307
126. Dilman VM; Anisimov VN: Hypothalamic mechanisms of ageing and of specific age pathology – I. Sensitivity threshold of hypothalamo-pituitary complex to homeostatic stimuli in the reproductive system. Exp. Gerontol 1979; 14: 161-174
127. Dilman VM; Anisimov VN: Potentiation of antitumor effect of cyclophosphamide and hydrazine sulfate by treatment with the antidiabetic agent, 1-phenylethylbiguanide (phenformin). Cancer Lett. 1979a; 7: 357-361
128. Dilman VM; Anisimov VN: Effect of treatment with phenofromin, dyphenylhydantoin or L-DOPA on life span and tumor incidence in C3H/Sn mice. Gerontology 1980; 26: 241-245
129. Rossmanith WG; Neuroendocrinology of aging in the reproductive system: gonadotropin secretion as an example. In: Kumar A.; Mukhopadhayay AK (eds). Follicular Growth, Ovulation and Fertilization: Molecular and Clinical Basis. Narosa Publ. House, New Dehli 2001;15-25
130. Hung AJ; Stanbury MG; Shanabrough M; Horvath TL; Garcia-Segura LM; Naftolin F: Estrogen, synaptoc plasticity and hypothalamic reproductive aging. Exp Gerontol 2003; 38:53-59
131. Awartani KA; Cheung AP: Metformin and polycystic ovary syndrome: a literature review. J Obstet Gynecol Can 2002; 24, 393-401
132. Fernandes ML; Saad MJ; Velloso LA: Effect of age on elements of insulin-signaling pathway in central nervous system of rats. Endocrine 2001;16: 227-234
133. Mattson MP; Duan W; Maswood N: How does the brain control lifespan? Ageing Res Rev 2002; 1: 155-165
134. McCarty MF; Longevity effect of chromium picolinate – 'rejuvenation' of hypothalamic function? Medical Hypotheses 1994; 3: 253-265
135. De Benedictis G; Tan Q; Jeune B; Christensen K; Ukraintseva SV; Bonafe M; Franceschi C; Vaupel JW; Yashin.AI: Recent advances in human gene-longevity association studies. Mech Ageing Dev 2001; 122:909-920
136. Huxtable SJ; Saker PJ; Haddad L; Walker M; Frayling TM; Levy JC; Hitman GA; O'Rahilly S; Hattersley AT; McCarthy MI: Analysis of parent-offspring trios provides evidence for linkage and association between the insulin gene and type 2 diabetes mediated exclusively through paternally transmitted class III variable number tandem repeat allels. Diabetes 2000; 49: 126-130
137. Weaver JU; Kopelman PG; Hitman GA: Central obesity and hyperinsulinemia in women are associated with polymorphism in the 5' flanking region of the human insulin gene. Eur. J. Clin. Invest 1992; 22: 265-270
138. Waterworth DM; Bennett ST; Gharani N; McCarthy MI.; Hague S; Batty S; Conway GS; White D; Todd JA; Franks S; Williamson R: Linkage and association of insulin gene

VNTR regulatory polymorphism with polycystic ovary syndrome. Lancet 1997; 349: 986-990

139. Tybaierg-Hansen A; Gerdes IU; Overgaard K; Ingerslev J; Faergeman O; Nerup J; Polymorphysm in 5' flanking region of human insulin gene. Relationships with atherosclerosis, lipid levels and age in three samples from Denmark. Arteriosclerosis 1990; 10: 372-378
140. Anisimov VN; Belous NM; Vasilyeva IA; Dilman VM: Inhibitory effect of phenformin on the development of mammary tumors induced by N-nitrosomethylurea in rats. Exp Onkol 1980 2(3): 40-43
141. Dilman VM; Sofronov BN; Anisimov VN; Nazarov PG; L'vovich EG: Phenformin elimination of the immunodepression caused by 1,2-dimethylhydrazine in rats. Vopr Onkol 1977; 23(8): 50-54
142. Wu Y; Yakar S; Zhao L; Hennighausen L; LeRoith D: Circulating insulin-like growth factor-1 levels regulate colon cancer growth and metastasis. Cancer Res. 2002; 62: 1030-1035
143. Alexandrov VA; Anisimov VN; Belous NM; Vasilyeva IA; Mazon VB: The inhibition of the transplacental blastomogenic effect of nitrosomethylurea by postnatal administration of buformin to rats. Carcinogenesis 1980; 1:975-978
144. Bespalov VG; Alexandrov VA: Influence of anticarcinogenic agents on the transplacental carcinogenic effect of N-nitroso-N-ethylurea. Bull Exp Biol Med 1985; 100:73-76
145. Schneider MB; Matsuzaki H; Harorah J; Ulrich A; Standlop J; Ding XZ; Adrian TE; Pour PM: Prevention of pancreatic cancer induction in hamsters by metformin. Gastroenterology 2001, 120, 1263-1270
146. Gargiulo P; Caccese D; Pignatelli P; Brufani C; De Vito F; Marino R; Lauro R; Violi F; Di Mario U; Sanguigni V: Metformin decreases platelet superoxide anion production in diabetic patients. Diabetes Metab Res Rev 2002; 18:156-159
147. Lee J; Chan SL; Lane MA; Mattson MP: Phenformin suppresses calcium responses to glutamate and protects hippocampal neurons against excitotoxicity. Exp Neurol 2002; 175:161-167
148. El Mir MY; Nogueira V; Fontaine E; Averet N; Rigoulet M; Leverve X: Dimethylbiguanide inhibits cell respiration via an indirect effect targeted on the respiratory chain complex I. J Biol Chem 2000; 275:223–228
149. Zhou G; Myers R; Li Y; Chen Y; Shen X; Fenyk-Melody J; Wu M; Ventre J; Doebber T; Fujii N; Musi N; Hirshman MF; Goodyear LJ; and Moller DE: Role of AMP-activated protein kinase in mechanism of metformin action. J Clin Invest 2001; 108:1167–1174
150. Paolisso G; Gambardella A; Ammendola S; D'Amore, A; Varrichio M: Glucose tolerance and insulin action in healthy centenarians. Am J Physiol 1996; 270:E890-E-896
151. Paolisso G; Amato L; Eccellente R; Gambardella A; Tagliamonte MR; Varricchio G; Carella C; Giugliano D; D'Onofrio F: Effect of metformin on food intake in obese subjects. Eur J Clin Invest 1998; 28:441–446
152. Fruehwald-Schultes B; Oltmanns KM; Toschek B; Sopke S; Kern W; Born J; Fehm HL; Peters A: Short-term treatment with metformin decreases serum leptin concentration without affecting body weight and body fat content in normal-weight healthy men. Metabolism 2002; 51:531–536
153. Mick GJ; Wang X; Ling FC; McCormick KL: Inhibition of leptin secretion by insulin and metformin in cultured rat adipose tissue. Biochim Biophys Acta 2000; 1502:426–432
154. Carrilo MC; Favre C; Carnovale CE et al: Involvement of μ class glutathione S-transferase subunit M_2 (rGST M_2) levels in the initiation and promotion of hepatocarcinogenesis in old rats. Exp Gerontol 2001; 36:255-265
155. Reuber MD; Glover EL: Hyperplastic and early neoplastic lesions of the liver in Buffalo strain rats of various ages given subcutaneous carbon tetrachloride. J Natl Cancer Inst 1967; 38:891-897

156. Youssef JA; Bouziane M; Badr MZ: Age-dependent effects of nongenotoxic hepatocarcinogens on liver apoptosis in vivo. Mech Ageing Dev 2003; 12
157. Anisimov VN; Sheiko EV; Zhukovskaya NV: Effect of age on development of tumours in the intrasplenic ovarian grafts in ovariectomized rats. J Cancer Res Clin Oncol 1992; 119:111-116

Chapter 3

REPLICATIVE SENESCENCE AND CANCER

Peter J. Hornsby

Department of Physiology and Sam and Ann Barshop Center for Longevity and Aging Studies, University of Texas Health Science Center, San Antonio, Texas

1. THE CAUSE OF REPLICATIVE SENESCENCE: TELOMERE SHORTENING

Since the pioneering experiments of Leonard Hayflick in the 1960s it has been known the limited replicative capacity of human cells in culture is very unlikely to be a experimental artifact, but is a reproducible biological phenomenon [1]. However, it was not until it was discovered that the limitation in replicative capacity directly correlates with shortening of telomeres that the notion that it might be a culture artifact was finally laid to rest [2,3]. Telomeres undergo shortening in most dividing human somatic cells because of the lack of telomerase activity that is required for telomere maintenance [4, 5]. The lack of telomerase activity results from the absence of expression of the reverse transcriptase subunit (TERT) of the telomerase ribonucleoprotein complex [6, 7]. When cells divide in the absence of telomerase activity about 40-100 bp of the terminal telomeric repeat DNA is not replicated [4, 5]. This amount is a constant for various types of human cells, thus providing a kind of mitotic counter [4, 5].

After a normal human cell has divided a certain number of times, further cell division is then blocked by inhibitors of cell proliferation such as $p21^{SDI1/WAF1/CIP1}$ and $p16^{INK4A}$ [8, 9]. When this checkpoint is abrogated by oncoproteins such as SV40 T antigen, which suppress the activity of p53 and pRb, this checkpoint ("Hayflick limit," also termed M1) is bypassed and cells eventually enter a second state, termed crisis or M2 [10]. In this state the much shorter telomeres undergo end-to-end fusions and initiate chromosomal breakage-fusion cycles that cause the cells to undergo apoptosis. There is massive loss of cells from the culture, whereas in replicative senescence (M1) cells do not die, and are in fact more resistant to apoptosis [11]. About 1 in 10^7 cells undergoes an unknown change that permits escape from crisis/M2 [12]. Such a cell line is said to be "immortal" in the jargon of cell culture, a term that should not be interpreted as implying the reversal of a cellular aging process. In most of these immortalized cell lines the TERT gene has become reactivated [13], but some activate a recombination-based process call ALT (alternative lengthening of telomeres) [14]. Although human fibroblasts can form immortal cell lines in this way by escaping from crisis, they never spontaneously immortalize by escaping from replicative senescence/M1. Most cancer cells that can be grown in culture are also immortal and express TERT. The mechanisms by which cancer cells reactivate or maintain expression of TERT or activate alternate mechanisms for avoiding telomere shortening are largely unknown.

The phenomenon of telomere shortening is clearly the result of the lack of expression of TERT in most normal human somatic cells. Initially it was thought that somatic human cells completely lack telomerase activity and that germ line cells, some stem cells and most cancer cells do have telomerase activity. Subsequently it has become clear that normal human cells do express TERT but that expression is tightly regulated, by processes not yet well understood [15-19]. In some cell types telomerase activity is induced when cells are first isolated from the body and stimulated to divide in culture [20-23]. Curiously, longer-term proliferation is associated with a decline in telomerase activity, sometimes very rapid, so that few long-term cultures of normal human cells have sufficient telomerase activity for telomere maintenance. One type of non-cancer cells that are believed to be immortal are human embryonic stem cells, when they are grown under conditions that prevent differentiation from occurring [24].

Proof that the limitation on indefinite cell division in most human cells results from lack of expression of TERT was obtained by showing that forced expression of hTERT is sufficient to immortalize normal human fibroblasts and retinal pigmented epithelial cells, and is required (although not sufficient by itself) to immortalize keratinocytes and mammary epithelial cells [25, 26]. Immortalization by hTERT is accompanied by increased or stabilized telomere length, but cells retain a normal karyotype [27, 28]. Conversely, some immortal cells suffer telomere shortening and eventual cessation of growth when telomerase is inhibited [29-31].

The second part of the phenomenon of replicative senescence is the state that cells enter as a result of telomere shortening. This state is characterized by altered patterns of gene expression. One well-established biochemical marker for senescent cells, although one of unknown biological significance, is the high level of β-galactosidase enzymatic activity with a pH optimum of 6.0, termed senescence-associated β-galactosidase (SA-β-gal) [32]. In fibroblasts the altered pattern of gene expression resembles that of fibroblasts in inflammation [33]. Of particular significance is the production of proteases that may erode the surrounding extracellular matrix and the production of cytokines that could have effects on neighboring cells [34-37]. Interestingly, other cell types (retinal pigmented epithelial cells and endothelial cells) show different patterns of alteration of gene expression when they reach replicative senescence [33]. The current data are consistent with the hypothesis that the triggering of the block to DNA synthesis that is characteristic of replicative senescence is accompanied by dysregulation of expression of various other genes, and that the pattern of dysregulation will be cell-type specific.

The term "replicative senescence" therefore encompasses two different phenomena: one is the process of telomere shortening, resulting from the lack of expression of TERT, and the second is the cell state that is produced when telomere shortening shuts off further cell division. It is important to distinguish these two processes because they may have quite different implications for the relationship of cancer to aging. One important reason for this statement is that the same set of gene expression changes and molecular markers that occurs in short-telomere senescent cells also occurs in nondividing cells under circumstances that do not involve telomere shortening or cell division. Oxidative stress, radiation, and the ectopic expression of some signal transduction molecules and cyclin-dependent kinase inhibitors can place cells into a senescent state [38-40]. This is often termed "stress-induced senescence." Although both telomere-dependent replicative senescence and stress-induced senescence are termed "terminally nondividing states," the re-initiation of cell division in such cells is possible when genetic interventions are made that can overcome the cell cycle blocks [41].

2. TELOMERE SHORTENING OCCURS IN VIVO IN HUMANS AND OTHER LONG-LIVED SPECIES

It is now well established that many human tissues show shortening of telomeres over the course of the life span. Although that conclusion is now based on direct measurements of telomere length in human tissue samples, it was earlier observed that proliferative potential in culture of cells from older donors was less than that of cells from younger donors. In the 1970s it was shown that the replicative capacity of human fibroblasts in culture decreases as a function of donor age [42]. It was well known even at the time of these initial observations that there was much variation within each decade of age in the maximal and minimal proliferative capacity of the different cell samples. Subsequently the generality of the observation was challenged by finding that the decrease as a function of donor age applied only to fibroblasts isolated from diabetic and "prediabetic" patients [43], and was not evident in fibroblasts obtained from non-sun exposed skin [44, 45]. However, other sets of data have upheld the original observations [3].

Fibroblasts from older donors also showed a higher level of expression of collagenase, characteristic of replicative senescent cells [46]. Fibroblasts are readily cultured and most cell culture data on the molecular basis for replicative senescence have come from studies on fibroblasts. Unfortunately, fibroblasts as a cell type are not ideal for these kinds of studies. First, the cell population that is isolated is hard to standardize. When fibroblasts are isolated by allowing cells to migrate out from an explant, there is a great deal of selection for what cells form the "starting" culture population (designated as population doubling level zero). Some of the lack of agreement among investigators could result from different isolation techniques, which have provided differing degrees of initial selection. Second, the biology of fibroblasts undoubtedly differs from one organ to another, and even from one part of the skin to another, but these distinctions have not always been considered. Third, most fibroblasts are probably proliferatively quiescent in vivo after maturity and undergo very low rates of cell division. Therefore it would not be surprising if little or no exhaustion of proliferative capacity were observed.

Less ambiguous data are obtained when studies of the effects of donor age on replicative capacity are performed in those cell types where pure populations can be reproducibly isolated from defined sites in the body, and where some cell turnover occurs throughout life. In such cell populations there would be at least the potential for exhaustion of proliferative capacity. Such studies become more powerful when there is an ability to correlate the donor-age cell culture data with direct in vivo data on replicative potential, although this is obviously difficult in humans when such data are from clinical observations rather than direct experimental intervention.

Studies that have been done on non-fibroblast cell populations have shown much larger decreases in proliferative capacity than was observed as a function of donor age in fibroblasts. In some non-fibroblast cell types, many cells in the population isolated from older donors have very limited or no proliferative capacity. Some examples are age-related decrements in proliferative potential in lens epithelial cells [47, 48], retinal pigmented epithelial cells [49], smooth muscle cells [50-52], osteoblasts [53-55] and adrenocortical cells [56].

Proliferative capacity is closely related to telomere length in endothelial cells. Telomere lengths in endothelial cells decreased as a function of donor age, with a greater decline being observed in cells isolated from the iliac artery in comparison to cells from the thoracic artery [57]. The greater decline in telomere length was observed in the cells had likely undergone more proliferation in vivo, because they resided in a part of the vascular system where blood flow might cause most chronic damage to the endothelium. Unfortunately, because the data are from human specimens, it is difficult to test this hypothesis directly. Skeletal muscle satellite cells can be isolated from human muscle samples and exhibit a limited replicative potential in culture. They show decreasing proliferative potential as a function of donor age and decreased telomere length but muscle fiber nuclei showed stable telomere length [58].

Telomere shortening is observed in bone marrow cells from adult humans in comparison to fetal liver and umbilical cord blood cells [59]. A population enriched in stem cells ($CD34^+$ $CD38^-$) also had shorter telomeres in adults [59]. Lymphocytes show a continuous decline in telomere length with age, consistent with a continuous decline in telomere length in stem cells [60, 61]. The loss of telomere DNA has been measured by a fluorescence technique in lymphocytes and granulocytes from a large number of human donors in the range of 0 to 90 years of age. There was a very striking continuous decline in telomere length, that fits a pattern of a somewhat more accelerated loss of telomere DNA in the age of up to about 1 year followed by a constant linear rate of loss up to the oldest ages studied [62, 63]. These data all suggest that telomerase in hematopoietic stem cells is insufficient to maintain telomere length. Direct data for this is difficult to obtain because of the fact that it is now understood that telomerase in many cell types is regulated, as discussed earlier. This fact means that very quiescent stem cells that are not stimulated to divide in culture might be capable of telomerase induction, but this cannot be proved until culture conditions are found that cause them to proliferate and retain stem cell properties [64, 65]. Patients with syndromes of increased replication of hematopoietic cells, such as aplastic anemia, including Fanconi's anemia, show variable increases in the rate of telomere shortening, sometimes quite dramatically elevated [66,67].

These examples are consistent with the hypothesis that cell proliferation occurring over the life span of the donor causes telomere shortening; and that cell cultures are then initiated with cells that have a lowered remaining proliferative potential because continued cell division in culture shortens telomeres to a point where replicative senescence occurs. Independent of the question of whether replicative senescent cells affect tissue function, it is clear that telomere shortening does occur in human tissues in vivo, potentially putting cells ever closer to replicative senescence. It is important to distinguish the phenomenon of telomere shortening from its significance. The significance is still under debate, but the fact that it does indeed occur should not be considered controversial.

The phenomenon of telomere shortening, leading to replicative senescence, has been described in some other mammalian species. For example, bovine cells lose telomeric DNA at each cell division and eventually enter replicative senescence. Expression of hTERT immortalizes bovine cells by preventing telomere erosion [68], as in human cells [25]. The discovery that animals can be cloned from nuclei of bovine cells close to senescence also shows that replicative senescence in this species is not associated with chromosomal abnormalities or other massive changes in the genome that would prevent the formation of a viable organism [69].

3. TELOMERES AND AGING IN RODENTS

Rodent cells differ from those of longer-lived mammals. Human cells have relatively short telomeres compared to those of mice and rats (although not all rodents have long telomeres) [70-72]. Whereas most somatic human tissues and cells are telomerase negative, many mouse and rat tissues and cells are telomerase positive [72]. Although rodent cells undergo replicative arrest or slowed growth after a limited period of proliferation in culture, this is not a telomere-based senescence process. In mouse cells, the arrest is caused by oxidative damage resulting from the exposure of cells to 20% O_2, the usual conditions under which cells are cultured [73]. Whereas the cause of the replicative arrest of mouse cells in culture is not the same as that for human cells, some of the biochemical features of the nonreplicating state in rodent cells are very similar to those of senescent human cells [74]. The function of p53, although not pRb, is required in mouse cells; the arrest is maintained by high levels of cell cycle inhibitory proteins; and SA-β-gal is induced. The frequency of escape from this period of slowed growth (spontaneous immortalization) is very high in mouse cells. This may be one manifestation of more general differences in the consequences of DNA damage between mouse and human cells, as reviewed below.

In wild type mice, cells have not been shown to undergo telomere shortening in tissues during aging. However, telomere shortening can be produced in mice by inactivation of the telomerase RNA gene (*Terc*$^{-/-}$ mice) [70]. After three generations, the normally long mouse telomeres have shortened in the *Terc*$^{-/-}$ animals, and these mice present a picture of a "segmental progeroid syndrome," i.e. some aspects of the phenotype resemble accelerated aging. They have premature graying and loss of hair, poor wound healing, gastrointestinal defects, infertility, decreased adipose tissue, and a shortened life span [75-77].

Terc$^{-/-}$ mouse embryonic stem cells show progressive telomere shortening in culture that eventually results in growth arrest [78]. As telomeres shorten in these cells there is an increasing frequency of chromosome aberrations. Like wild-type mouse cells, *Terc*$^{-/-}$ fibroblasts undergo a high rate of spontaneous immortalization, but in this case this is via the ALT pathway [79]. These observations lead to the tentative conclusion that the short-telomere checkpoint that leads to G1 arrest (i.e. replicative senescence or M1) is lacking in mouse cells. The chromosomal abnormalities seen in *Terc*$^{-/-}$ mouse cells as telomeres shorten, leading eventually to impaired cell division, indicate that the growth arrest is a form of crisis/M2 rather than replicative senescence. The important distinction is that cell cycle arrest in *Terc*$^{-/-}$ mouse cells appears to be directly related to chromosomal dysfunction, whereas human cells arrest in G1 at a telomere length that is still much longer than the length seen in human cells that have bypassed M1 and are in M2/crisis.

These differences in the behavior of human and mouse cells may be examples of a more general species difference in the late consequences of DNA damage [80]. Human cells may have a more efficient arrest following chromosome damage than mouse cells. In cells that survive an insult that causes DNA damage, the damage may become fixed in the form of mutations and chromosome aberrations. When cells with chromosome damage continue clonal expansion, there has been a failure of the checkpoints that would normally eliminate such cells by apoptosis or senescence.

In a population of irradiated human cells, many clones with chromosome aberrations disappear in the first few divisions after radiation exposure [81]. On the other hand, the frequent spontaneous immortalization of primary mouse cell cultures, with the production of cell lines that are often aneuploid [82], may be an example of the failure of a checkpoint that should eliminate such cells by apoptosis or senescence.

There is clearly a close relationship between the checkpoints that operate to eliminate cells with chromosome damage and the replicative senescence checkpoint, in the form in which it operates in human cells [83]. Telomere-based replicative senescence itself, as it occurs in human cells, could in fact be an example of the difference in the reaction of human and mouse cells to chromosome damage. As reviewed above, most evidence suggests that both human and bovine fibroblasts, cells that show telomere-based replicative senescence, arrive at senescence with a near-normal karyotype. However, it is possible that the last cell division that takes place before one or both daughter cells become terminally senescent creates a chromosome fusion or break that triggers senescent growth arrest [83]. If so, arrest would appear to occur efficiently in human cells, whereas in mouse cells chromosome aberrations that should cause growth arrest often fail to do so and become stably propagated in descendant cells. The basis for these differences requires more study [80].

4. THE FUNCTION (EVOLUTIONARILY CONSERVED SELECTIVE VALUE) OF REPLICATIVE SENESCENCE: AN ANTI-CANCER MECHANISM

Because TERT appears to be re-expressed in the majority of human cancers [13], it is been hypothesized that the process by which TERT is repressed in most somatic cells is an anti-cancer mechanism. The best evidence that TERT repression is indeed an anti-cancer mechanism in human cells comes from data showing that the well-known oncoproteins Ras and SV40 T antigen cannot transform a normal human cell into a tumor cell unless they are also expressed together with TERT [84]. Presumably, the reason that TERT can co-operate with other oncogenes is that, during the process by which a normal cell and its descendants become fully malignant tumor cells, many cell divisions must take place and telomeres would become critically short, unless the cell activates telomerase or other mechanisms to prevent telomere shortening.

Thus the combination of initially short telomeres, suppression of TERT expression, and a checkpoint that triggers replicative senescence in response to short telomeres, together provide an anti-cancer mechanism. The existence of this anti-cancer mechanism in humans might contribute to the large difference in susceptibility to cancer (calculated on a per cell basis) between mice and humans. Suppose that mice and humans have the same risk of dying of cancer over their life spans (approximately true at least for some strains of mice [85]. However, a human being is about 3,000 times heavier than a 25-gram mouse and lives about 30 times as long. Consider also that cells are about the same size in mice in humans and that cell turnover occurs at about same rate. All these assumptions may not be entirely correct but this does not substantially affect the basic validity of this argument. Then it is evident that human cells are approximately 90,000 times more resistant to tumorigenic conversion per unit of time than are mouse cells. Presumably, as part of the evolution of the life history of the human species, anti-cancer mechanisms evolved that were not present in short-lived ancestors. In this case the anti-cancer process may provide an example of antagonistic pleiotropy, the genetic event (repression of TERT) having beneficial effects in early life span and possibly negative effects in late life span [86, 87].

In mice, such anti-cancer strategies are unnecessary for their life history. Their small size and short life span means that they are not more likely than humans to die of cancer before being able to reproduce. Thus there has not been an evolutionary selective pressure to repress TERT expression in this species (and presumably in other similar small short-lived mammals, although this has not yet been well studied). Presumably there are similar arguments that can be made in terms of trade-offs between the advantages and disadvantages of long and short telomeres [74]. Evidently, however, an organism that adopts TERT repression as an evolutionary anti-cancer strategy must also have short telomeres, or TERT repression becomes irrelevant to suppression of malignant transformation.

If suppression of TERT/short telomeres is a strategy that has evolved as an anti-cancer mechanism we are left with a puzzle. The senescent state appears to be a universal process, present in both human and mouse cells that is a reaction to certain kinds of DNA damage. The kinds of damage that cause cells to enter this state are very similar to those types of damage that cause other cells to enter apoptosis. From the point of view of the organism and the genome, making cells undergo apoptosis makes sense because the damaged cell and its progeny, carrying potentially damaged copies of the genome, are removed from the body. One may consider cells to be very cheap in terms of the overall economy of the body – millions of cells are born and die every day and there would seem to be no reason why cells should be preserved via the "replicative senescence" process, rather than killed off via apoptosis.

Therefore, one must ask the question, does replicative senescence occur in tissues in vivo? There is much evidence that telomere shortening occurs in tissues, but very little evidence directly addresses the question of whether telomere shortening causes cells to reach the same state in the body as it does in cell culture. In a recent review, Hanahan and Weinberg state: "The above-cited observations [on replicative senescence] might argue that senescence, much like apoptosis, reflects a protective mechanism that can be activated by shortened telomeres or conflicting growth signals that forces aberrant cells irreversibly into a G0-like state, thereby rendering them incapable of further proliferation. If so, circumvention of senescence in vivo may indeed represent an essential step in tumor progression that is required for the subsequent approach to and breaching of the crisis barrier. But we consider an alternative model equally plausible: senescence could be an artifact of cell culture that does not reflect a phenotype of cells within living tissues and does not represent an impediment to tumor progression in vivo. *Resolution of this quandary will be critical to completely understand the acquisition of limitless replicative potential.*" [emphasis added] [88].

To state the problem in another way, the short telomere/TERT repression combination is generally accepted to be an anti-cancer mechanism, but we do not know if the anti-cancer effect is mediated through the replicative senescence/M1 cell cycle block, as it is observed in cell culture.

5. BY WHAT MECHANISMS CAN REPLICATIVE SENESCENCE ACT TO SUPPRESS CANCER?

As reviewed above, and more extensively elsewhere [89], there is considerable evidence that telomere shortening occurs in tissues in vivo and one might expect therefore that short-telomere cells in tissues would stop dividing when they reach the M1 telomere length. However, observations made in the human genetic disease dyskeratosis congenita (DKC) suggest that perhaps this does not occur in vivo. DKC is a disease of impaired telomerase activity and shortened telomeres [90-92]. In one form of the disease (X-linked) the DKC1 gene is defective; its protein product, dyskerin, is required for proper RNA processing, including the RNA of the telomerase ribonucleoprotein complex. In an autosomal dominant form of DKC, telomerase RNA is mutated. In these syndromes there are proliferative defects in tissues known to have telomerase-positive stem cells (hematopoietic system and skin). DKC patients have very short telomeres in fibroblasts and white blood cells. They usually die of bone marrow failure at a young age. However, the disease is also associated with chromosomal abnormalities and early death from some cancers. Whether replicative senescence accounts for some of the pathology in DKC is unknown, but the chromosomal instability and increased cancer suggest that shortening telomeres in human tissues in vivo might lead to crisis rather than replicative senescence.

If so, to some extent this resembles the situation in *Terc*$^{-/-}$ mice [70], where chromosomal aberrations cause defects in proliferation. As reviewed above, these mice lack telomerase activity and undergo generation-dependent telomere shortening. Moreover cells from these mice lack an M1/replicative senescence arrest in culture. They also appear to lack this form of growth arrest in vivo. *Terc*$^{-/-}$ mice are viable to the sixth generation, when infertility prevents a seventh generation. Well before this point, increased numbers of end-to-end chromosome fusions are observed (0/metaphase in wild type; 0.26 in generation 2; 0.56 in generation 4; and 1.93 in generation 6) [70]. Regeneration of the liver after partial hepatectomy is impaired in G6 *Terc*$^{-/-}$ mice [93]. Flow cytometry shows that many hepatocytes have a 4N DNA content. Thus cells do not arrest in G1, as expected if the short telomeres trigger replicative senescence, but instead hepatocytes have impaired progress through mitosis. Many aberrant mitotic figures are observed. In G6 *Terc*$^{-/-}$ mice, excess apoptosis of germ cells is observed, providing an explanation for infertility. Apoptosis was blocked, and fertility restored, when G6 *Terc*$^{-/-}$ mice were generated in a p53$^{-/-}$ background [94]. Therefore, at least in germ cells, short telomeres appear to trigger p53-dependent

Figure 1. Replicative senescence and crisis. In germ cells telomere length is maintained by telomerase, but most human somatic cells do not have sufficient telomerase activity to maintain telomere length and undergo telomere shortening with each cell division. Stem cells have telomerase activity but may not maintain full telomere length. When telomeres reach a certain length (point "M1") they enter replicative senescence. The expression of oncoproteins such as SV40 T antigen enables cells to bypass the point by inactivation of pRB/p16 or p53. Such cells continue to undergo telomere shortening to the "M2" point, or crisis. Rare cells in crisis cultures activate telomerase by unknown mechanisms and thereby are able to grow indefinitely with a stabilized telomere length. When cells are cultured in adequate conditions, ectopic expression of hTERT allows cells maintain telomere length greater than the M1 length. Reproduced with permission from Cong et al., 2002.

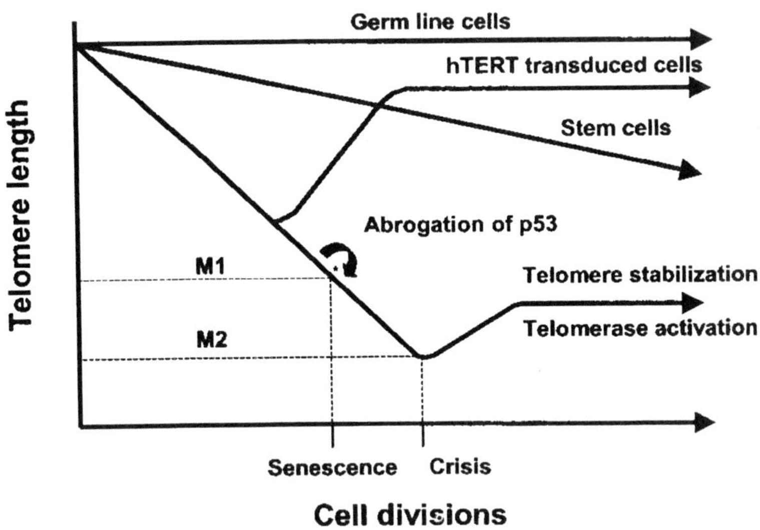

apoptosis. When this block is bypassed in the $p53^{-/-}$ background, two more generations of *Terc*$^{-/-}$ mice are possible before a non-p53 dependent "genetic catastrophe" occurs [94].

Figure 2. The "telomere paradox": short telomeres may both suppress cancer formation and promote cancer formation. Reproduced with permission Masutomi and Hahn, 2003.

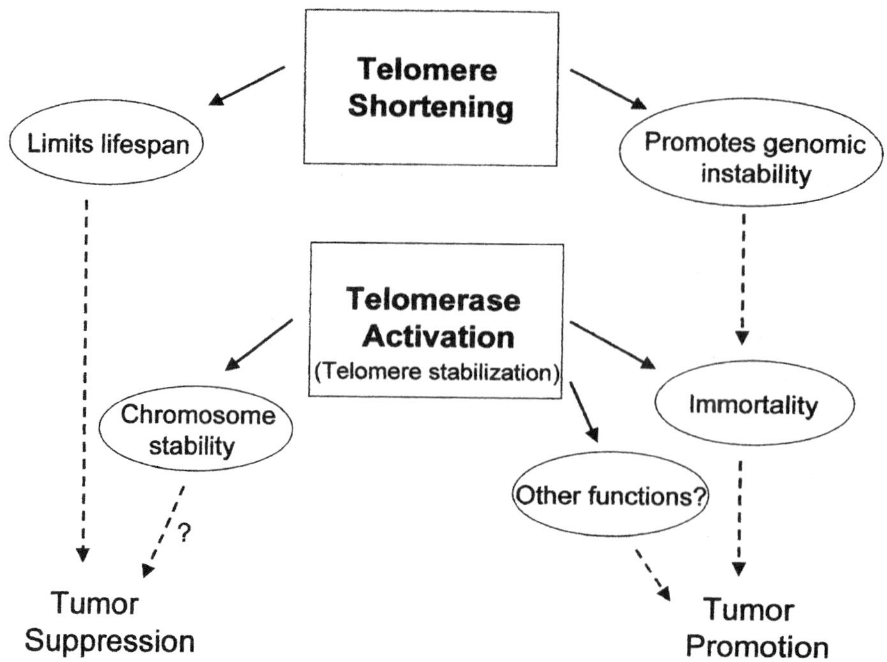

Late generation *Terc*$^{-/-}$ mice with short telomeres also show increased cancer incidence [73], as do human DKC patients. However, when G6 *Terc*$^{-/-}$ were generated on the cancer-prone *INK4A*$^{-/-}$ background cancer incidence was reduced in comparison with telomerase-positive *INK4A*$^{-/-}$ mice [95].

Thus, the data point to a telomere paradox (Figure 2). If short telomeres/repression of TERT is an anti-cancer mechanism, why does a disease in which these traits are exaggerated display an increased cancer risk? This paradox currently lacks a satisfactory explanation. As it is evident that humans as a species have a greater need for anti-cancer mechanisms than rodents, the conclusion that short telomeres/repression of TERT is an anti-cancer mechanism seems inevitable, yet the means by which the anti-cancer effects are exerted remain unresolved.

6. CAN REPLICATIVE SENESCENCE ACT TO PROMOTE CANCER?

If cells that reach the M1 telomere length truly "senesce" in vivo, and then undergo the same kinds of changes in gene expression as they do in culture, this process could certainly have adverse effects on tissue function. In this regard one can pose a series of related questions: (i) Do cells undergo telomere shortening to the extent of reaching the M1 telomere length? (ii) If so, is the consequence of this the same as it is in culture, i.e. the generation of senescent cells, or do they suffer some other fate (e.g. crisis)? (iii) If they become senescent, do such cells accumulate in tissues, or are they eliminated by some part of either the acquired or innate immune system? (iv) If they do accumulate in tissues, do they exert a pro-carcinogenic effect because they secrete proteases and cytokines?

The most significant evidence for the occurrence of senescent cells in aging tissues is the occurrence of cells that stain for senescence-associated β-galactosidase (SA-β-gal) in tissues as a function of age. The presence of SA-β-gal$^+$ cells was first reported for human skin [32] and was subsequently shown in the rhesus monkey in retinal pigmented epithelium [96] and in the epidermis [97]. In these studies the number of SA-β-gal$^+$ cells increased as a function of donor age. These intriguing observations raise several questions. First, we do not know the mechanism by which such cells are formed; if their existence has consequences for tissue function, the mode by which they become senescent should be understood, so that appropriate interventions (both experimental and clinical) can be designed and tested. Second, whether such cells in vivo actually have the same range of changes in gene expression observed in replicative senescent cells in culture is also unknown. This is important, because it has been speculated that these changes may result in a pro-carcinogenic state in tissues that could aid the growth of pre-malignant cells and provide a permissive environment for tumor progression [98, 99] (Figure 3). It is conceivable that many properties of aging tissues, including an increased rate of neoplastic conversion, might result from the presence of relatively small numbers of replicative senescent cells.

Figure 3. Hypothetical scheme by which the presence of senescent cells in tissue during aging could exert a pro-neoplastic effect. In the young tissue, a cell with potentially oncogenic mutations ("initiated") is prevented from uncontrolled growth by neighboring cells. In the old tissue, senescent cells secrete enzymes and cytokines that enable the initiated cell to grow into a cancer. Reproduced with permission from Campisi, 2003.

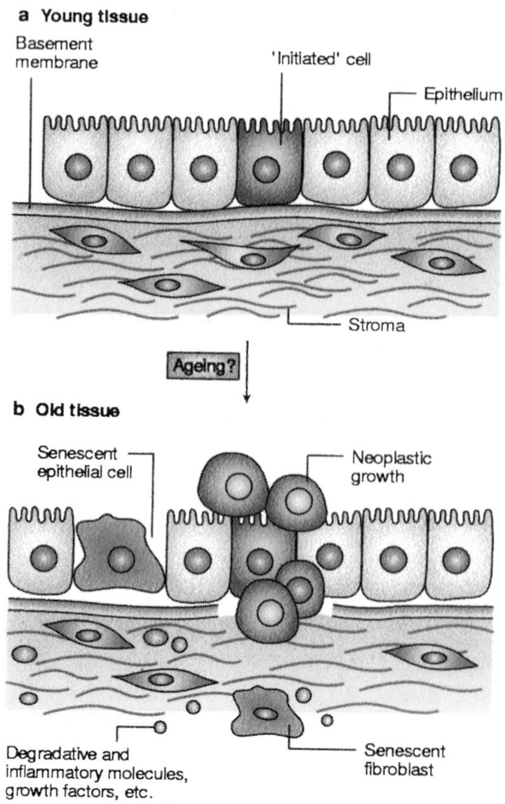

Many more studies are needed in this area. First, the variety of tissues and the range of donor ages that have been surveyed so far is very small, and it is not possible yet to determine whether the occurrence of SA-β-gal⁺ cells is an inevitable part of normal aging or alternatively evidence of a pathological process. Studies in the prostate, liver, and vascular endothelium are suggestive of an accumulation of SA-β-gal⁺ cells in disease states [100-102]. Second, more studies are needed to show whether SA-β-gal⁺ cells are generated by telomere shortening or by some other process. The suspicion that in some cases telomere shortening is not involved exists for retinal pigmented epithelial cells, because these cells are mostly postmitotic in adult life [103]. These cells may have entered the senescent state as a form of stress-induced senescence as a result of exposure to oxidative damage.

Conversely, more studies are needed to show the fate of cells with shortening telomeres in tissues. One consequence of our lack of knowledge in this area is that SA-β-gal$^+$ staining cannot be used as an *in situ* assay for cells that have exhausted their replicative capacity in vivo by telomere shortening.

One final point is there has not yet been enough consideration given to alternate fates of cells that have undergone telomere shortening in vivo and whose telomeres have reached the M1/senescent length. The possibility should be considered that their changes in gene expression might become so marked that they are no longer recognized as "self" and are eliminated by either acquired or innate immune functions, much as incipient cancer cells are eliminated by immune surveillance [104].

5. CONCLUSIONS

Replicative senescence appears to be a form of protection against cancer, but the means by which it may have this action are not yet clear. More research is needed to understand the fate of cells with short telomeres in tissues during aging, to understand the effects on neoplasia of telomere shortening in tissues in vivo, to understand whether telomere shortening results in the accumulation of senescent cells in tissues, and, if so, what effects this may have on tissue function.

ACKNOWLEDGEMENTS

Research mentioned in this chapter from the author's laboratory was supported by grants from the National Institute on Aging (AG 12287 and AG 20752) and by a Senior Scholar Award from the Ellison Medical Foundation.

REFERENCES

1. Hayflick L: Cell aging. Annu Rev Gerontol Geriatr 1980, 1: 26-67
2. Harley CB; Futcher AB; Greider CW: Telomeres shorten during ageing of human fibroblasts. Nature 1990, 345: 458-460
3. Allsopp RC; Vaziri H; Patterson C; Goldstein S; Younglai EV; Futcher AB; Greider CW; and Harley CB: Telomere length predicts replicative capacity of human fibroblasts. Proc Natl Acad Sci USA, 1992, 89: 10114-10118
4. Greider CW: Telomeres, telomerase and senescence. Bioessays 1990, 12: 363-369
5. Harley CB: Telomere loss: Mitotic clock or genetic time bomb? Mutat Res 1991, 256: 271-282
6. Lingner J; Hughes TR; Shevchenko A; Mann M; Lundblad V; Cech TR: Reverse transcriptase motifs in the catalytic subunit of telomerase. Science 1997, 276: 561-567

7. Meyerson M; Counter CM; Eaton EN; Ellisen LW; Steiner P; Caddle SD; Ziaugra L; Beijersbergen RL; Davidoff MJ; Liu Q; Bacchetti S; Haber DA; Weinberg RA: hEST2, the putative human telomerase catalytic subunit gene, is up-regulated in tumor cells and during immortalization. Cell 1997, 90: 785-95
8. Noda A; Ning Y; Venable SF; Pereira-Smith OM; Smith JR: Cloning of senescent cell-derived inhibitors of DNA synthesis using an expression screen. Exp Cell Res 1994, 211: 90-98
9. Smith JR; Pereira-Smith OM: Replicative senescence: Implications for in vivo aging and tumor suppression. Science 1996, 273: 63-67
10. Cong YS; Wright WE; Shay JW: Human telomerase and its regulation. Microbiol Mol Biol Rev 2002, 66: 407-25
11. Wang E: Senescent human fibroblasts resist programmed cell death, and failure to suppress bcl2 is involved. Cancer Res 1995, 55: 2284-2292
12. Shay JW; Wright WE: Quantitation of the frequency of immortalization of normal human diploid fibroblasts by SV40 large T-antigen. Exp Cell Res 1989, 184: 109-118
13. Holt SE; Wright WE; Shay JW: Multiple pathways for the regulation of telomerase activity. Eur J Cancer 1997, 33: 761-6
14. Reddel RR; Bryan TM: Alternative lengthening of telomeres: dangerous road less travelled. Lancet 2003, 361: 1840-1
15. Belair CD; Yeager TR; Lopez PM; Reznikoff CA: Telomerase activity: a biomarker of cell proliferation, not malignant transformation. Proc Natl Acad Sci USA 1997, 94: 13677-82
16. Ramakrishnan S; Eppenberger U; Mueller H; Shinkai Y; Narayanan R: Expression profile of the putative catalytic subunit of the telomerase gene. Cancer Res 1998, 58: 622-5
17. Wu K-J; Grandori C; Amacker M; Simon-Vermot N; Polack A; Lingner J; Dalla-Favera R: Direct activation of TERT transcription by c-MYC. Nature Genet 1999, 21: 220-4
18. Hodes RJ: Telomere length, aging, and somatic cell turnover. J Exp Med 1999, 190: 153-6
19. Masutomi K; Yu EY; Khurts S; Ben-Porath I; Currier JL; Metz, GB; Brooks MW; Kaneko S; Murakami S; DeCaprio JA; Weinberg RA; Stewart SA; Hahn WC: Telomerase maintains telomere structure in normal human cells. Cell 2003, 114: 241-53
20. Yasumoto S; Kunimura C; Kikuchi K; Tahara H; Ohji H; Yamamoto H; Ide T; Utakoji T: Telomerase activity in normal human epithelial cells. Oncogene 1996, 13: 433-439
21. Hsiao R; Sharma HW; Ramakrishnan S; Keith E; Narayanan R: Telomerase activity in normal human endothelial cells. Anticancer Research 1997, 17: 827-32
22. Kunimura C; Kikuchi K; Ahmed N; Shimizu A; Yasumoto S: Telomerase activity in a specific cell subset co-expressing integrin β1/EGFR but not p75NGFR/bcl2/integrin β4 in normal human epithelial cells. Oncogene 1998, 17: 187-97
23. Suwa T; Yang L; Hornsby PJ: Telomerase activity in primary cultures of normal adrenocortical cells. J Endocrinol 2001, 170: 677-684
24. Thomson JA; Itskovitz-Eldor J; Shapiro SS; Waknitz MA; Swiergiel JJ; Marshall VS; Jones, JM: Embryonic stem cell lines derived from human blastocysts. Science 1998, 282: 1145-7
25. Bodnar AG; Ouellette M; Frolkis M; Holt SE; Chiu CP; Morin GB; Harley CB; Shay JW; Lichtsteiner S; Wright WE: Extension of life-span by introduction of telomerase into normal human cells. Science 1998, 279: 349-52
26. Kiyono T; Foster SA; Koop JI; McDougall JK; Galloway DA; Klingelhutz AJ: Both Rb/p16INK4a inactivation and telomerase activity are required to immortalize human epithelial cells. Nature 1998, 396: 84-8

27. Jiang XR; Jimenez G; Chang E; Frolkis M; Kusler B; Sage M; Beeche M; Bodnar AG; Wahl GM; Tlsty TD; Chiu CP: Telomerase expression in human somatic cells does not induce changes associated with a transformed phenotype. Nature Genet 1999, 21: 111-4
28. Morales CP; Holt SE; Ouellette M; Kaur KJ; Yan Y; Wilson KS; White MA; Wright WE; Shay JW: Absence of cancer-associated changes in human fibroblasts immortalized with telomerase. Nature Genet 1999, 21: 115-8
29. Hahn WC; Counter CM; Lundberg AS; Beijersbergen RL; Brooks MW; Weinberg RA: Creation of human tumour cells with defined genetic elements. Nature 1999, 400: 464-468
30. Zhang X; Mar V; Zhou W; Harrington L; Robinson MO: Telomere shortening and apoptosis in telomerase-inhibited human tumor cells. Genes Dev 1999, 13: 2388-99
31. Shammas MA; Simmons CG; Corey DR; Shmookler Reis RJ: Telomerase inhibition by peptide nucleic acids reverses 'immortality' of transformed human cells. Oncogene 1999, 18: 6191-200
32. Dimri GP; Lee XH; Basile G; Acosta M; Scott C; Roskelley C; Medrano EE; Linskens M; Rubelj I; Pereira-Smith OM; Peacocke M; Campisi J: A biomarker that identifies senescent human cells in culture and in aging skin in vivo. Proc Natl Acad Sci USA 1995, 92: 9363-9367
33. Shelton DN; Chang E; Whittier PS; Choi D; Funk WD: Microarray analysis of replicative senescence. Curr Biol 1999, 9: 939-45
34. Sottile J; Mann DM; Diemer V; Millis AJ: Regulation of collagenase and collagenase mRNA production in early- and late-passage human diploid fibroblasts. J Cell Physiol 1989, 138: 281-290
35. West MD; Pereira-Smith OM; Smith JR: Replicative senescence of human skin fibroblasts correlates with a loss of regulation and overexpression of collagenase activity. Exp Cell Res 1989, 184: 138-147
36. Kumar S; Millis AJT; Baglioni C: Expression of interleukin 1-inducible genes and production of interleukin 1 by aging human fibroblasts. Proc Natl Acad Sci USA 1992, 89: 4683-4687
37. Millis AJ; Hoyle M; McCue HM; Martini H: Differential expression of metalloproteinase and tissue inhibitor of metalloproteinase genes in aged human fibroblasts. Exp Cell Res 1992, 201: 373-379
38. Robles SJ; Adami GR: Agents that cause DNA double strand breaks lead to p16(INK4A) enrichment and the premature senescence of normal fibrolasts. Oncogene 1998, 16: 1113-1123
39. Serrano M; Lin AW; Mccurrach ME; Beach D; Lowe SW: Oncogenic ras provokes premature cell senescence associated with accumulation of p53 and p16 INK4A. Cell 1997, 88: 593-602
40. Zhu J; Woods D; McMahon M; Bishop JM: Senescence of human fibroblasts induced by oncogenic Raf. Genes Dev 1998, 12: 2997-3007
41. Beausejour CM; Krtolica A; Galimi F; Narita M; Lowe SW; Yaswen P Campisi J: Reversal of human cellular senescence: roles of the p53 and p16 pathways. EMBO J 2003, 22: 4212-22
42. Martin GM; Sprague CA; Epstein CA: Replicative life-span of cultivated human cells: Effects of donor's age, tissue and genotype. Lab. Invest 1970, 23: 86-92
43. Goldstein S; Moerman EJ; Soeldner JS; Gleason RE; Barnett DM: Chronologic and physiologic age affect replicative life-span of fibroblasts from diabetic, prediabetic, and normal donors. Science 1978, 199: 781-782
44. Gilchrest BA: Prior chronic sun exposure decreases the lifespan of human skin fibroblasts in vitro. J Gerontol 1980, 35: 537-41

45. Cristofalo VJ; Allen RG; Pignolo RJ; Martin BG; Beck JC: Relationship between donor age and the replicative lifespan of human cells in culture: a reevaluation. Proc Natl Acad Sci USA 1998, 95: 10614-9
46. Burke EM; Horton WE; Pearson JD; Crow MT; Martin GR: Altered transcriptional regulation of human interstitial collagenase in cultured skin fibroblasts from older donors. Exp Gerontol 1994, 29: 37-53
47. Tassin J; Malaise E; Courtois Y: Human lens cells have an in vitro proliferative capacity inversely proportional to the donor age. Exp Cell Res 1979, 123: 388-392
48. Power W; Neylan D; Collum L: Growth characteristics of human lens epithelial cells in culture. Effect of media and donor age. Doc Ophthalmol 1993, 84: 365-372
49. Flood MT; Gouras P; and Kjeldbye H: Growth characteristics and ultrastructure of human retinal pigment epithelium in vitro. Invest Ophthalmol Visual Sci 1980, 19: 1309-20
50. Bierman EL: The effect of donor age on the in vitro life span of cultured human arterial smooth-muscle cells. In Vitro 1978, 14: 951-955
51. Start RD; Loomes RS; Shortland JR: The relationship between donor age and the growth characteristics of human smooth muscle cultures of aorta and stomach. Int J Exp Pathol 1991, 72: 647-654
52. Ruiz-Torres A; Gimeno A; Melon J; Mendez L; Munoz FJ; Macia M. Age-related loss of proliferative activity of human vascular smooth muscle cells in culture. Mech Aging Dev 1999, 110: 49-55
53. Koshihara Y; Hirano M; Kawamura M; Oda H; Higaki S: Mineralization ability of cultured human osteoblast-like periosteal cells does not decline with aging. J Gerontol 1991, 46: B201-B206
54. Kasse M; Ankersen L; Eriksen EF; Clark BFC; Rattan SIS: Demonstration of cellular aging and senescence in serially passaged long-term cultures of human trabecular osteoblasts. Osteoporos Int. 7: 1997, 514-24
55. D'Ippolito G; Schiller PC; Ricordi C; Roos BA; Howard GA: Age-related osteogenic potential of mesenchymal stromal stem cells from human vertebral bone marrow. J Bone Mineral Res 1999, 14: 1115-22
56. Yang L; Suwa T; Wright WE; Shay JW; Hornsby PJ: Telomere shortening and decline in replicative potential as a function of donor age in human adrenocortical cells. Mech Ageing Dev 2001, 122: 1685-1694
57. Chang E; Harley CB: Telomere length and replicative aging in human vascular tissues. Proc Natl Acad Sci USA 1995, 92: 11190-11194
58. Decary S; Mouly V; Hamida CB; Sautet A; Barbet JP; Butler-Browne GS: Replicative potential and telomere length in human skeletal muscle: implications for satellite cell-mediated gene therapy. Hum Gene Ther 1997, 8: 1429-38
59. Vaziri H; Dragowska W; Allsopp RC; Thomas TE; Harley CB; Lansdorp PM: Evidence for a mitotic clock in human hematopoietic stem cells: Loss of telomeric DNA with age. Proc Natl Acad Sci USA 1994, 91: 9857-9860
60. Hastie ND; Dempster M; Dunlop MG; Thompson AM; Green DK; Allshire RC: Telomere reduction in human colorectal carcinoma and with ageing. Nature 1990, 346: 866-868
61. Vaziri H; Schachter F; Uchida I; Wei L; Zhu X; Effros R; Cohen D; Harley CB: Loss of telomeric DNA during aging of normal and trisomy 21 human lymphocytes. Am J Hum Genet 1993, 52: 661-667
62. Frenck RW Jr; Blackburn EH; Shannon KM: The rate of telomere sequence loss in human leukocytes varies with age. Proc Natl Acad Sci USA 1998, 95: 5607-10
63. Rufer N; Brummendorf TH; Kolvraa S; Bischoff C; Christensen K; Wadsworth, L., Schulzer M; Lansdorp PM: Telomere fluorescence measurements in granulocytes and T

lymphocyte subsets point to a high turnover of hematopoietic stem cells and memory T cells in early childhood. J Exp Med 190: 157-67
64. Yui J; Chiu CP; Lansdorp PM: Telomerase activity in candidate stem cells from fetal liver and adult bone marrow. Blood 1998, 91: 3255-62
65. Glimm H; Eaves CJ: Direct evidence for multiple self-renewal divisions of human in vivo repopulating hematopoietic cells in short-term culture. Blood 1999, 94: 2161-8
66. Ball SE; Gibson FM; Rizzo S; Tooze JA; Marsh JC; Gordon-Smith EC: Progressive telomere shortening in aplastic anemia. Blood 1998, 91: 3582-92
67. Leteurtre F; Li X; Guardiola P; Le Roux G; Sergere JC; Richard P; Carosella ED; Gluckman E: Accelerated telomere shortening and telomerase activation in Fanconi's anaemia. Br J Haematol 1999, 105: 883-93
68. Thomas M; Yang L; Hornsby PJ: Formation of functional tissue from transplanted adrenocortical cells expressing telomerase reverse transcriptase. Nature Biotechnol 2000, 18: 39-42
69. Lanza RP; Cibelli JB; Blackwell C; Cristofalo VJ; Francis MK; Baerlocher GM; Mak J; Schertzer M; Chavez EA; Sawyer N; Lansdorp PM; West MD: Extension of cell life-span and telomere length in animals cloned from senescent somatic cells. Science 2000, 288: 665-9
70. Blasco MA; Lee HW; Hande MP; Samper E; Lansdorp PM; DePinho RA; Greider CW: Telomere shortening and tumor formation by mouse cells lacking telomerase RNA. Cell 1997, 91: 25-34
71. Coviello-McLaughlin GM; Prowse KR: Telomere length regulation during postnatal development and aging in Mus spretus. Nucleic Acids Res 1997, 25: 3051-8
72. Prowse KR; Greider CW: Developmental and tissue-specific regulation of mouse telomerase and telomere length. Proc Natl Acad Sci USA 1995, 92: 4818-22
73. Parrinello S; Samper E; Krtolica A; Goldstein J; Melov S; Campisi J: Oxygen sensitivity severely limits the replicative lifespan of murine fibroblasts. Nature Cell Biol 2003, 5: 741-7
74. Wright WE; Shay JW: Telomere dynamics in cancer progression and prevention: Fundamental differences in human and mouse telomere biology. Nature Med 2000, 6: 849- 851
75. Rudolph KL; Chang S; Lee HW; Blasco M; Gottlieb GJ; Greider C; DePinho RA: Longevity, stress response, and cancer in aging telomerase-deficient mice. Cell 1999, 96: 701-12
76. Herrera E; Samper E; Martin-Caballero J; Flores JM; Lee HW; Blasco MA: Disease states associated with telomerase deficiency appear earlier in mice with short telomeres. EMBO J 1999, 18: 2950-60
77. Kipling D; Faragher RG: Telomeres. Ageing hard or hardly ageing? Nature 1999, 398: 191
78. Niida H; Shinkai Y; Hande MP; Matsumoto T; Takehara S; Tachibana M; Oshimura M; Lansdorp PM; Furuichi Y: Telomere maintenance in telomerase-deficient mouse embryonic stem cells: Characterization of an amplified telomeric DNA. Mol Cell Biol 2000, 20: 4115-27
79. Hande PM; Samper E; Lansdorp PM; Blasco MA: Telomere length dynamics and chromosomal instability in cells derived from telomerase null mice. J Cell Biol 1999, 144: 589-601
80. Hornsby PJ: Mouse and human cells versus oxygen. Sci Aging Knowl Environ 2003: PE21
81. Kano Y; Little JB: Persistence of X-ray-induced chromosomal rearrangements in long-term cultures of human diploid fibroblasts. Cancer Res 1984, 44: 3706-11
82. Worton RG; Duff C: Karyotyping. Meth Enzymol 1979, 58: 322-44
83. Artandi SE; and DePinho RA: A critical role for telomeres in suppressing and facilitating carcinogenesis. Curr Opin Genet Dev 2000,10: 39-46

84. Hahn WC; Stewart SA; Brooks MW; York SG; Eaton E; Kurachi A; Beijersbergen RL; Knoll JH; Meyerson M; Weinberg RA: Inhibition of telomerase limits the growth of human cancer cells. Nature Med 1999, 5: 164-70
85. Peto R.; Parish SE; Gray RG: There is no such thing as aging and cancer is not related to it. In: *Age-Related Factors in Carcinogenesis* Likhachev A.; Anisimov VN; Montesano R (eds.) International Agency for Research on Cancer, Lyon, 1985, 43-53
86. Williams GC: Pleiotropy, natural selection, and the evolution of senescence. Evolution 1957, 11: 389-411
87. Campisi J: Aging and cancer: The double-edged sword of replicative senescence. J Am Geriatr Soc 1997, 45: 482-488
88. Hanahan D; Weinberg RA: The hallmarks of cancer. Cell 2000, 100: 57-70
89. Hornsby PJ: Cell proliferation in mammalian aging. In: *Handbook of the Biology of Aging (Fifth Edition)* Masoro EJ; Austad SN (eds). Academic Press, San Diego 2001, 207-266
90. Mitchell JR; Wood E; Collins K: A telomerase component is defective in the human disease dyskeratosis congenita. Nature 1999, 402: 551-5
91. Vulliamy T; Marrone A; Goldman F; Dearlove A; Bessler M; Mason PJ; Dokal I: The RNA component of telomerase is mutated in autosomal dominant dyskeratosis congenita. Nature 2001, 413: 432-5
92. Marciniak RA; Johnson FB; Guarente L: Dyskeratosis congenita, telomeres and human ageing. Trends Genet 2000, 16: 193-5
93. Rudolph KL; Chang S; Millard M; Schreiber-Agus N; DePinho RA: Inhibition of experimental liver cirrhosis in mice by telomerase gene delivery. Science 2000, 287: 1253-8
94. Chin L; Artandi SE; She Q; Tam A; Lee SL; Gottlieb GJ; Greider CW; DePinho RA: p53 deficiency rescues the adverse effects of telomere loss and cooperates with telomere dysfunction to accelerate carcinogenesis. Cell 1999, 97: 527-38
95. Greenberg RA; Chin L; Femino A; Lee KH; Gottlieb GJ; Singer RH; Greider CW; DePinho RA: Short dysfunctional telomeres impair tumorigenesis in the INK4a(Δ2/3) cancer-prone mouse. Cell 1999, 97: 515-25
96. Mishima K; Handa JT; Aotaki-Keen A.; Lutty GA; Morse LS; Hjelmeland LM: Senescence-associated β-galactosidase histochemistry for the primate eye. Invest Ophthalmol Vis Sci 1999, 40: 1590-3
97. Pendergrass WR; Lane MA.; Bodkin NL; Hansen BC; Ingram DK; Roth GS; Yi L; Bin H; Wolf NS: Cellular proliferation potential during aging and caloric restriction in rhesus monkeys (Macaca mulatta). J Cell Physiol 1999, 180: 123-30
98. Krtolica A; Parrinello S; Lockett S; Desprez PY; Campisi J: Senescent fibroblasts promote epithelial cell growth and tumorigenesis: A link between cancer and aging. Proc Natl Acad Sci USA 2001, 98: 12072-7
99. Campisi J. Cancer and aging: rival demons? Nature Rev Cancer 2003, 3: 339-49
100. Choi J; Shendrik I; Peacocke M; Peehl D; Buttyan R; Ikeguchi EF; Katz AE; Benson MC: Expression of senescence-associated β-galactosidase in enlarged prostates from men with benign prostatic hyperplasia. Urology 2000, 56: 160-6
101. Paradis V; Youssef N; Dargere D; Ba N; Bonvoust F; Deschatrette J; Bedossa P: Replicative senescence in normal liver, chronic hepatitis C, and hepatocellular carcinomas. Hum Pathol 2001, 32: 327-32
102. Vasile E; Tomita Y; Brown LF; Kocher O; Dvorak HF: Differential expression of thymosin β-10 by early passage and senescent vascular endothelium is modulated by VPF/VEGF: Evidence for senescent endothelial cells in vivo at sites of atherosclerosis. FASEB J 2001, 15: 458-66

103. Hjelmeland LM: Senescence of the retinal pigmented epithelium. Invest Ophthalmol Vis Sci 1999, 40: 1-2
104. Nossal GJ: Life, death and the immune system. Sci Am 1993, 269(3): 52-62
105. Masutomi K; Hahn WC: Telomerase and tumorigenesis. Cancer Lett 2003, 194: 163-72

Chapter 4

THE INFLUENCE OF ADVANCED AGE ON CANCER OCCURRENCE AND GROWTH

William B. Ershler

Institute for Advanced Studies in Aging & Geriatric Medicine, Washington, DC.

Recently there has been an increased awareness of the overlapping biologic pathways operant in the processes of aging and carcinogenesis. Coincidently, there has been increased interest in both basic and clinical research pertaining to cancer and aging. There remain many unanswered questions about cancer management in geriatric patients, in part, due to the lack of understanding of the influence of age on tumor biology. This review will attempt to establish a framework around themes in aging biology that are relevant to the development and progression of cancer.

1. NORMAL AGING

It is a central gerontologic principle that aging is not a disease. The functional declines that accompany normal aging have been well characterized [1], but under normal circumstances do not account for symptoms or disease. For example, kidney function declines with age [2], and, in fact, has proven to be a useful biological marker of aging (see below). Yet, clinical consequences of this change in renal function, in the absence of a disease or the exposure to an exogenous nephrotoxic agent, do not occur commonly. Similarly, the bone marrow changes with age (discussed elsewhere in this volume).

Aging is not a disease but the consequences of aging may make an individual susceptible to disease. For example, changes in the immune system may render an individual susceptible to reactivation of tuberculosis [3,4] or herpes zoster [5] and less capable of responding to influenza vaccine with protective titers of antibody [6-8]. The immune decline, however, is not of sufficient magnitude or duration to account for the increased incidence of cancer in old people [9]. In fact, based upon findings in experimental animals, it has been postulated that immune senescence may contribute to the observed reduced tumor growth and spread in a variety of tumors (discussed below).

2. LIFESPAN AND MAXIMUM SURVIVAL

From the perspective of those who study aging, there is an important distinction made between median (life expectancy) and maximum life span. Over the past several decades, with the advent of modern sanitation, refrigeration and other public health measures including vaccination and antibiotics, there has been a dramatic increase in median survival [10]. Early deaths have been diminished and more individuals are reaching old age. In the United States today, life expectancy now approaches 80 years [11]. Median survival is what concerns public health officials and health care providers but for those studying the biology of aging, it is maximum survival that is the focus of greatest attention. It is worthwhile to note that it has been estimated that if atherosclerosis and cancer were eliminated from the population as a cause of death, about ten years would be added to the average life span, yet there would be no change in maximum life span [12].

The oldest human being alive today is approximately 120 years old. What is intriguing is that the record has remained stable, unchanged by the public health initiatives mentioned above. In fact, there has been some recent data presented that the maximum survival is actually declining in the United States [13,14]. In the laboratory, similar limits have been established for a variety of species. Drosophila, free of predators, can live 30 days, whereas C57BL/6 mice in a laboratory environment and allowed to eat a healthy diet ad libitum, may survive 40 months. What is interesting is that, unlike the public health initiatives in humans, experimental interventions in lower species have been associated with a prolongation of maximum survival. In Drosophila, for example, transgenic offspring producing extra copies of the free radical scavenging enzymes superoxide dismutase and catalase survived about 33% longer than controls [15]. However, there has been some criticism of this work based on the claim that the controls were unusually short lived. In mammalian species, the only experimental intervention that characteristically prolongs maximum survival is the restriction of caloric intake. In fact, dietary restriction (DR) has become a common experimental paradigm exploited in the investigation of primary processes of aging (for a review see reference 16).

3. CELLULAR VERSUS ORGANISMAL AGING

There has been much written about cellular senescence and the events that lead up to cell death (reviewed in reference17). After a finite number of divisions, normal somatic cells invariably enter a state of irreversibly arrested growth, a process termed replicative senescence [18]. In fact, it has been proposed that escape from the regulators of senescence is the antecedent of malignant transformation. However, the role of replicative senescence as an explanation of organismal aging remains the subject of vigorous debate. The controversy relates, in part, to the fact that certain organisms (e.g., Drosophila, C. elegans) undergo an aging process, yet all of their adult cells are post replicative.

What is clear is that the loss of proliferative capacity of human cells in culture is intrinsic to the cells and not dependent on environmental factors or even culture conditions [18]. Unless transformation occurs, cells age with each successive division. The number of divisions turns out to be more important than the actual amount of time passed. Thus, cells held in a quiescent state for months, when allowed back into a proliferative environment, will continue approximately the same number of divisions as those that were allowed to proliferate without a quiescent period [19].

The question remains whether this in vitro phenomenon is relevant to animal aging. One suggestive observation is that of fibroblasts cultured from samples of old skin undergoes fewer cycles of replication than those from young [20]. Furthermore, when various species are compared, replicative potential is directly and significantly related to life span [21]. An unusual β-galactosidase with activity peaks at pH6 has proved to be a useful biomarker of in vitro senescence because it is expressed by senescent but not presenescent or quiescent fibroblasts [22]. This particular β-galactosidase isoform was found to have the predicted pattern of expression in skin from young and old donors with measurably increased levels in dermal fibroblasts and epidermal keratinocytes with advancing age [22]. The nature of the expression of this in vivo biomarker of aging in other tissues will be important to discern.

4. IMMUNITY AND AGING

There is a well-characterized deficit in immune function with advancing age, but the consequences are not fully established. It is apparent that otherwise healthy older individuals are more susceptible to reactivation of tuberculosis [3,4] or Herpes zoster [5], and responses to vaccines, such as the commercially available and widely used influenza hemagglutinin, are lower [23-25]. However, it has been postulated that other age-associated diseases, such as cancer [26], atherosclerosis [27,28], diabetes [29], and even Alzheimer's disease [30,31] have been related to the immune decline with age. Yet more recent evidence would argue that inflammation may contribute to Alzheimer's disease (see below).

What can be said with confidence is that there are changes in T cell function with age that result in decreased proliferation when measured in vitro [32]. When studied as a population, there appears to be an accumulation of T cells with cell surface characteristics of memory cells, whereas in contrast, there is a relative decrease in naïve T cells [33]. B cell function, including the capacity to make antibody remains intact, although certain intrinsic alterations have been noted [34]. Immunoregulatory functions are affected by the aging process and paraproteinemia, and autoantibody is observed with increasing frequency with each advancing decade. In general, the paraproteinemia is an indicator of dysregulated immunity, but it is considered not to be the antecedent of multiple myeloma [35-37]. However, myeloma does increase in incidence in geriatric populations and it must be distinguished from the benign paraproteinemia of aging. Typically, this is accomplished by examination of bone marrow, skeletal x-rays and renal function and serial (e.g., every 3 months) determination of paraprotein level [38].

Another indication of dysregulated immune function is the alterations in certain key cytokines, measured in plasma, culture supernatants, or in the appropriate tissue microenvironment. Notably and consistently interleukin-2 (IL-2) levels and function decrease with age [39], and IL-6 levels increase [40]. The decline in IL-2 may account for a significant component of the measured decline in T cell function and the increased IL-6 has been implicated in the pathogenesis of certain age-associated diseases (osteoporosis, Alzheimer's disease and cancer and the syndrome of frailty [41,42]).

5. IMMUNESENESCENCE AND CANCER

Proponents of an immune explanation point to experiments in which outbred strains of mice with heterogeneous immune functions were followed for their life span [45]. Those who demonstrated better functions early in life (as determined by a limited panel of assays available at the time on a small sample of blood) were found to have fewer spontaneous malignancies and a longer life than those estimated to be less immunologically competent. Recently, a report from Japan [46] in which a cohort of individuals, on whom lymphocyte (specifically NK cell function) measures were obtained decades earlier, demonstrated a reduced incidence of cancer in those who had better lymphocyte functions. These and other similar observations do support the notion of immune surveillance and indicate the potential importance of immunesenescence in explaining the great rise in incidence of cancer with age.

Despite the controversy regarding the importance of immune surveillance, there is much greater consensus on the importance of the immunodeficiency of aging in the clinical management of cancer, eluding the problems associated with infection and disease progression.

6. THE AGING HOST AND THE DEVELOPMENT OF CANCER

Carcinogenesis is a multistage process involving serial alterations of cellular genes. These include oncogenes and antiproliferative genes (antioncogenes), which modulate cell proliferation and genes which prevent apoptosis (programmed cell death). It is now understood that oncogenes encode proteins with a myriad of functions including growth factors, growth factor receptors, enzymes involved in the transduction of proliferative signals, DNA synthesis and replication (for a review, see reference 47). Similarly, antioncogenes encode cell proliferation or DNA-replication inhibiting proteins and apoptosis-preventing genes encode proteins that inhibit the activation of endonucleases which would otherwise disrupt the template function of DNA and result in cell death [48].

The multistage nature of carcinogenesis has been demonstrated in experimental models with strong circumstantial support in human cancers. For example, for the case of colorectal cancer, Vogelstein and colleagues [49] described a sequence of genetic alterations leading from normal mucosal epithelium to invasive carcinoma. One step, the loss of the Familial Adenomatous Polyposis (FAP) gene on the 5th chromosome, is associated with hyperproliferation of the mucosal cells and formation of adenomatous polyps. Additional changes in the expression of the p53 gene on chromosome 18 and the DCC gene on chromosome 17 may lead to a more malignant phenotype. Likewise, in the case of brain tumors, loss of a portion of the 17th chromosome (17p) is seen in malignancy of all grades, whereas loss of chromosome 10 and of the genes encoding interferon receptors was found only in glioblastoma multiforme [50]. These changes may provide the genetic basis for the transformation from indolent to more aggressive disease. Sequential genetic changes leading to more aggressive neoplasms have been reported in many other diseases, including breast, cervical, renal and lung cancer [51-57].

6.1 Serial Stochastic Events

The interpretation of carcinogenesis as a multistage process presents at least two non-mutually exclusive explanations for the increasing incidence of cancer with age. The first and simplest is that the tissues of an older person will have, over time, sustained the serial stochastic events involved in carcinogenesis. Accordingly, the cancers more prevalent among the aged, such as prostate, colon or breast cancer, are those involving a greater number of steps. In contrast, this hypothesis would predict that tumors more common in young people (lymphoma, leukemia, neuroblastoma, etc.) would require fewer steps in the progression from normal to the malignant state.

6.2 Age as a Risk Factor

The second hypothesis holds that age itself is a risk factor for cancer because the process of aging involves genetic events that are similar to those occurring during early carcinogenesis. Thus, the number of cells that would be susceptible to the effects of late-stage carcinogens increases with age. Both experimental and clinical evidence support this theory. Cytogenetic and molecular changes observed in early carcinogenesis are also seen in cells maintained in long-term culture. These changes include formation of DNA adducts, DNA hypomethylation, chromosomal breakage and translocation [58,59]. Also, the accumulation of iron commonly observed in some aging cells, may cause oncogene activation and antioncogene suppression [59-61]. The likelihood of neoplastic transformation after exposure to late-stage carcinogens is higher in tissues from older animals than in those of younger animals, both in tissue culture and in cross-transplant experiments [62-65].

Epidemiological data for some cancers suggest that the susceptibility to late-stage carcinogens increases with age [66]. The comparison between the incidence of melanoma and of squamous cell carcinoma (SCC) of the skin is particularly illustrative [67,68]. Whereas, in the United States the incidence of melanoma plateaus at age 45 for women and 61 for men, the incidence of SCC continues to rise even beyond age 85. This is what might be predicted if there were more steps in the generation of SCC than in melanoma. However, the increased number of steps is not the total explanation because the incidence of SCC increases logarithmically with age [68]. This suggests either the association of longevity with a genetic predisposition to SCC (unlikely) or, the increased susceptibility with age to late-stage carcinogens. It should be underscored that both basic and clinical data suggest that there is an increased susceptibility and it may be tissue and organ specific. For example, skin epithelium, liver and lymphoid tissues, but not nervous or muscular tissues, show increased susceptibility to late-stage carcinogens in older rodents [69]. Similarly, the incidence of melanoma and mesothelioma in humans demonstrates an age-related plateau, suggesting that these tissues are not more susceptible to late-stage carcinogens [66-68].

Other age-related factors that may increase the risk of cancer include reduced DNA repairing ability and decreased carcinogen catabolism [70]. It has been proposed that these lead to an accelerated carcinogenic process with more rapid generation of cells susceptible to late-stage carcinogens (promoters) [71].

7. TUMOR AGGRESSIVENESS IN THE AGING HOST

There has been a long-held but incompletely documented clinical notion that cancers in older people are "less aggressive" (Table 1). However, epidemiological data from tumor registries or large clinical trials have not been supportive. This may be because this type of data is confounded by special problems common to geriatric populations (e.g., comorbidity, "poly-pharmacy," physician or family bias regarding diagnosis and treatment in the elderly, and age-associated life stresses) and these factors may counter any primary influence that aging might have on tumor aggressiveness. However, there is experimental support for the contention that there is reduced tumor aggressiveness with age. Data obtained from laboratory animals with a wide range of tumors under highly controlled circumstances demonstrate slower tumor growth, fewer experimental metastases, and longer survival in old mice [72-75].

What accounts for the age-associated changes observed in these experimental systems? One explanation derives from the understanding that the tumors, although histologically quite similar, may be biologically very different in old patients. For example, breast cancer cells are more likely to contain estrogen receptors, and leukemic cells have cytogenetic abnormalities in elderly patients with those disorders. Each of these

Table 1. Cancers Reported to Have Reduced or Altered Patterns of Growth with Age

Breast
Colon
Lung
Prostate
Renal

Tumors originating in these organs have been reported to have reduced tumor growth rates or longer survival in older patients. For a review of these reports, see reference 75.

Figure 1. One explanation for varying tumor aggressiveness with age. Rates of tumor proliferation may play a role in the apparent slower growth of tumors. For example, if two tumors, one fast growing and one slow both arise at the same stage of life, the faster growing tumor would present clinically at a younger age. This model might explain why tumors arising in younger patients tend to be more aggressive, and why there is such great heterogeneity in tumor characteristics (such as aggressiveness) in older individuals.

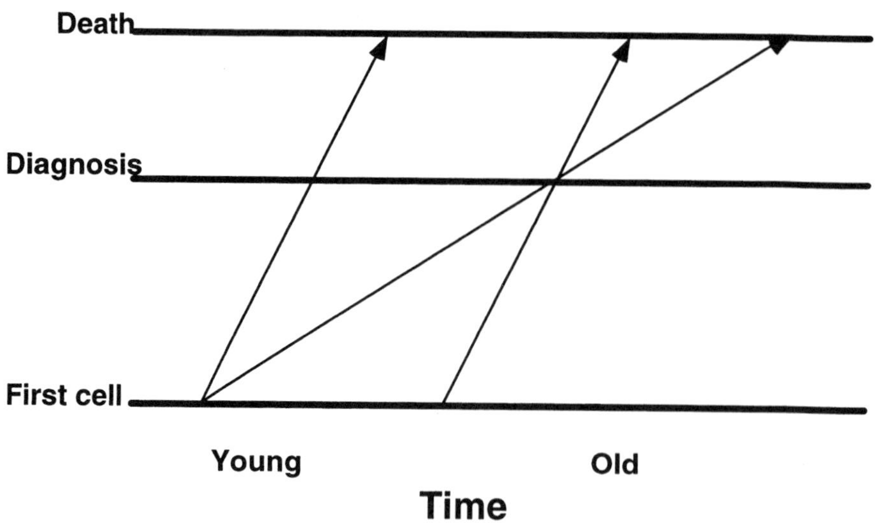

associations has prognostic significance. Furthermore, there is the issue of the "time line" artifact (Figure 1) that implies that old patients (more so than young) may develop slow growing tumors on the basis of time required to develop such slow tumors. Such is, of course, consistent with the multistep hypothesis as discussed above.

It is probable that certain factors that influence tumor growth change with age. With this in mind, various endocrine, nutritional, wound healing, and angiogenesis factors have been explored. For some tumors, age-associated changes in these factors have been correlated with reduced tumor growth [76-80]. However, several early observations led to the seemingly paradoxical conclusion that immune senescence accounted for a large component of the observed reduced tumor growth with age. For example, B16 melanoma grows less well in congenitally immune deficient mice [81] and in young mice rendered T-cell deficient [119]. Furthermore, when young, thymectomized, lethally irradiated mice received bone marrow or splenocytes from old donor mice, tumor growth was less than when the spleen or bone marrow was from young donor mice [73,74].

It is believed that competent immune cells provide factors that augment tumor growth under certain circumstances. If a tumor is only weakly antigenic, non-specific growth stimulatory factors provided by lymphocytes or monocytes may actually counteract the inhibitory forces provided by those same cells (because of the lack of tumor antigen). In this situation immune deficiency does not render a host more susceptible to aggressive tumor growth and spread; in fact immune deficiency renders a host more resistant because those cells are less likely to provide the non-specific stimulatory factors. This hypothesis is akin to the immune enhancement theory promoted several decades ago by Prehn and colleagues [82]. Briefly stated in the context of cancer and aging; the positive growth, angiogenic and other tumor stimulatory signals produced nonspecifically by cells considered part of the immune system will be less by cells from old animals. In other words, the "soil" is less fertile for aggressive tumor growth

8. CONCLUSIONS

It has been said that all medical oncologists, with the exception of those who restrict their practice to pediatric patients, are 'geriatric oncologists'. This, of course, because the average age of cancer is in excess of 65 years and the median age of most common adult tumors approaches 70 years. Similarly, scientists studying the mechanisms of cancer development and growth are uncovering and elucidating some of the basic molecular and cellular processes of aging. These include the controls of cellular proliferation, mechanisms of DNA repair, and programmed cell death. There are striking voids in our understanding of the basic mechanisms of aging, but one can not help but have the sense that the advances in this field will have the added value of enhancing our understanding of tumor development and growth.

REFERENCES

1. Duthie EH: Physiology of aging: relevance to symptoms, perceptions and treatment tolerance in Comprehensive Geriatric Oncology L. Balducci , G. Lyman and W.B. Ershler (eds). Harwood Academic, Amsterdam, pp 247-262, 1998
2. Lindeman RD: Overview: renal physiology and pathophysiology of aging. Am J Kidney Dis 1990, 16(4):275-82
3. Dubrow EL: Reactivation of tuberculosis; a problem of aging. J Am Geriatr Soc 1976; 24(11):481-7
4. Nagami PH, Yoshikawa TT: Tuberculosis in the geriatric patient. J Am Geriatr Soc 1983; 31(6):356-63
5. Gelato MC: Aging and immune function: a possible role for growth hormone. Hormone Res 1996; 45:46-9

6. Arden NH, Patriarca PA, Kendal AP: Experiences in the use and efficacy of inactivated influenza vaccine in the nursing home in Kendal AP, Patriarca PA, eds, Options for the Control of Influenza. New York. Alan Liss, Inc, 1986; 155-68
7. Powers DC, Sears SD, Murphy BR, Thurmar B, Clements ML: Systemic and local antibody responses in elderly subjects give live or inactivated influenza A virus vaccines. J Clin Microbiol 1989; 27:2666-71
8. Hilleman, RM: Realities and enigmas of human viral influenza: pathogenesis, epidemiology and control. Vaccine 2002; 19;20(25-26):3068-87
9. Kaesberg PR, Ershler WB: The importance of immune senescence in the incidence and malignant properties of cancer in hosts of advanced age. J Gerontology 1989; 44:63-6
10. Christensen K, Vaupel JW: Determinants of longevity: genetic, environmental and medical factors. J Intern Med 1996; 240(6):333-41
11. Guyer B, Strobino DM, Ventura S.J., MacDorman M., Martin JA: Annual summary of vital statistics 1995. Pediatrics 1996; 98(6):1007-19
12. Greville TNE: U.S. life tables by cause of death: 1969-1971. U.S. Decennial Life Tables for 1969-1971 1971; 1:5-15
13. Riggs JE: Longitudinal Gompertzian analysis of adult mortality in the U.S., 1900-1986. Mech Ageing Dev 1990; 54(3):235-47
14. Hirsch HR: Can an improved environment cause maximum survival to decrease? Comments on lifespan criteria and longitudinal Gompertzian analysis. Exp Gerontol 1994; 29(2):119-37
15. Orr WC, Sohal RS: Extension of life-span by overexpression of superoxide dismutase and catalase in Drosophila melanogaster. Science 1994; 263(5150):1128-30
16. Weindruch R: Caloric restriction and aging. Scientific American 1996; 274:46-52.
17. Cristofalo VJ, Pignolo, RJ: Replicative senescence of human fibroblast-like cells in culture. Physiol Rev 1993;73:617-38
18. Hayflick L: The limited in vitro lifetime of human diploid cell strains. Exp Cell Res 1965; 37:614-36
19. Cristofalo VJ, Palazzo, R., Charpentier, R.L: Limited lifespan of human fibroblasts in vitro: metabolic time or replications? In Adelman RC, Roberts, J., Baker, G.T., ed., Neural Regulatory Mechanisms During Aging. New York: Alan R. Liss, 1980
20. Schneider EL, Mitsui, Y: The relationship between in vitro cellular aging and in vivo human age. Proc Natl Acad Sci USA 1976; 73:3584-88
21. Rohme D: Evidence for a relationship between longevity of mammalian species and lif-spans of normal fibroblasts in vitro and erythrocytes in vivo. Proc Natl Acad Sci USA 1976; 78:5009-13
22. Dimri GP, Lee, X., Basile, G., Acosta, M., Scott, G., Roskelley, C., Medrano, EE, Linskens, M., Rubelj, I., Pereira-Smith, O, Peacocke, M, Campisi, J: A biomarker that identifies senescent human cells in culture and in aging skin in vivo. Proc Natl Acad Sci USA 1995; 92(20):9363-7
23. Stjernsward J: Age-dependent tumor host barrier and effect of carcinogen-induced immunodepression on rejection of isografted methylcholanthrene-induced sarcoma cells. J Natl Cancer Inst 1966; 37:505-12
24. Yuhas JM, Pazmino NH, Proctor JO, Toya RE: A direct relationship between immune competence and the subcutaneous growth rate of a malignant murine lung tumor. Cancer Res 1974; 34:722-28
25. Rockwell SC: Effect of host age on transplantation, growth and radiation response of EMT6 tumors. Cancer Research 1981; 41:527-31
26. Gatti RQ, Good RA: Aging, immunity and malignancy. Geriatrics 1979; 25:158-68
27. Bulychev VV: Longevity, atherosclerosis and cellular immunity. Klin Med (Mosk) 1993; 71(5):51-4
28. Hansson GK, Libby P, Schonbeck U, Yan ZQ: Innate and adaptive immunity in the pathogenesis of atherosclerosis. Circ Res 2002 23;91:281-91

29. Lehuen A, Bendelac A, Bach JF, Carnaud C: The nonobese diabetic mouse model. Independent expression of humoral and cell mediated autoimmune features. J Immunol 1990; 144(6):2147-51
30. Hull M, Strauss S, Berger M, Volk B, Bauer J: The participation of interleukin-6, a stress-inducible cytokine, in the pathogenesis of Alzheimer's disease. Behav Brain Res 1996; 78(1):37-41
31. Hull M, Fiebich BL., Lieb S, Berger SS, Volk B, Bauer J: Interleukin-6-associated inflammatory processes in Alzheimer's disease: New therapeutic options. Neurobiol Aging 1996; 17(5):795-800
32. Gillis S, Kozak R, Durante M, Weksler ME: Decreased production and response to T cell growth factor by lymphocytes from aged humans. J Clin Invest 1981; 67:937-42.
33. Miller RA: The aging immune system: primer and prospectus. Science 1996; 273(5271):70-4
34. Stephan RP, Sanders VM, Witte PL: Stage-specific alterations in murine lymphopoiesis with age. Int Immunol 1996; 8(4):509-18
35. Radl J, Sepers JM, Skvaril F: Immunoglobulin patterns in humans over 95 years of age. Clin Exp Immunol 1975; 22:84-90
36. Radl J: Animal model of human disease. Benign monoclonal gammopathy (idiopathic paraproteinemia). Am J Pathol 1981; 105(1):91-3
37. Radl J: Age-related monoclonal gammopathies: Clinical lessons from the aging C57BL/6 mouse. Immunol Today 1990; 11:234-6
38. Kyle RA: Monoclonal gammopathy of undetermined significance and solitary plasmacytoma. Implications for progression to overt myeloma. Hematol Oncol Clin North Am 1997; 11(1):71-87
39. Thoman M, Weigle WO: Lymphokines and aging: Interleukin-2 production and activity in aged animals. J Immunol 1981; 127:2102-6
40. Ershler WB, Sun WH, Binkley N: Interleukin-6 and aging: Blood levels and mononuclear cell production increase with advancing age and in vitro production is modifiable by dietary restriction. Lymphokine Cytokine Res 1993; 12:225-30
41. Ershler WB: Interleukin-6: a cytokine for gerontologists. Journal of the American Geriatrics Society 1993; 41(2):176-81
42. Ershler WB, Keller ET: Age-associated increased IL-6 gene expression, late-life diseases and frailty. Ann Rev Med 2000;51:245-270
43. Ershler WB: The influence of an aging immune system on cancer incidence and progression. J Gerontol 1993;48:B3–B7
44. Miller RA: Aging and cancer: another perspective. J Gerontol 1993;48:B8–B10
45. Covelli V, Mouton D, Mojo V et al: Inheritance of immune responsiveness, life span and disease incidence in interline crosses of mice selected for high or low multispecific antibody production. J Immunology 1989;142:1224–1234
46. Imai K, Matsuyama S, Miyake S, Suga K, Nakachi K: Natural cytotoxic activity of peripheral-blood lymphocytes and cancer incidence: an 11-year follow-up study of a general population. Lancet 2000;356:1795-99
47. Weinberg RA: Oncogenes and the Molecular Origins of Cancer. Cold Spring Harbor Laboratory Press. 1989
48. Korsemeyer SJ: Programmed cell death: Bcl-2. In: DeVita V.T.; Hellman S.; Rosenberg S.A.: Important Advances in Oncology, 1993. J.B. Lippincott, 1993, 19-28
49. Vogelstein B, Fearon ER, Hamilton SR et al: Genetic alterations during colorectal tumor development. N Engl J Med 1988; 319: 525-532
50. James CD, Carlbom E, Dumanskji JP, et al: Clonal genomic alterations in glioma malignancy stages. Cancer Res 1988; 48: 5546-5551
51. Boyle P, Leake R: Progress in understanding breast cancer: Epidemiological and biological interactions. Breast Cancer Res Treat 1988; 11: 91-112

52. Harris JR, Lippman ME, Veronesi U, Willett W: Breast cancer. N Engl J Med 1992; 327: 319-328, 390-398, 473-480
53. Carney DN: Biology of small cell lung cancer. Lancet 1992; 339: 843-846
54. Correa P: Biochemical and molecular methods in cancer epidemiology and prevention: the path between the laboratory and the population. Cancer Epidem Biomark Prev 1993; 2:85-88
55. Vineis P: Epidemiological models of carcinogenesis: the example of bladder cancer. Cancer Epidem Biomark Prev 1992; 1:149-154
56. el Azouzi M, Chung RY, Farmer GE, et al: Lost of distinct regions on the short arm of chromosome 17 associated with tumorigenesis of human astrocytomas. Proc Natl Acad Sci USA 1989; 86: 7186-7190
57. Linehan WM, Gnarra JR, Lerman MI, et al: Genetic bases of renal cell cancer. In: DeVita VT; Hellman S.; Rosenberg S.A.: Important Advances in Oncology, 1993. J.B. Lippincott, 1993, 47-70
58. Franco EL: Prognostic value of human papillomavirus in the survival of cervical cancer patients: an overview of the evidence. Cancer Epidemiol Biomark Prev 1992; 1: 499-504
59. Anisimov VN: Age as a factor of risk in multistage carcinogenesis. In Balducci L, Lyman GH, Ershler WB, eds: Geriatric Oncology, J.B. Lippincott, 1992, 53-60
60. Fernandez-Pol JA: Growth factors, oncogenes, antioncogenes and aging. In Balducci L, Lyman GH, Ershler WB, eds: Comprehensive Geriatric Oncology, Harcourt, 1998, 179-196
61. Stevens RG, Jones DY, Micozzi MS, Taylor PR: Body iron stores and the risk of cancer. N Engl J Med 1988; 319: 1047-1052
62. Anisimov VN: Effect of age on dose-response relationship in carcinogenesis induced by single administration of N-methynitrosourea in female rats. J Cancer Res Clin Oncol 1988; 114: 628-635
63. Ward JM, Lynch P, Riggs C: Rapid development of hepatocellular neoplasms in aging male C3H/HeNcr mice given phenobarbital. Cancer Lett 1988; 39:9-18
64. Ebbesen P: Reticulosarcoma and amyloid development in BALB/c mice inoculated with syngeneic cells from young and old donors. J Natl Cancer Inst 1971; 47: 1241-1245
65. Anisimov VN, Loktionov AS, Khavinson VK, Morozov VG: Effect of low molecular weight factors of thymus and pineal gland on life span and spontaneous tumor development in female mice of different age. Mech Ageing Dev 1989; 49: 245-257
66. Kaldor JM, Day NE: Interpretation of epidemiological studies in the context of the multistage model of carcinogenesis. In Barrett JC: Mechanisms of Environmental Carcinogenesis, Vol 2, CRC press, 1987, 21-57
67. Tantranond P, Karam F, Wang TY, et al: Management of cutaneous squamous cell carcinoma in an elderly man. J Am Ger Soc 1992; 40: 510-512
68. Glass AG, Hoover RN: The emerging epidemic of melanoma and squamous cell carcinoma of the skin. JAMA 1989; 262: 2097-2100
69. Matoha MF, Cosgrove JW, Atak JR, Rappoport SI: Selective elevation of the c-myc transcript levels in the liver of the aging Fischer 344 rat. Biochem Biophys Res Commun 1987; 147:1-7
70. Bohr VA, Evans MK, Fornace AJ: Biology of disease: DNA repair and its patogenetic implications. Lab Invest 1989; 61:143-161
71. Randerath K, Reddy MV, Disher RM: Age- and tissue-related DNA modifications in untreated rats: Detection by ^{32}P-post-labeling assay and possible significance for spontaneous tumor induction and aging. Carcinogenesis 1986; 7:1615-1617
72. Ershler WB, Stewart JA, Hacker MP, Moore AL, Tindle BH: B16 murine melanoma and aging: Slower growth and longer survival in old mice, JNCI 1984; 72:161-165
73. Ershler WB, Moore AL, Shore H, Gamelli RL: Transfer of age-associated restrained tumor growth in mice by old to young bone marrow transplantation. Cancer Research 1984; 44:5677-81

74. Tsuda T, Kim YT, Siskind GW, DeBlasio A, Schwab R, Ershler WB, Weksler ME: Role of the thymus and T-cells in slow growth of B16 melanoma in old mice. Cancer Research 1987; 47:3097-3103
75. Ershler WB, Guest Editorial: Why tumors grow more slowly in old people. JNCI 77 1986;837-839
76. Simon SR, Ershler WB: Hormonal influences on growth of B16 murine melanoma. JNCI 1985; 74:1085-1088
77. Ershler WB, Berman E, Moore AL: B16 melanoma growth is slower, but pulmonary colonization is greater in calorie restricted mice. J Natl Cancer Inst 1986; 76:81-5
78. Ershler WB, Gamelli RL, Moore AL, Hacker MP, and Blow AJ: Experimental tumors and aging: Local factors that may account for the observed age advantage in the B16 murine melanoma model. Exp Gerontol 1984 19:367-375
79. Hadar E, Ershler WB, Kreisle R.A, Ho S-P, Volk MJ, Klopp RG: Lymphocyte-induced angiogenesis factor is produced by L3T4+ murine T lymphocytes, and its production declines with age. Cancer Immunol. Immunother 1988; 26:31-37
80. Kreisle RA, Stebler B, Ershler WB: Effect of host age on tumor associated angiogenesis in mice. JNCI 1990; 82:44-47
81. Fidler IJ, Gersten DM, Riggs CW: Relationship of host immune status to tumor cell arrest, distribution and survival in experimental metastases. Cancer 1977 40:46-55
82. Prehn RT, Lappe, MA: An immunostimulation theory of tumor development. Transplant Rev 1971; 7:26-30

Chapter 5

AGE AND CO-MORBIDITY IN CANCER PATIENTS: A POPULATION-BASED APPROACH

Maryska L.G. Janssen-Heijnen, Saskia Houterman, Valery E.P.P. Lemmens, Marieke W.J. Louwman, Jan Willem W. Coebergh

Maryska L.G. Janssen-Heijnen, Senior Researcher, Saskia Houterman, Staff Researcher, Valery E.P.P. Lemmens, Junior Researcher, Marieke W.J. Louwman, Senior Researcher, Eindhoven Cancer Registry at Comprehensive Cancer Center South (IKZ), 5600 AE Eindhoven, The Netherlands. Jan Willem W. Coebergh, Head of Research, Department of Public Health, Professor, Erasmus University Medical Centre Rotterdam, 3000 DR Rotterdam, The Netherlands.

The mean age of patients diagnosed with cancer is increasing in western countries due to rising incidence rates of most cancers with age and ageing of the population. In most European countries more than 40% of all new patients with cancer are over the age of 70, which implies that they increasingly suffer from one or more other serious (chronic) diseases and from interactions with and side effects from their treatment. Besides affecting the life expectancy co-morbid conditions and their treatment may complicate the clinical management of cancer patients, especially when they are frail. Since they are often excluded from clinical trials, little is known about treatment outcome, such as complications, quality of life and survival. Choice of curative treatment of cancer for older patients may be influenced by the physical condition of the patient (co-morbidity, reduced functional reserves, interaction between medications, performance status), the psychological condition (depression, dementia) and social parameters (informal care, mobility) [1-3].

This chapter focuses on the role of age and co-morbidity in cancer patients. The value of studying co-morbidity is demonstrated by data of the population-based Eindhoven Cancer Registry [4]. We were looking for answers on questions on guideline adherence from local clinicians who increasingly experienced problems with an increasing number of elderly patients. The clinical context is one of community hospitals only, within the framework of the Comprehensive Cancer Centre [5]. We give insight in the prevalence of co-morbidity in unselected cancer patients, and the effects of co-morbidity on treatment and prognosis.

1. METHODS

The Eindhoven Cancer Registry records data on all patients newly diagnosed with cancer in the southern part of the Netherlands, an area with now 2.3 million inhabitants and only general hospitals. Since 1993 serious co-morbidity with prognostic impact has been recorded for all patients. The Charlson Co-morbidity Index is most widely used for recording co-morbidity and was validated in various studies [6]. We used a slightly adapted version of this index for recording co-morbidity (Table 1). Co-morbidity was defined as life-shortening diseases that were present at the time of cancer diagnosis and/or received some treatment or surveillance.

Table 1. Classification of co-morbidity, according to an adapted version of the list of Charlson et al. (1987)

Chronic Obstructive Pulmonary Diseases (COPD)
Cardiovascular disease: myocardial infarction, cardiac insufficiency, angina pectoris, CABG (coronary artery bypass graft)
Peripheral arterial disease: intermittent claudication, abdominal aneurysm, surgical intervention
Cerebrovascular diseases (cerebrovascular accident, hemiplegia)
Other malignancies (except basal cell skin carcinoma)
Hypertension
Diabetes mellitus
Other:

- autoimmune diseases: sarcoidosis, Wegener's disease, SLE (systemic lupus erythematosis)
- rheumatoid arthritis (only severe)
- kidney diseases: glomerulonephritis, pyelonephritis
- gastrointestinal: stomach ulcer & resection, colitis
- liver diseases: cirrhosis, hepatitis
- dementia
- chronic infection

The data were extracted from the medical records between 6 and 18 months after diagnosis, when the trained registry personnel does its routine view. Previous admissions, letters from and to general practitioners (every patient has his GP in the Netherlands) and other specialists, the medical history and preoperative screening were used as sources. On average, it takes about 5 minutes per patient to record co-morbidity. The medical record is generally regarded as the most complete source of information on the patient's past and current health status [7].

Patients with cancer of the esophagus, stomach, colon or rectum, pancreas, lung, breast, cervix uteri, corpus uteri, ovary, prostate, bladder, kidney, and non-Hodgkin's lymphoma, newly diagnosed between 1995 and 2001 (N=48,030), were included for this overview. Patients with cancer diagnosed at autopsy (N=447 or 1%) were excluded. Treatment was classified as surgery (resection), radiotherapy, chemotherapy, hormonal therapy (or combinations) and 'other or none'. Surgery did not comprise diagnostic operations.

Survival analyses were restricted to patients with cancer of the colon or rectum, lung, breast, prostate or non-Hodgkin's lymphoma diagnosed between 1995 and 1999 (N=21,984). Vital status was available up to 1 April 2002. In addition to passive follow-up via the hospitals, this information was also obtained from the municipal registries in the area of the Eindhoven Cancer Registry and the Central Bureau for Genealogy. The latter is an institution that collects data on all deceased Dutch citizens via the civil municipal registries. In this way, information on patients who moved outside the registry area was also obtained. Patients who died outside the Netherlands were lost-to follow-up. The estimated proportion of these patients was less than 1%.

Survival time was defined as the time from diagnosis to death or the end of the study. Survival generally decreases with age, because other causes-of-death also take their share. The prevalence of co-morbidity increases with age. Therefore, we calculated relative survival rates which are an estimation of disease-specific survival. Survival of cancer patients is adjusted for mortality from all causes of death in the background population with the same age structure. Relative survival is calculated as the ratio of the observed to the expected rates [8]. Expected survival rates were estimated from life tables for regional male and female populations.

2. RESULTS

2.1 Prevalence

The prevalence of co-morbidity usually increased with age (Table 2), but remained stable or decreased above age 80 for some tumours. About 60% of all new cancer patients older than 65 also suffered from at least one other serious disease. The most frequent concomitant diseases were previous cancers, heart disease, hypertension, COPD, and diabetes mellitus, with prevalence rates up to 20%, 23%, 26%, 17%, and 16%, respectively. The prevalence of co-morbidity was highest for patients with lung cancer (over 70% for men aged 65 or older) and lowest for patients with breast cancer (about 55% for women aged 65 or older) (Table 3). The prevalence of cardiovascular diseases was higher among men compared to women, and was up to 35% of male and 28% of female patients with cancer of the digestive tract, lung, and kidney, and non-Hodgkin's lymphoma (Table 4). The prevalence of COPD was relatively high among older patients with lung cancer (31% of males and 24% of females), and also among men with esophageal and bladder cancer (20%). The prevalence of hypertension was highest among women with gynaecological tumors (38%) or adenocarcinoma of the kidney (up to 45%). High prevalence rates of diabetes in older patients were observed for cancer of the pancreas (up to 27%), cervix uteri (32%), corpus uteri (25%) and kidney (22%). The prevalence of diabetes in women with cervical cancer was twice as high among those with squamous cell than with adenocarcinoma, being 16% and 7% respectively (not shown).

The higher prevalence rates of digestive tract conditions among males compared to females were largely due to concomitant stomach ulcers (3.5% versus almost 2%) and previous gastrectomy (2.7% versus 0.6%), whereas the prevalence of colitis was about similar with 0.3%.

2.2 Treatment (see overview in Table 5)

Patients with colon cancer underwent surgery regardless of age or the number of co-morbid conditions: more than 95% with Dukes A-C did so and about 75% of patients with Dukes D. However, patients with Dukes C received less adjuvant chemotherapy with the rise of age: from 65% of patients at middle age to 33% of patients aged 65 or older (data 1997-2001). The proportion of patients with Dukes D receiving adjuvant chemotherapy decreased from 56% at middle age to 20% of patients aged 65 or older. The proportion receiving adjuvant chemotherapy also decreased from 27% of patients without co-morbidity to 17% of those with co-morbidity. The proportion of rectal cancer patients receiving adjuvant radiotherapy decreased from 53% of patients younger than 65 to 37% of patients aged 65 or older, and also decreased with co-morbidity from 51% of patients without co-morbidity to 39% in case of co-morbidity.

Table 2. Age-specific prevalence (%) of serious concomitant diseases among newly diagnosed cancer patients in southeastern Netherlands, 1995-2001.

	MEN Age (years)			WOMEN Age (years)		
	50-64	65-79	80+	50-64	65-79	80+
Concomitant disease	(n = 8294)	(n = 14,593)	(n = 3362)	(n = 8210)	(n = 9621)	(n = 3623)
Other cancers[a]	8.2	15	20	8.3	13	16
Heart disease	11	22	23	3.6	12	19
Peripheral vascular disease	4.4	8.8	7.4	1.4	3.1	3.2
COPD	9.5	17.1	17	5.7	8.4	7.1
Hypertension	12	16.2	12	14	26	24
Diabetes mellitus	5.7	9.3	11	5.2	14	16
Cerebrovascular disease	2.3	5.7	6.7	1.2	4.3	7.1
Autoimmune	0.7	1.0	0.9	0.9	1.6	1.8
Chronic infection	1.3	2.3	1.7	1.0	2.1	1.9
Central nervous system	0.1	0.5	2.5	-	0.8	4.1
Liver disease	0.9	0.7	0.5	0.5	0.5	0.3
Urinary	0.5	0.5	0.5	0.3	0.4	0.4
Gastro-intestinal	4.7	6.4	6.0	1.8	2.5	3.9
Connective tissue	0.3	0.1	-	0.3	0.2	0.3
Together[b]	**43**	**63**	**64**	**34**	**56**	**63**

Source: Eindhoven Cancer Registry; [a] also in same organ (but not metastasis of primary tumor), excluding basal cell skin Carcinoma; [b] more conditions per patient

Table 3. Age-specific prevalence (%) of the number of serious concomitant diseases among newly diagnosed patients with 13 major cancers in southeastern Netherlands, 1995-2001 Source: Eindhoven Cancer Registry.

				number of co-morbid conditions			
tumor site	sex	age (years)	N	None %	1 %	≥ 2 %	unknown %
All cancers	Men	50-64	8294	42	28	15	15
		65-79	14593	25	33	30	12
		80+	3362	20	32	33	16
	Women	50-64	8170	52	25	9	14
		65-79	9587	33	31	24	11
		80+	3618	23	31	32	14
Esophagus	Men	50-64	200	42	28	23	8
		65-79	216	24	33	39	4
		80+	57	21	35	37	7
	Women	50-64	73	48	30	11	11
		65-79	100	40	30	24	6
		80+	50	18	42	34	6
Stomach	Men	50-64	356	41	30	18	11
		65-79	619	26	32	34	7
		80+	171	18	32	40	10
	Women	50-64	132	51	27	16	7
		65-79	284	35	29	27	9
		80+	196	24	29	39	7
Colon/rectum	Men	50-64	1254	50	26	14	11
		65-79	2029	28	33	31	7
		80+	522	22	33	37	8
	Women	50-64	916	53	27	10	10
		65-79	1733	35	32	24	9
		80+	773	25	30	35	10
Pancreas	Men	50-64	156	35	32	18	15
		65-79	274	27	30	35	8
		80+	45	27	31	33	9
	Women	50-64	105	47	28	12	13
		65-79	255	29	34	27	9
		80+	85	24	31	34	12

Table 3 continued

Lung	Men	50-64	1945	39	32	21	8
		65-79	3478	22	35	38	5
		80+	518	21	31	40	8
	Women	50-64	673	45	32	15	8
		65-79	741	27	33	33	8
		80+	94	32	27	33	9
Breast	Women	50-64	3247	60	21	7	12
		65-79	2655	37	31	22	10
		80+	824	25	33	33	9
Cervix uteri	Women	50-64	125	57	26	9	8
		65-79	87	44	32	18	6
		80+	37	27	30	32	11
Corpus uteri	Women	50-64	507	54	27	10	9
		65-79	490	31	34	28	7
		80+	126	19	34	42	5
Ovary	Women	50-64	380	57	26	8	9
		65-79	386	36	33	24	7
		80+	102	29	36	25	9
Prostate	Men	50-64	1158	45	27	11	18
		65-79	3316	30	33	22	15
		80+	784	27	32	25	16
Bladder	Men	50-64	350	39	30	16	16
		65-79	804	22	38	31	9
		80+	248	18	35	38	9
	Women	50-64	87	30	38	14	18
		65-79	186	32	30	31	8
		80+	109	22	31	29	17
Kidney	Men	50-64	263	42	32	16	10
		65-79	315	22	34	34	10
		80+	50	8	34	44	14
	Women	50-64	157	42	31	13	13
		65-79	241	23	35	32	10
		80+	58	17	31	43	9
NHL	Men	50-64	268	50	24	15	11
		65-79	335	29	36	31	5
		80+	63	14	41	33	11
	Women	50-64	201	54	24	10	12
		65-79	280	36	33	26	6
		80+	98	32	30	36	3

Table 4. Age-specific prevalence (%) of the most common serious concomitant diseases among newly diagnosed patients with 13 major cancers, 1995-2001. Source: Eindhoven Cancer Registry.

		other cancers			heart /vascular disease			COPD			hypertension			diabetes		
age (yrs)		50-64	65-79	80+	50-64	65-79	80+	50-64	65-79	80+	50-64	65-79	80+	50-64	65-79	80+
tumor	Sex	%	%	%	%	%	%	%	%	%	%	%	%	%	%	%
Esophagus	M	7	19	26	15	35	32	12	16	23	15	20	9	5	11	16
	W	11	16	16	4	16	16	14	9	8	10	17	24	4	13	14
Stomach	M	6	12	20	19	33	26	7	14	16	15	15	19	6	9	12
	W	10	13	15	8	15	25	4	9	7	14	26	29	7	14	20
Colon/rectum	M	7	15	22	13	28	31	6	15	16	16	20	15	7	10	12
	W	10	14	16	5	14	24	5	8	9	15	25	25	6	14	16
Pancreas	M	6	13	13	22	26	33	5	17	16	12	18	18	13	20	22
	W	8	9	7	8	15	27	3	9	6	15	27	28	11	27	25
Lung	M	9	16	17	18	33	31	20	29	31	10	15	10	6	10	11
	W	9	15	14	11	21	21	21	24	14	12	22	18	5	12	10
Breast	W	6	10	14	4	12	21	4	6	7	13	29	26	5	13	16
Cervix uteri	W	5	8	11	6	16	22	5	6	3	13	21	27	9	15	32
Corpus uteri	W	8	10	19	3	12	23	4	6	12	23	38	33	8	22	25
Ovary	W	12	13	15	4	15	16	5	7	5	13	26	26	4	12	12
Prostate	M	6	9	14	12	23	27	6	12	14	13	17	11	5	8	9
Bladder	M	19	24	30	16	28	28	8	15	21	9	16	13	4	11	11
	W	24	23	17	8	13	24	9	7	8	11	31	18	7	17	15
Kidney	M	12	16	28	15	32	34	6	15	16	16	25	18	8	10	20
	W	7	18	17	6	18	28	8	6	3	27	32	45	9	18	22
NHL	M	5	13	17	14	28	35	4	15	10	12	18	11	5	10	11
	W	6	15	15	6	11	24	2	8	4	15	25	21	7	11	13

Table 5. Influence of age and co-morbidity on primary treatment, according to tumor type and/or stage

Tumor	Stage	Influence of rising age (> 60 yrs)	Influence of co-morbidity
Colon	Dukes A/B	None	None
	Dukes C/D	Less adjuvant CT, none >80yrs	Age 65-79: less adjuvant CT
Rectum	Dukes B/C	Less adjuvant RT	Less adjuvant RT
NSCLC*	I/II	Less surgery, more RT alone	Age 60-79: less surgery
	III/IV	Less CT	None
SCLC**	Limited	Less CT+RT, more CT alone	Age 70-79: less CT+RT
	Extensive	Less CT, more abstinence	None
Breast		Less surgery, more endocrine	Less adjuvant RT, more endocrine
Prostate		Less prostatectomy, more endocrine	Age 60-79: less prostatectomy, more endocrine
NHL***	Indolent	Less CT, more RT and wait & see	None
	Aggressive	Less CT, more abstinence	Age 70+: less CT

* Non-small cell lung cancer

** Small cell lung cancer

*** Non-Hodgkin's lymphoma

CT=chemotherapy

RT=radiotherapy

Source: Eindhoven Cancer Registry

The proportion of patients with localized non-small cell lung cancer who underwent surgery with or without radiotherapy was only 9% of those aged 80 or older versus 92%, 79% and 61% of the age groups <60, 60-69 and 70-79, respectively. Patients aged 60-69 and 70-79 received less surgery in the presence of co-morbidity. Most patients with non-localized non-small cell lung cancer received only radiotherapy. The proportion receiving chemotherapy (with or without radiotherapy) was considerably higher among patients younger than 60 (24%) than among those aged 80 or older (2%). Older patients more often did not receive oncological treatment. The number of co-morbid conditions had no substantial influence on treatment chosen for patients with non-localized disease. Elderly patients with limited small cell lung cancer received less adjuvant radiotherapy and more chemotherapy alone. Among patients aged 70-79 with limited small cell lung cancer the proportion receiving adjuvant radiotherapy also decreased in the presence of co-morbidity.

Among patients with breast cancer younger than 80 years over 90% underwent surgery, compared with only 74% of those aged 80 or older. The proportion receiving systemic treatment (mostly chemotherapy for those below 50 years and endocrine treatment for those aged 50 or older) increased from about 40% of those younger than 80 to 57% of patients aged 80 or older. In the presence of co-morbidity less patients received adjuvant radiotherapy (50% of patients with co-morbidity compared to 65% of those without co-morbidity) and more older women received endocrine treatment only.

The number of prostate cancer patients undergoing prostatectomy decreased with increasing age, from 42% of patients younger than 60 to 1% of patients aged 80 or older. The proportion of patients receiving curative radiotherapy also decreased from 17% among those at middle age to 4% of those aged 80 or older. With the rise of age prostate cancer patients received more often hormonal therapy: from 19% of patients below 60 to 59% of patients aged 80 or older. Among patients aged 60-69, the proportion who underwent prostatectomy decreased significantly with co-morbidity from 31% of patients without co-morbidity to 18% of patients with two or more comorbid conditions. In those aged 70-79, these percentages were 8% and 3% respectively. The proportion of patients aged 60-69 receiving hormonal therapy increased from 22% of patients without co-morbidity to 27% of those with two or more co-morbid conditions. In those aged 70-79, these proportions were 36% and 41%, respectively. In the other age groups (< 60 years and 80+ years) there was no significant influence of co-morbidity on treatment choice.

Among patients with non-Hodgkin's lymphoma the proportion receiving chemotherapy decreased with age. For patients with indolent disease the proportion receiving chemotherapy decreased from 60% of patients younger than 70 to 40% of those aged 70 or older. For patients with aggressive disease the proportion receiving chemotherapy decreased from about 80% to about 60%. Among patients with aggressive disease aged 70 or older the proportion receiving chemotherapy also decreased with co-morbidity.

2.3 Prognosis (see Table 6)

Five-year relative survival rates for colon cancer patients aged 70 or older without co-morbidity exceeded those of patients younger than 70: 75% versus 61%. Relative survival decreased in the presence of co-morbidity, especially for patients aged 70 or older and in case of COPD. Rectal cancer patients younger than 70 exhibited a 5-year survival rate of 65%, which amounted to 62% for patients aged 70 or older. For the latter, the presence of diabetes and cardiovascular diseases lowered 5-survival to 34%. One-year relative survival rates of patients with localized non-small cell lung cancer (NSCLC) were clearly lower for older patients: a 1-year survival rate of 81% for patients younger than 70 and 62% for patients aged 70 or older. The presence of COPD and diabetes affected survival negatively. Survival of non-localised NSCLC was mostly affected by the presence of diabetes. Although survival of small cell lung cancer was strongly related to age at diagnosis, co-morbidity did not seem to have a clear prognostic impact. Breast cancer patients without co-morbidity exhibited 5-year relative survival rates of 86% (when younger than 70) and even 90% (aged 70 or older). But the presence of diabetes and cardiovascular diseases lowered 5-year survival rates of patients aged 70 or older substantially: 56% and 58%, respectively. Prostate cancer patients without co-morbidity had a 5-year survival rate of 88% (no difference between younger and older patients), whereas diabetes and COPD had a negative impact on survival of patients aged 70 or older. Indolent non-Hodgkin's lymphoma patients younger than 70 without co-morbidity had a 1-year survival rate of 94%, versus 80% of patients aged 70 or older. One-year survival of aggressive non-Hodgkin's lymphoma without concomitant diseases at diagnosis was 80% for patients younger than 70 and 73% for patients aged 70 or older. The presence of cardiovascular diseases lowered 1-year survival to 51% for patients younger than 70 and to 43% for patients aged 70 or older.

		Relative survival (SE)			
		<70 years		>70 years	
Tumor type	**Co-morbidity**	1-year	5-year	1-year	5-year
Colon	None	0.82 (1)	0.59 (2)	0.82 (2)	0.75 (4)
	Diabetes	0.77 (4)	0.51 (6)	0.67 (3)	0.50 (5)
	COPD	0.73 (4)	0.47 (6)	0.68 (4)	0.41 (6)
	Cardiovascula	0.74 (4)	0.54 (5)	0.68 (3)	0.45 (4)
Rectum	None	0.89 (1)	0.65 (2)	0.80 (3)	0.62 (5)
	Diabetes	0.78 (5)	0.46 (8)	0.73 (5)	0.34 (7)
	COPD	0.87 (4)	0.53 (8)	0.68 (5)	0.40 (7)
	Cardiovascula	0.80 (4)	0.55 (6)	0.72 (4)	0.34 (6)
NSCLC* localised	None	0.81 (3)	*0.68 (3)*	0.62 (6)	*0.46 (6)*
	Diabetes	0.75 (6)	*0.59 (7)*	0.57 (7)	*0.29 (7)*
	COPD	0.77 (3)	*0.60 (4)*	0.53 (4)	*0.29 (4)*
	Cardiovascula	0.76 (4)	*0.65 (4)*	0.59 (5)	*0.39 (5)*
NSCLC* non-local	None	0.29 (2)	*0.13 (1)*	0.21 (3)	*0.10 (2)*
	Diabetes	0.29 (5)	*0.16 (4)*	0.11 (4)	*0.03 (2)*
	COPD	0.26 (3)	*0.10 (2)*	0.22 (3)	*0.09 (2)*
	Cardiovascula	0.26 (3)	*0.11 (2)*	0.21 (3)	*0.07 (2)*
SCLC**	None	0.41 (3)	*0.10 (2)*	0.15 (4)	*0.05 (2)*
	Diabetes	0.28 (6)	*0.06 (3)*	0.15 (7)	*0.04 (4)*
	COPD	0.33 (4)	*0.17 (4)*	0.19 (4)	*0.06 (2)*
	Cardiovascula	0.31 (4)	*0.10 (3)*	0.18 (4)	*0.09 (3)*
Breast	None	0.99 (0)	0.86 (1)	0.98 (0)	00.. (3)
	Diabetes	0.95 (2)	0.82 (4)	0.88 (2)	0.56 (5)
	COPD	0.97 (2)	0.82 (4	0.92 (3)	0.71 (8)
	Cardiovascula	0.93 (2)	0.76 (4)	0.91 (2)	0.58 (5)
Prostate	None	0.99 (1)	0.88 (2)	0.99 (1)	0.89 (4)
	Diabetes	0.92 (3)	0.74 (7)	0.93 (3)	0.64 (7)
	COPD	0.92 (30	0.81 (5)	0.86 (3)	0.63 (5)
	Cardiovascula	0.95 (2)	0.78 (4)	0.90 (2)	0.70 (4)
NHL*** indolent	None	0.94 (2)	*0.90 (3)*	0.80 (9)	*0.78 (10)*
	Diabetes	0.88 (11)	*0.77 (16)*	0.73 (17)	*0.79 (19)*
	COPD	0.92 (9)	*0.84 (12)*	0.86 (19)	*0.46 (25)*
	Cardiovascula	0.95 (6)	*0.71 (12)*	0.79 (12)	*0.78 (14)*
NHL*** aggressive	None	0.80 (3)	*0.68 (3)*	0.73 (7)	*0.61 (8)*
	Diabetes	0.64 (11)	*0.65 (11)*	0.70 (11)	*0.58 (13)*
	COPD	0.80 (11)	*0.81 (11)*	0.56 (12)	*0.38 (12)*
	Cardiovascula	0.51 (9)	*0.41 (9)*	0.43 (8)	*0.42 (8)*

Table 6. Relative 1- and 5-year survival rates, according to age and co-morbidity. Source: Eindhoven Cancer Registry. SE= standard error. * Non-small cell lung cancer. ** Small cell lung cancer. *** Non-Hodgkin's lymphoma. # *2-year survival*

3. DISCUSSION

3.1 Validity of Data

Co-morbidity is a multidimensional variable with a variation in severity. Diseases that influence mortality may not be the same as those influencing function or tolerance to treatment. Although there is general agreement about the importance of co-morbidity for cancer management and prognosis, there is no consensus about the types of diseases that should be included, nor about the weighing of the conditions. There are several methods for determining the total score of diseases. The most global measure is the sum of the number of conditions present. Secondly, a severity score can be assigned to each condition and the total score is the summation of all the severity scores present in a patient at a certain moment. A third method is to assign a severity score to each condition and the total severity is based on the most severe condition present in a patient. When a patient has more than one disease, there may also be a multiplicative or synergistic effect on outcomes, and grading severity according to only the sum of diseases or scores or to only the single most severe condition may miss the burden that multiple chronic diseases can place on an individual. Several systems have been proposed, each with its own classification and scoring system. The choice of the classification system is dependent on the aim of the study, the clinical problem to be explored. The five most widely used systems are: the indexes of Kaplan-Feinstein [9], Charlson [6], and of the National Institute of Ageing/National Cancer Institute (NIA/NCI) [10], the Cumulative Illness Rating Scale-Geriatric (CIRS-G) [11], and the Index of Co-Existent Diseases (ICED) [12]. In the Eindhoven Cancer Registry an adapted version of the Charlson co-morbidity index was chosen for the following reasons: it was the most widely used validated classification system at the time and it is relatively easy to use [4, 13]. We wanted to avoid the plethora of minor conditions, each with their classification problems and changes in the natural history. Scoring needed to be done by cancer registry personnel trained in oncological diagnoses who could only spend a limited amount of time on this.

For the assessment of co-morbidity several sources can be used. Although the medical record is generally regarded as the most complete source of information on the patient's past and current health status, there may be some limitations in using medical records, such as differences in information in the records between hospitals or specialists, or possible selection bias due to differences in the number of physician visits. Data on co-morbidity can also be gathered from administrative medical record databases or discharge data. In a comparison between the Charlson co-morbidity index derived from medical records with that derived from databases of administrative medical records, the data derived from the medical records had a better predictive value than the administrative disease data [7].

Between 2001 and 2003 the completeness and accuracy of our data on co-morbidity in the Eindhoven Cancer registry were validated in a random sample of 2607 patients with colorectal, lung, breast and prostate cancer and non-Hodgkin's lymphoma aged 40 and older and diagnosed between 1995 and 1999. Co-morbidity scored by the registry team was compared with that scored by a team of a surgeon and an epidemiologist. Recording of co-morbidity proved to be entirely correct for almost 70% (ranging from 59% to 72%) of patients. Some under-registration occurred especially of cardiovascular conditions (Internal report, 2002). This appeared to be mainly due to the use of unknown terminology, unknown abbreviations or illegible handwriting of the specialist. Although the unregistered conditions were at the time not very severe, this would imply that the real effects of co-morbidity on treatment and survival are probably stronger than those presented in this chapter and in our publications.

3.2 Prevalence

The higher prevalence of co-morbidity among older patients was expected, because the prevalence of chronic diseases generally increases with age. The prevalence of co-morbidity among older patients may even be underestimated due to ascertainment bias. Younger patients underwent surgery more often and received chemotherapy more often. The prevalence of co-morbidity reported by the treating physician might then be more elevated among younger patients, due to the required screening examinations before treatment.

The high risk of cardiovascular diseases and chronic obstructive pulmonary diseases for patients with cancer of the esophagus, stomach, lung, bladder and kidney can be explained by the high proportion of smokers among these patients, especially men [14, 15]. That diabetes mellitus occurred in a high proportion of patients with cancer of the pancreas is not surprising [16, 17]. A history of diabetes has been consistently associated with a two-fold increased risk for endometrial cancer [18], probably because both are related with obesity. The increased prevalence of diabetes among patients with cervical cancer was more strongly related to squamous cell carcinoma than to adenocarcinoma. Kidney cancer has been associated with hypertension, although it is unknown whether this results from the hypertension itself or from the anti-hypertensives [19]. Previously, we also found an association of hypertension with the incidence of gliomas [20]. The risk of renal cancer is also elevated among patients with diabetes [21].

The prevalence of cardiovascular diseases and pulmonary diseases was higher among men compared to women, which can be largely explained by a higher prevalence of smoking among men in the past. By contrast, the prevalence of hypertension (a less serious condition) and diabetes was higher among women.

3.3 Treatment

If alternative treatment strategies were available, older patients were often treated less aggressively than younger patients. After stratification for age, the influence of age and co-morbidity on treatment choice differed, according to tumor type.

When surgery is inevitable like in patients with colorectal cancer, higher age or the prevalence of co-morbidity did not have any influence on the resection rate. On the other hand, older patients with non-small cell lung cancer (with serious co-morbidity) more often received radiotherapy instead of surgery [22]. Surgical mortality increases markedly with age and is especially high for pneumonectomy [23, 24]. The resection rate also declined with co-morbidity, probably because of the expected higher incidence of postoperative complications and mortality [25]. However, in everyday practice the resectability is not determined primarily by co-morbid conditions, but by its effects on lung function and cardiac function. The resection rate for prostate cancer also decreased with co-morbidity, whereas the proportion receiving hormonal treatment increased [26].

Administration of adjuvant chemotherapy markedly decreased with rising age and co-morbidity for patients with Dukes C or D colon cancer [27], probably because of the higher rate of hematological complications [28, 29, 30]. Administration of primary chemotherapy also decreased with age and co-morbidity in patients with non-Hodgkin's lymphoma [31].

Administration of adjuvant radiotherapy decreased with age and co-morbidity in patients with rectal cancer, limited small cell lung cancer or breast cancer [13, 27, 32]. However, we did not find that the rate of expected complications of radiotherapy was higher for older patients with co-morbidity. Therefore, the reluctance of offering adjuvant radiotherapy might be related to practical reasons like the distance to a radiotherapy institute or the burden of the 20 to 30 visits to the radiotherapy institute.

Several authors also found less aggressive treatment of patients with co-morbidity in case of breast cancer, colorectal cancer, or prostate cancer [33, 34, 26, 35, 36].

Age seemed to have more influence on treatment chosen than co-morbidity. Apparently, co-morbidity alone does not entirely explain why elderly non-small cell lung cancer patients and prostate cancer patients underwent surgery less often and why those with colon cancer, rectal cancer, small cell lung cancer and breast cancer received less (adjuvant) chemotherapy or adjuvant radiotherapy. Performance status, the psychological condition of the patient, social factors and patient's decision, families decision or doctor's decision may also play a role [33, 2]. The lower proportion of elderly patients undergoing surgery or receiving chemotherapy also appeared in another area of the Netherlands [37].

3.4 Survival

For most tumor types relative survival for those without co-morbidity did not decrease with age, except for patients with lung cancer or non-Hodgkin's lymphoma. The outcome of patients without co-morbidity could be comparable to the outcome of patients in clinical trials, because those with co-morbidity are often excluded from clinical trials.

For patients with lung cancer co-morbidity had no independent prognostic effect [22]. This contradicts some other studies [38-41], but they were not population-based. They also used other scales for measuring co-morbidity: the Kaplan-Feinstein Index [9] and the Cumulative Illness Rating Scale-Geriatric (CIRS-G) [11]. In one of the studies, co-morbidity affected overall survival in surgically resected stage I NSCLC patients, when co-morbidity was rated according to CIRS-G, but not according to the Charlson scale [39]. In another American study co-morbidity count and the Charlson index were significant predictors for lung cancer survival, but only explained 2.5% and 2.0% of the survival variation, respectively [42]. Probably the influence of co-morbidity on survival is of less importance in the case of a lethal disease such as lung cancer. Most of these patients die from lung cancer, before they become at risk of dying from the co-morbid condition.

For the other tumors, co-morbidity had an independent prognostic effect. This negative influence of co-morbidity on survival of cancer patients might be due to several mechanisms: the increased risk of death due to the co-morbid condition itself, more contra-indications for anti-cancer treatment, more indications for dose reduction and a higher rate of treatment-related complications such as infections and cardiovascular events. In several of our recent studies the adverse effects of co-morbidity on survival appeared to be independent of treatment, so less aggressive treatment could not (fully) account for the observed differences in survival between patients with and without co-morbidity [22, 27, 32, 31]. The minor effects of cardiovascular conditions on relative survival of lung or colon cancer may be explained by earlier detection of the cancer through surveillance (X-thorax) or early bleeding of polyps by thrombolytic therapy. Some studies have shown that performance status and co-morbidity are both independent prognostic factors [1, 2], which therefore may need to be included in future prognostic studies, supplemented by the psychological or mental condition of the patient, and the patient's and/or family decision or even doctor's decision should be included.

4. CONCLUSIONS

There is now clear evidence that the prevalence of co-morbidity among older cancer patients is high and that older patients (with co-morbidity) are often treated less aggressively, which seems to have a negative influence on survival. However, would outcomes really improve if more patients were treated, according to the guidelines that were developed on the basis of results in groups of younger patients without co-morbidity? Would more complications occur in older patients with co-morbidity? If that is the case, is it possible to develop special treatment regimens for older cancer patients with co-morbidity and adapt the guidelines? It remains relevant to study the influence of age and co-morbidity on toxicity from treatment, quality of life and prognosis in unselected groups of patients.

REFERENCES

1. Extermann M; Overcash J; Lyman GH; Parr J; Balducci L: Comorbidity and functional status are independent in older cancer patients. J Clin Oncol, 1998, 16:1582-1587
2. Repetto L; Fratino L; Audisio RA; Venturino A; Gianni W; Vercelli M; Parodi S; Dal Lago D; Gioia F; Monfardini S; Aapro MS; Serraino D; Zagonel V: Comprehensive geriatric assessment adds information to Eastern Cooperative Oncology Group performance status in elderly cancer patients: an Italian Group for Geriatric Oncology Study. J Clin Oncol, 2002, 20:494-502
3. Yancik R; Ganz PA; Varricchio CG; Conley B: Perspectives on comorbidity and cancer in older patients: approaches to expand the knowledge base. J Clin Oncol, 2001, 19:1147-1151
4. Coebergh JWW; Janssen-Heijnen MLG; Post PN; Razenberg PPA: Serious co-morbidity among unselected cancer patients newly diagnosed in the southeastern part of the Netherlands in 1993-1996. J Clin Epidemiol, 1999, 52:1131-1136
5. Coebergh JWW; Janssen-Heijnen MLG; Louwman WJ; Voogd AC eds: Cancer incidence, care and survival in the South of the Netherlands, 1955-1999: a report of the Eindhoven Cancer Registry with cross-border implications. Eindhoven: Comprehensive Cancer Centre South (IKZ), 2001
6. Charlson ME; Pompei P; Ales KL; MacKenzie CR: A new method of classifying prognostic comorbidity in longitudinal studies: development and validation. J Chronic Dis, 1987, 40:373-383
7. Kieszak SM; Flanders WD; Kosinski AS; Shipp CC; Karp H: A comparison of the Charlson comorbidity index derived from medical record data and administrative billing data. J Clin Epidemiol, 1999, 52:137-142
8. Hakulinen T; Abeywickrama KH: A computer program package for relative survival analysis. Comput Programs Biomed, 1985, 19:197-207
9. Kaplan MH; Feinstein AR: The importance of classifying initial co-morbidity in evaluating the outcome of diabetes mellitus. J Chronic Dis, 1974, 27:387-404
10. Yancik R; Wesley MN; Ries LA; Havlik RJ; Long S; Edwards BK; Yates JW: Comorbidity and age as predictors of risk for early mortality of male and female colon carcinoma patients: a population-based study. Cancer, 1998, 82:2123-2134
11. Miller MD; Paradis CF; Houck PR; Mazumdar S; Stack JA; Rifai AH; Mulsant B; Reynolds CF, 3rd: Rating chronic medical illness burden in geropsychiatric practice and

research: application of the Cumulative Illness Rating Scale. Psychiatry Res, 1992, 41:237-248

12. Greenfield S; Blanco DM; Elashoff RM; Ganz PA: Patterns of care related to age of breast cancer patients. JAMA, 1987, 257:2766-2770
13. Janssen-Heijnen MLG; Smulders S; Lemmens VEPP; Smeenk FWJM; Coebergh JWW: Do age and comorbidity in unselected patients with small cell lung cancer influence treatment chosen and prognosis? Submitted
14. Koppert LB; Janssen-Heijnen MLG; Louwman WJ; Lemmens VEPP; Wijnhoven BPL; Tilanus HW; Coebergh JWW: Comparison of comorbidity prevalence in oesophageal and gastric carcinoma patients: a population-based study. Eur J Gastrol Hepatol (2004 in press)
15. Janssen-Heijnen MLG; Schipper RM; Razenberg PPA; Crommelin MA; Coebergh JWW: Prevalence of co-morbidity in lung cancer patients and its relationship with treatment: a population-based study. Lung Cancer, 1998, 21:105-113
16. Jain M; Howe GR; St Louis P; Miller AB: Coffee and alcohol as determinants of risk of pancreas cancer: a case-control study from Toronto. Int J Cancer, 1991, 47:384-389
17. Kalapothaki V; Tzonou A; Hsieh CC; Toupadaki N; Karakatsani A; Trichopoulos D: Tobacco, ethanol, coffee, pancreatitis, diabetes mellitus, and cholelithiasis as risk factors for pancreatic carcinoma. Cancer Causes Control, 1993, 4:375-382
18. Parazzini F; La Vecchia C; Bocciolone L; Franceschi S: The epidemiology of endometrial cancer. Gynecol Oncol, 1991, 41:1-16
19. McLaughlin JK; Chow WH; Mandel JS; Mellemgaard A; McCredie M; Lindblad P; Schlehofer B; Pommer W; Niwa S; Adami HO: International renal-cell cancer study. VIII. Role of diuretics, other anti-hypertensive medications and hypertension. Int J Cancer, 1995, 63:216-221
20. Houben MP; Louwman WJ; Tijssen CC; Teepen JL; Coebergh JW: Hypertension a risk factor for glioma? Evidence from a population-based study of comorbidity in glioma patients. Submitted
21. Lindblad P; Chow WH; Chan J; Bergstrom A; Wolk A; Gridley G; McLaughlin JK; Nyren O; Adami HO: The role of diabetes mellitus in the aetiology of renal cell cancer. Diabetologia, 1999, 42:107-112
22. Janssen-Heijnen MLG; Smulders S; Lemmens VEPP; Smeenk FWJM; van Geffen HJAA; Coebergh JWW: Elderly non-small cell lung cancer patients with comorbidity are treated less aggressively, whereas comorbidity has little effect on prognosis. Submitted
23. Damhuis RA; Schutte PR: Resection rates and postoperative mortality in 7,899 patients with lung cancer. Eur Respir, 1996, J 9:7-10
24. Finlayson EV; Birkmeyer JD: Operative mortality with elective surgery in older adults. Eff Clin Pract, 2001, 4:172-177
25. Bolliger CT; Jordan P; Soler M; Stulz P; Gradel E; Skarvan K; Elsasser S; Gonon M; Wyser C;Tamm M; et al: Exercise capacity as a predictor of postoperative complications in lung resection candidates. Am J Respir Crit Care Med, 1995, 151:1472-1480
26. Post PN; Kil PJ; Hendrikx AJ; Janssen-Heijnen ML; Crommelin MA; Coebergh JW: Comorbidity in patients with prostate cancer and its relevance to treatment choice. BJU Int, 1999, 84:652-656
27. Lemmens VEPP; Janssen-Heijnen MLG; Verheij CDGW; Houterman S; Repelaer van Driel OJ; Coebergh JWW: Comorbidity leads to altered treatment and worse survival of elderly colorectal cancer patients: a population-based study. Submitted
28. Forman WB: The role of chemotherapy and adjuvant therapy in the management of colorectal cancer. Cancer, 1994, 74:2151-2153
29. Stein BN; Petrelli NJ; Douglass HO; Driscoll DL; Arcangeli G; Meropol NJ: Age and sex are independent predictors of 5-fluorouracil toxicity. Analysis of a large-scale phase III trial. Cancer, 1995, 75:11-17

30. Zalcberg J; Kerr D; Seymour L; Palmer M: Haematological and non-haematological toxicity after 5-fluorouracil and leucovorin in patients with advanced colorectal cancer is significantly associated with gender, increasing age and cycle number. Tomudex International Study Group. Eur J Cancer, 1998, 34:1871-1875
31. van Spronsen DJ; Janssen-Heijnen MLG; Lemmens VEPP; Peters WG; Coebergh JWW: The independent prognostic effect of co-morbidity in lymphoma patients: results from the population-based Eindhoven Cancer Registry. Submitted
32. Louwman WJ; Janssen-Heijnen MLG; Houterman S; Voogd AC; Coebergh JWW: Less extensive treatment and lower survival in breast cancer patients with comorbidity: a population-based study. Submitted
33. Ayanian, JZ; Zaslavsky AM; Fuchs CS; Guadagnoli E; Creech CM; Cress RD; O'Connor LC; West DW; Allen ME; Wolf RE; Wright WE: Use of adjuvant chemotherapy and radiation therapy for colorectal cancer in a population-based cohort. J Clin Oncol, 2003, 21:1293-1300
34. Lash TL; Thwin SS; Horton NJ; Guadagnoli E; Silliman RA: Multiple informants: a new method to assess breast cancer patients' comorbidity. Am J Epidemiol, 2003, 157:249-257
35. Satariano WA; Ragland DR: The effect of comorbidity on three-year survival of women with primary breast cancer. Ann Intern Med, 1994, 120:104-110
36. van Spronsen DJ; Janssen-Heijnen ML; Breed WP; Coebergh JW: Prevalence of co-morbidity and its relationship to treatment among unselected patients with Hodgkin's disease and non-Hodgkin's lymphoma, 1993-1996. Ann Hematol, 1999, 78:315-319
37. de Rijke JM; Schouten LJ; Schouten HC; Jager JJ; Koppejan AG; van den Brandt PA: Age-specific differences in the diagnostics and treatment of cancer patients aged 50 years and older in the province of Limburg, The Netherlands. Ann Oncol, 1996, 7:677-685
38. Battafarano RJ; Piccirillo JF; Meyers BF; Hsu HS; Guthrie TJ; Cooper JD; Patterson GA: Impact of comorbidity on survival after surgical resection in patients with stage I non-small cell lung cancer. J Thorac Cardiovasc Surg, 2002, 123:280-287
39. Firat S; Bousamra M; Gore E; Byhardt RW: Comorbidity and KPS are independent prognostic factors in stage I non-small-cell lung cancer. Int J Radiat Oncol Biol Phys, 2002, 52:1047-1057
40. Firat S; Byhardt R; Gore E: Comorbidity and Karnofksy performance score are independent prognostic factors in stage III non-small-cell lung cancer: an institutional analysis of patients treated on four RTOG studies. Radiation Therapy Oncology Group. Int J Radiat Oncol Biol Phys, 2002, 54:357-364
41. Piccirillo JF: Importance of comorbidity in head and neck cancer. Laryngoscope, 2000, 110:593-602
42. Tammemagi CM; Neslund-Dudas C; Simoff M; Kvale P: Impact of comorbidity on lung cancer survival. Int J Cancer, 2003, 103:792-802
43. Post PN; Hansen BE; Kil PJ; Janssen-Heijnen ML; Coebergh JW: The independent prognostic value of comorbidity among men aged < 75 years with localized prostate cancer: a population-based study. BJU Int, 2001, 87:821-826.

Chapter 6

HEMOPOIESIS AND AGING

Lodovico Balducci, Cheryl L Hardy, Gary H Lyman

Lodovico Balducci, Program Leader, Senior Adult Oncology Program, H. Lee Moffitt Cancer Center and Research Institute, Tampa, Florida, Professor of Oncology and Medicine, University of South Florida College of Medicine, Tampa, Florida. Cheryl L. Hardy, Associate Professor of Medicine, University of Mississippi Medical Center, Jackson, Mississippi. Gary H Lyman, Professor of Medicine, University of Rochester Medical Center, Rochester, New York.

Hemopoiesis is central to the study of cancer and aging for the following reasons: (1) to some extent, hemopoiesis is a sensor of physiologic aging. In particular, hemopoiesis may be inhibited by the same catabolic cytokines that accumulate in the circulation with aging and predict functional decline and death, [1-4] (2) hemopoiesis is one of the main targets of cytotoxic chemotherapy [1,5]. A decline in hemopoietic reserve may compromise the ability to administer chemotherapy in adequate doses to older individuals [6]. In addition, anemia is an independent risk factor for chemotherapy-induced myelosuppression, [7-10] and, (3) anemia has a number of detrimental effects on the older person that include increased risk of mortality [11-14] and disabilities [15-18]. Thus, anemia may lessen the benefits and enhance the risk of cancer treatment.

In this chapter we examine the influence of aging on hemopoiesis, the risk of myelosuppression following cytotoxic chemotherapy in the older aged person, the prevalence, incidence, mechanisms and consequences of anemia in the older person, and the management of anemia and of hemopoietic complications of cancer treatment.

1. AGE AND HEMOPOIESIS

Hemopoiesis is compartmentalized (Figure 1)[1] The homeostasis of the peripheral blood, that is a balance between losses and production of circulating blood elements involves the integrity and the coordination of a number of serial processes. The pluripotent hemopoietic stem cells (PHSC) need commit into hemopoietic progenitors and at the same time maintain their own population by self-replication. The high plasticity of the PHSC that may give origin to different lines of blood elements while replicating themselves is largely lost by the committed progenitors which do differentiate only into one hemopoietic line, giving origin to the recognizable marrow precursors that mature into circulating blood elements[1]. Commitment, differentiation, and maturation are modulated by hemopoietic cytokines and made possible by the hemopoietic stroma. The roles of the stroma include homing of PHSC and committed progenitors, and production of some of the cytokines that modulate growth and differentiation. Hemopoietic insufficiency may be caused by one or more of these mechanisms: exhaustion of PHSC, inadequate production of growth factors or excess production of inhibitory substances, decreased sensitivity of PHSC and hemopoietic progenitors to the growth factors and disruption of the hemopoietic microenvironment.

1.1 Aging and PHSC Reserve

The influence of aging on PHSC reserve is controversial. Both experimental and clinical observations suggest the self-renewal of PHSC is exhaustable. In the murine model the ability of forming hemopoietic colonies in the spleen declined with serial stem cell transplants [19]. Telomere length and telomerase activity of PHSC underwent a progressive decline with age, [20] and hemopoietic stress was associated with a reduction in the concentration of PHSC of older, but not of younger animals [21-22]. Hemopoietic stress consisted of isolation [21] or of sepsis [22]. In humans, the hemopoietic tissue becomes progressively reduced with age, [23] while mortality from infection increases, which suggests decline in neutrophil reserve [24]. The number of CD 34+ cells, that may reflect the reserve of pluripotent hemopoietic progenitors [25] and the self-replicative ability of these elements appear to decline with age [26]. Hemopoietic stress in human reveals some degree of hemopoietic insufficiency: the injection of granulocyte-macrophage colony stimulating factors (GM-CSF) in healthy individuals aged 70 and older and 30 and younger, produced a much lower increment in

Figure 1. Overview of hemopoiesis as a compartmental process.

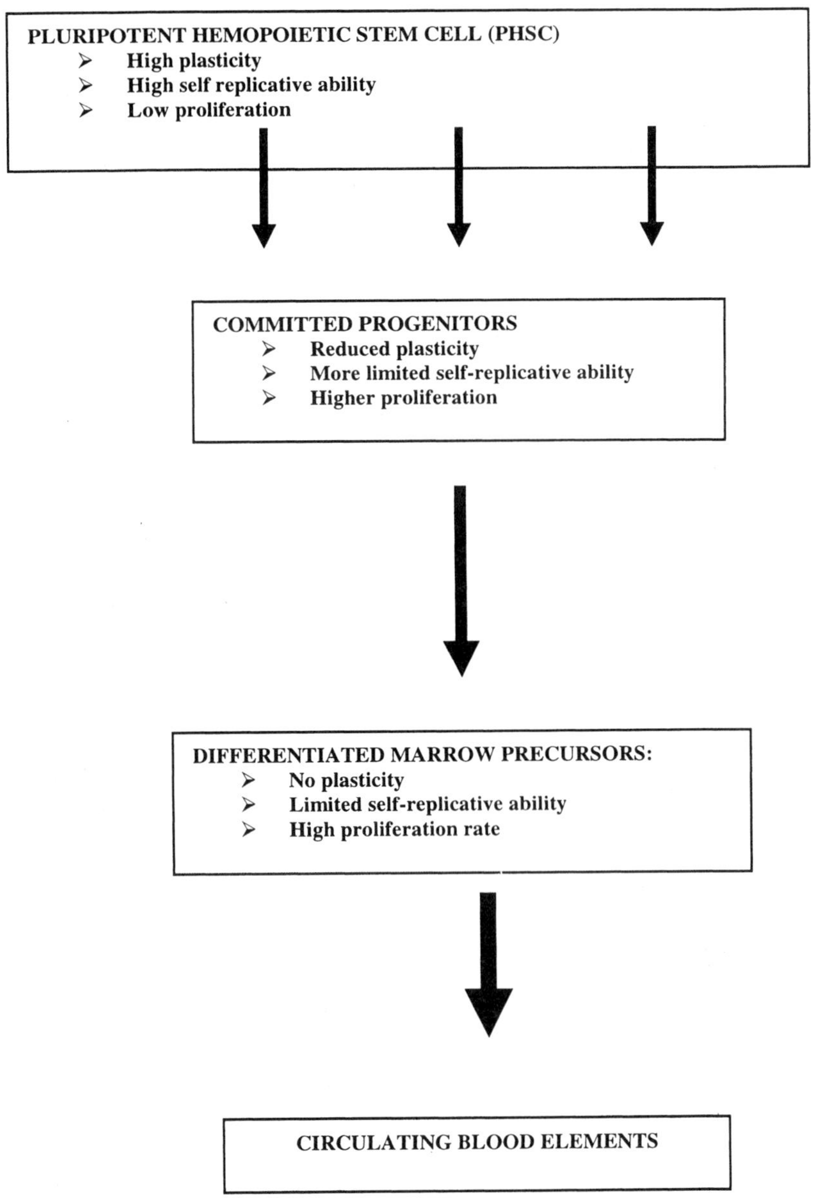

the concentration of pluripotent hemopoietic progenitors in the circulation of the aged, despite that the baseline concentrations of these elements were the same in both groups, [27] and the risk of neutropenia, neutropenic infections and thrombocytopenia following cytotoxic chemotherapy increased after age 60 [28-39]. The fact that the prevalence and incidence of anemia of unknown causes increase with age may also be construed as evidence of progressive hemopoietic insufficiency [40-43].

These observations support an age-related decline in hemopoietic reserve that may be of consequence in the presence of severe and prolonged hemopoietic stress. In condition of homeostasis, the hemopoietic activity appears adequate to preserve a normal peripheral blood count throughout a person's lifetime, in the majority of individuals [44-45]. Even among the oldest old, it should not be assumed that anemia, neutropenia, thrombocytopenia or pancytopenias are a natural consequence of age.

1.2 Age and Production of Hemopoietic Cytokines

The relationship between age and production of hemopoietic cytokines is not clear. In the murine model, utilizing transgenic mice undergoing early senescence (senescence-accelerated mice or SAM), some authors reported increased production of colony inhibiting activity (CIA) in response to lypopolysaccaride [46]. Of interest, lypopolysaccaride induced production of colony stimulating activity, followed by CIA in young animals. This observation suggests that age may lead to a loss in ability to produce hemopoietic growth factors, while the ability to produce CIA is unaffected and maybe enhanced.

In humans the data are inconclusive. Whereas the production of GM-CSF from monocytes grown "in vitro" seem to decline with the age of the cell, [47] recent studies demonstrated a decline in GM-CSF production following exposure to phytohemagglutinines only by monocytes obtained from healthy centenarians [25]. An age effect was not observed in younger subjects up to age 73.

Several studies explored the production of erythropoietin in the aged, with conflicting results. In some cases of anemia of unknown causes in older individuals, the circulating levels of erythropoietin were inadequate for the degree of anemia; [40, 48-52] but the Glomerular Filtration Rate (GFR) of these patients had not been measured. It is reasonable to expect that [54-61] reduction in GFR, common with aging [53] might have accounted for the poor erythropoietin response to anemia. In other studies comparing the concentration of circulating erythropoietin in younger and older individuals with sideropenic anemia the level of erythropoietin were normal and even increased among the old ones [54, 55]. In a rare form of age-related anemia (dysautonomic anemia) [52] the production of erythropoietin is decreased.

The production of hemopoietic cytokines in the aged should be seen in the context of the increased concentration of catabolic cytokines in the circulation of some elderly individuals. Recent studies demonstrated that increased concentrations of Interleukin 6 are associated with functional decline, increased risk of geriatric syndromes and of death [2, 54-61]. Increased levels of IL-6 are also present in patients with anemia and IL6 appears to inhibit both the response of erythropoietic progenitors to erythtopoietin and the production of erythropoietin [3, 62]. IL-6 and possibly other catabolic cytokines such as tumor necrosis factor (TNF), interleukin 1 (IL1) and Interleukin 10 (IL10) may be responsible of a relative hemopoietic insufficiency by reducing both the production of growth factors and the sensitivity of hemopoietic progenitors to these factors [3, 22, 46, 63, 64]. The catabolic effects of these cytokines may be enhanced by reduced secretion of Growth Hormone [63, 64].

1.3 Aging and Sensitivity to Hemopoietic Cytokines

The information related to this issue is very limited and circumstantial. The age-related progressive loss in ability to respond to hemopoietic stress might be explained in part by a loss of sensitivity to hemopoietic cytokines. It is also well known that catabolic cytokines and in particular IL-6 and TNF blunt the response of erythropoietic progenitors to erythropoietin [3, 61]. Other observations supporting a reduced sensitivity to hemopoietic growth factors include the fact that erythropoietic enhancement observed "in vitro" with addition of indocin to the culture appears diminished in the marrow from older individuals, [65, 66] that the generation of the same reticulocyte response requires higher levels of erythropoietin in anemic older than in younger patients [67-68]. Contrasting with these findings, Bagnara et al [25] found that *in vitro* responsiveness of pluripotent hemopoietic precursors to erythopoietin, G-CSF and GM-CSF was well maintained even in persons aged 100 and older. While there are circumstances that may reduce the sensitivity of erythopoietic progenitors to hemopoietic cytokines, this does not appear a generalized occurrence with aging. From a clinical standpoint it is important to realize that a good response to pharmacological doses of G-CSF, GM-CSF (69), Interleukin 11, [70] megakaryocite growth stimulating factors (M-CSF) [71] and erythropoietin [72] may be seen irrespective of the age of the patient.

1.4 Aging and Hemopoietic Microenvironment

The consequences of aging on the function of the hemopoietic microenvironment are largely unknown. As autologous stem cell rescue after high dose chemotherapy has been carried on successfully in persons aged 70

and older with multiple myeloma, [73, 74] it is reasonable to assume that the ability to home stem cells persists to some extent beyond age 70.

2. AGE AND HEMOPOIETIC COMPLICATIONS OF CYTOTOXIC CHEMOTHERAPY

At this point it is legitimate to ask whether myelosuppression following cytotoxic chemotherapy becomes more prolonged and severe with age, as a consequence of progressive reduction in hemopoietic reserve and whether the risk of increased toxicity may be ameliorated, in order of preserving the full dose and the full benefits of chemotherapy.

The risk and severity of myelotoxicity was not increased in patients aged 65-70 and older in at least six large clinical trials (Table 1) [75-80]. While these studies demonstrate that the risk of myelosuppression is not increased in all older individuals, they shed little light on the risks of chemotherapy in the general aged population. The percentage of patients aged 80 and older was negligible, and also patients aged 70 and
older were underrepresented: whereas 40% of cancers occur in these age group, older individuals made up only 10-15% of patients enrolled in these clinical trials. Clearly, the older patients were highly selected as it is to be expected in studies conducted in major cancer centers or by cooperative oncology groups. Furthermore, the retrospective nature of these studies may have prevented the detection of small age-related differences.

Several other studies support increased risk of myelodepression among the elderly [29-32]. The risk of neutropenia was increased for women 65 and older receiving adjuvant chemotherapy for breast cancer with doxorubicin and cylophosphamide [32]. Of special interest, myelodepression was cumulative in the older but not the younger patients, suggesting impairment of hemopoietic reserve with age [32]. A review of the experience of the South West Oncology Group (SWOG) [29] and of the International Breast Cancer Study Group [30] showed that age 65 and older was a risk factor both for myelotoxicity and lower chemotherapy dose intensity. The once popular regimen MACOP-B (methotrexate, adriamycin, cyclophosphamide, oncovin prednisone and bleomycin) for Large cell Non-Hodgkin's Lymphoma has produced increased incidence of neutropenia, neutropenic infections, and infectious mortality in patients aged 60 and older [33]. Armitage et al reported a

30% mortality rate among individuals aged 70 and over treated with CHOP for non-Hodgkin's lymphoma [28].

A number of prospective trials exploring different forms of chemotherapy in elderly Non-Hodgkin's lymphoma patients (Table 2) [28, 31, 34-39, 81-82] reported a risk of severe neutropenia around 50% and a risk of

Table 1. Age and myelotoxicity of cancer chemotherapy: results of five retrospective trials.

Author	Patients #	Patients ≥ 70 (%)	Source
Begg & Carbone, 1983 (75)	5459	780 (13%)	ECOG data base
Gelman & Taylor, 1984 (76)	231	31 (13%)	Dana Farber Cancer center: Patients over 65 had been treated prospectively with dose-adjustment for cyclophosphamide and methotrexate and 2/3 FU dose And results compared with 161 fully evaluable younger patients. Patients over 80 experienced shortened survival
Christman et al, 1992 (77)	170	70 (42%)	Piedmont Oncology Group database; high degree of patients selection
Giovannazzi-Bannon et al, 1994 (78)	672	65: 271 (40.3%) 70: ? (25%)	Illinois cancer center phase II trials.
Ibrahim et al, 1996 (79)	1011	65: 244 (24%) 70: ? (,20%)	MD Anderson Hospital patients with metastatic breast cancer aged 50 and older
Ibrahim et al, 2000 (80)	390	65: 65 (18%) 70: ? (< 10%)	M D Anderson hospital patients with breast cancer receiving anthracycline-containing adjuvant chemotherapy

neutropenic infection around 25% among patients aged 60 and older treated with CHOP or CHOP-like regimens. The only exception to theses finding was the study of Doorduijn et al [83] in which the incidence of neutropenic infection was 10%. The difference may probably be accounted in terms of patient selections. In the majority of studies the risk of death varied between 5-15%. Age 60 and over is a risk factor for more prolonged neutropenia, neutropenic infections and infectious death also in the management of Acute Myelogenous Leukemia (AML) [84]. In this case the disease itself may compromise the patient's hemopoietic reserve, because in the elderly with AML the PHSC is involved by the disease in approximately 60% of the times [84, 85].

The risk of chemotherapy-induced thrombocytopenia and anemia in older individuals is less well known. It is important to remember however that anemia may be very deleterious in elderly cancer patients, because anemia by itself is a risk factor for myelosuppression [7-10]. This phenomenon may be accounted for by the pharmacokinetics of different cancer agents that are heavily bound to red blood cells [7, 10]. In presence of anemia the concentration of free drug in the circulation and the risk of toxicity may be increased. Furthermore, anemia is associated with fatigue that in older individuals is a risk factor for functional dependence [15-18, 86].

Several strategies have been proposed to reduce the risk of chemotherapy-induced neutropenia in the aged. These include dose-reduction, prophylactic oral antibiotics, prophylactic use of hemopoietic growth factors, and correction of anemia.

Dose reduction appears ill advised when dealing with curable cancer. In the case of large cell lymphoma, dose reduction has resulted in inferior outcome [36, 38, 40, 87, 88]. A recent study showing that dose-dense CHOP (every two weeks) was superior in terms of response rate and survival to classical CHOP every three weeks in lymphoma patients aged 60-75, further emphasizes the importance of the dose even in older patients [89]. In adjuvant treatment of breast cancer the importance of the dose was initially reported by Bonadonna et al, who demonstrated that older women had received lower total doses of CMF than younger women and experienced lower benefits [90]. The CALGB

Table 2. Incidence of life-threatening neutropenia; neutropenic infections and death in older individuals with large cell Non-Hodgkin's Lymphomas treated with CHOP-like regimens.

Author (s)	Patient #	Regimen	Age	Neutropenia	Neutropenic Fever	Treatment-related Deaths	Growth Factor
Zinzani (34)	161	VNCOP-B	60+	44%	32%	1.3%	-
Sonneveld (35)	148	CHOP CNOP	60+ 60+	NR NR	NR NR	14% 13%	- -
Gomez (31)	26	CHOP	60+ 70+	24% 73%	8% 42%	0 20%	GM-CSF GM-CSF
Tirelli (36)	119	VMP CHOP	70 + 70+	50% 48%	21% 21%	7% 5%	- -
Bastion (37)	444	CVP CTVP	70+ 70+	9% 29%	7% 13%	12% 15%	- -
Doorduijn (83)	152	CHOP	65+	21%	10%	5%	-
Osby (39)	455	CHOP CNOP	60+	91%	47%	n.r	-

study also showed that the dose of doxorubicin was critical to outcome [91] and recent studies showed that dose intense treatment was superior to standard treatment in terms of survival and recurrence [92]. In AML the importance of the dose of cytarabine in the consolidation phase has been well established [93, 94]. More controversial is the importance of the doses of anthracyclines in induction, but at least in patients with favorable cytogenetics 60mg /m2 of daunorubicin appear superior to 45 mg/m2 [95-98].

The adjustment of the dose of agents excreted from the kidney to the Glomerular Filtration Rate of individuals patients seems to reduce the toxicity without compromising the outcome of treatment [99] and is a reasonable approach for patients aged 65 and older, in whom a compromise of GFR is more likely. Given the variability of drug pharmakcokinetcs, it should also be recommended that the doses of treatment be increased in the absence of toxicity.

Though the prophylactic use of sulfametoxazol/trimetrophrin resulted in reduction in infection from gastrointestinal pathogens in patients with prolonged neutropenia [100], this strategy appears complementary rather than alternative to the use of hemopoietic growth factors. There is no proof that prophylactic antibiotics may also prevent pseudomonas, staphylococcal, fungal and viral infections. Furthermore, this practice may result in the emergence of resistant bacterial strains.

3. AGE AND ANEMIA

The incidence and prevalence of anemia increase with age [14, 40, 101]. The consequences of anemia are twofold: anemia may herald a serious underlying disease, and anemia itself may have serious health consequences including, death, functional dependence, dementia, cardiac failure, and increased risk of complications of pharmacotherapy [7-10].

3.1 Definition of Anemia

The definition of anemia by the World Health Organization (WHO) as hemoglobin levels of less than 13 g/dL in men and less than 12 g/dL in women [40], may be outdated in view of new evidence. A Cohort study of home dwelling women aged 65 and older, the Women's Health and Aging Study, showed hemoglobin levels below 13 gm/dl are independent risk factors for mortality [13] and disability [17]. A correlation between disability and hemoglobin levels below 13gm/dl was also shown by a cohort Italian study of healthy older individuals [16], whereas the EPESE study [15], and a cross-sectional study of 3,946 New Englanders (102) showed that declining hemoglobin is associated with declining function in home dwelling persons aged 70 and older. Prospective studies of cancer patients treated with erythropoietin showed reduction in fatigue and improvement in energy levels when hemoglobin levels rose above 12 g/dL [103-107].

3.2 Epidemiology of Anemia

The prevalence of anemia increases markedly after age 60 [14, 40, 101, 102]. Among the residents of Olmsted County, Minnesota, USA, both prevalence and incidence of anemia started rising by age 65 and rose more steeply after age 80 (Figure 2) [14, 108]. Despite these findings, anemia cannot be considered a common consequence of aging, as the average hemoglobin levels of older individuals without serious conditions, remained stable between ages 60 -98, according to longitudinal and cross-sectional studies [101, 102, 109, 112]. Seemingly, the increased prevalence of anemia reflects increased prevalence of comorbidity and of functional decline. Given a more limited hemopoietic reserve, older individuals may become more susceptible to anemia when faced by hemopoietic stress, such as bleeding, myelosuppressive substances, acute or chronic diseases [2, 113].

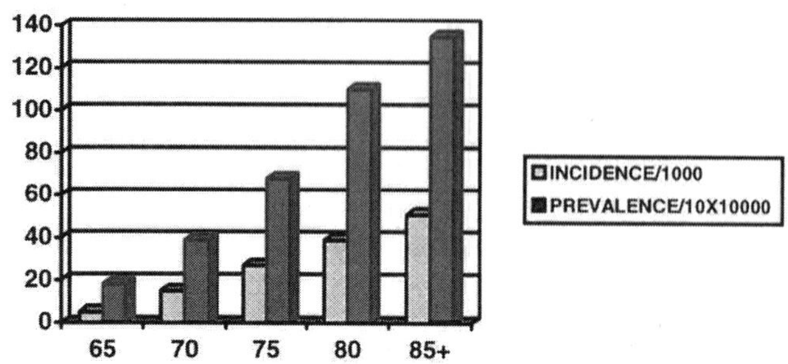

Figure 2. Age-related prevalence and incidence of Anemia in Olmstead County, Minnesota.

One should also remember that qualitative changes of hemopoiesis, such as myelodysplasia, are more common with age [1, 3].

The common causes of anemia in the elderly are shown in Table 3, derived from an outpatient [14] and an "in hospital" [42] study. The high prevalence of anemia of unknown causes, reported also by others [41] may reflect inadequate diagnostic work up, early myelodysplasias and absolute or relative erythropoietin deficiency. Absolute erythropoietin deficiency may result from some degree of renal insufficiency, progressively more common with age [53]. The construct of relative erythropoietin deficiency is illustrated by the comparison of the erythropoietin response to anemia in patients with iron deficiency and in those with chronic disease anemia [48-50, 55, 62, 68, 114, 115]. While baseline erythropoietin levels are similar in the two groups of patients for values of hemoglobin higher than 12 gm/dl, for anemic values of hemoglobin, they are lower in anemia of chronic diseases. Impaired erythropoietin secretion and reduced sensitivity to erythropoietin may both contribute to relative erythropoietin deficiency in this condition.

Anemia of chronic disease is probably the most common form of anemia in the elderly [14, 41, 42], and is characterized by low serum iron, low or normal TIBC, normal or high serum ferritin levels, and low concentrations of soluble transferrin receptor [115-117].

Table 3. Primary causes of anemia
(From Joosten, E., et al., Gerontology 1992;38:111–117.
with permission from S. Karger AG, Basel).

Cause	Prevalence (%) Joosten (Source: hospital discharges)	Anemia Source: Olmsted County Records
Chronic disease	35	17
Unexplained causes	17	36
Iron deficiency	15	15
Post-hemorrhagic	7	7
Renal failure, liver, and endocrine disease	6.5	8
Myelodysplasia or acute leukemia	5.5	-
Chronic leukemia or lymphoma	5.5	-
Vitamin B_{12} or folate deficiency	5.5	-
Other hematological disease	3	17

Patients with this condition cannot mobilize and utilize iron, which is stored in excess in the reticulo-endothelial system. The sensitivity to erythropoietin is reduced in all forms of anemia of chronic diseases, but varies from case to case. Anemia associated with rheumatoid arthritis generally responds to lower doses of erythropoietin than that associated with cancer, [115] suggesting different pathogenesis. In the "cancer type" of anemia an earlier erythropoietic progenitor may be involved. In addition, red blood cell survival is reduced [115]. Clearly, older individuals appear at increased risk for this form of anemia, due to increased concentration of catabolic cytokines in the circulation, and decline in GFR, that together may conjure relative erythropoietin insufficiency. While this hypothesis has not been completely proved yet, it is clear that the production of erythropoietin in response to anemia is inadequate in some older individuals [46-50].

Iron Deficiency Anemia is due to chronic blood loss whose possibility should always be investigated. Especially among oldest individuals a source of blood loss may not be found and the possibility of inadequate iron absorption should be entertained [41, 42, 117]

Figure 3. Pathogenesis of relative erythropoietin insufficiency

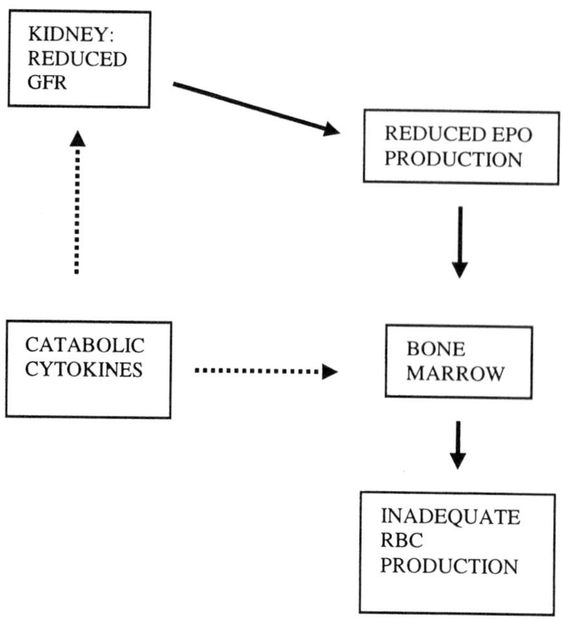

This appears particularly likely in individuals with lower iron stores, such as women, vegans, and individuals who had experienced multiple bleeding episodes earlier in life.

Iron deficiency is documented by low serum ferritin levels, high total iron binding capacity (TIBC) and transferrin levels, low transferrin saturation, high concentration of free transferrin receptor, and absent bone marrow iron stores [117].

Anemia of Renal Insufficiency is also likely in some older individuals, given a progressive decline in GFR with age [53]. As already discussed in the case of anemia of chronic disease, renal insufficiency may contribute to anemia, rather than being the only cause.

A deficiency in vitamin B_{12} should be suspected in all elderly individuals with circulating levels of cobalamine within the lower limits of normal but equal to or lower than 300 pg/ml [118-120]. In these cases elevated circulating levels of methyl malonic acid or histidine, indicate B_{12} deficiency [118]. The prevalence of B_{12} deficiency may be as high as 15% after age 60 and is rarely due to pernicious anemia: in the majority of cases it results from decreased digestion of food bind vitamin B_{12} due to increased gastric pH and reduced pepsin production [118-120]. In the majority of elderly individuals B12 deficiency may be present in the absence of anemia, if folate levels are normal and is manifested by neurological findings including peripheral neuropathy, posterior column dysfunction and reduced cognition [120].

3.3 Clinical Implications of Anemia

At least five studies have shown that anemia is an independent risk factor of mortality [11-14, 121]. Of these the report of Chaves et al is particularly provocative [13] as the risk of mortality started increasing for hemoglobin levels lower than 13.4 gm/dl among home dwelling women 65 and older. Based on these data, the author proposed that the current definition of anemia by the WHO be revisited. These authors also found the risk of dying decreased 0.76 times for every increase of 1 g/dL in hemoglobin between 8 and 12 g/dL. Common complications of anemia are listed in Table 3.

The most common and disabling chronic symptom of cancer and cancer treatment, [18, 86, 122] fatigue is particularly common after age 65 [18]. In these subjects, it may lead to progressive functional decline, delayed cancer treatment, suboptimal cancer control and substantial increase in the cost of managing these patients [86 18, 122]. Even in the absence of cancer anemia has been associated with functional decline among older individuals [15-17]. Of special interest, in the study of Ferrucci et al, an inverse correlation between hemoglobin and function was present also for hemoglobin levels above 12 gm/dl [16].

In patients with chronic renal failure anemia was associated with increased prevalence of congestive heart failure and coronary deaths, [123-126] neurologic symptoms and cognitive decline, [127-130] and correction of anemia prevented or reversed these complications. A recent review of Medicare patients admitted to a coronary care units showed that a hematocrit lower than 33% (grossly corresponding to hemoglobin levels of 10 gm/dl) was associated with enhanced risk of coronary deaths [126].

Anemia may increase the risk of adverse drug reaction, by a reduction of percentage of drugs bound to red blood cells and increased concentration of free drug in the circulation and by hypoxia that increases the susceptibility of these tissues to therapeutic complications [131]. In post-operative hospitalized patients over 70, anemia was associated with increased risk of delirium [130]. At least four studies showed that the risk of complications of cytotoxic chemotherapy, especially myelosuppression, increases in the presence of anemia [7-10].

3.4 Management of Anemia

Clearly anemia has a number of complications that may be particularly deleterious to older individuals and appear preventable with the correction of anemia. The treatment of underlying causes is the mainstay of management. In some forms of anemia of chronic diseases such as cancer and rheumatoid arthritis, correction of anemia resulted in improved quality of life and function and possibly in improved survival [103-107]. Ongoing studies explore the treatment of all forms of anemia of chronic diseases with erythropoietin in older individuals. It is tantalizing to hypothesize that the correction of anemia may result in improved function, cognition, lesser co-morbidity and possibly improved survival and active life-expectancy.

4. AGE AND THERAPEUTIC EFFECTIVENESS OF HEMATOPOIETIC GROWTH FACTORS

The effectiveness of filgrastim, sarmograstin and erythropoietin in therapeutic doses is well established in older individuals.

4.1 Myelopoietic Growth Factors

A number of studies documented the effectiveness of these substances in older individuals. A retrospective study of the English literature until 1991 demonstrated that the effectiveness of filgrastim and sarmograstim was similar in individuals younger than 65 and those older [132]. In healthy volunteers aged 70 and older, filgrastim induced the same increment in neutrophil count and neutrophil mitotic pool as seen in younger individuals [133]. In four randomized controlled trials (Table 3), filgrastim reduced the incidence of grade four neutropenia and neutropenic infections for patients with large cell lymphoma aged 70 and older [34, 39, 134, 135].

In Acute Myelogenous Leukemia both sargromostin and filgrastim reduced the risk of neutropenic infections and the duration of neutropenia in patients aged 60 and older [84, 136-139]. From this review there is definitive evidence of effectiveness for filgrastim, whereas the effectiveness of sarmograstin is suggested only in AML. The recent introduction of PEG-filgrastim requiring only one injection after chemotherapy appears particularly beneficial to older individuals both in terms of convenience and cost.

4.2 Erythropoietin

In patients of all ages, erythropoietin relieves anemia associated with renal insufficiency, [140] anemia of chronic diseases [115], cancer- and chemotherapy- related anemia [103-107]. Prophylactic use of erythropoietin in women receiving adjuvant chemotherapy for breast cancer reduced the risk of anemia and fatigue in a randomized-controlled study [141]. Improvement of anemia was associated with improved energy levels in patients receiving cytotoxic chemotherapy, and the highest incremental energy improvement was obtained when hemoglobin rose from 11 to 13 gm/dl [105, 107]. Erythropoietin α may be administered weekly [105], whereas the new compound, darbepoietin α may be administered every two or every three weeks.

Of special interest, recent studies both in experimental animals and in humans suggested that erythropoietin α may protect the brain from different forms of injuries, including ischemia, degenerative disease and toxins (it is not clear whether this effect is independent from the correction of anemia) [142].

Erythropoietin appears to hold a number of important promises in the management of older patients with and without cancer, to be tested in randomized controlled studies. These include improved function by reversing anemia of chronic disease, prevention of fatigue and functional dependence in older individuals receiving cancer chemotherapy with prophylactic erythropoietin, and preservation of cognitive function in older individuals treated with chemotherapy.

4.3 Other Hemopoietic Cytokines

Data on the effectiveness of growth factors for megakaryocytes are very limited. The activity of Interleukin-11 (oprevelkin) does not appear age-related [70]. Clincal trials with recombinant megakaryocytic growth factors are ongoing [71].

4.4 Recommendations for the Treatment of Elderly Cancer Patients with Hemopoietic Growth Factors

Clearly age is a risk factor for chemotherapy-induced myelotoxicity. Based on the evidence reviewed so far it is reasonable to recommend that Filgrastim or pegfilgrastim be used prophylacticly in older individuals receiving moderately toxic chemotherapy (CHOP and CHOP-like regimens). The hemoglobin of these patients should be maintained at levels of 12 gm/dl or higher for the duration of chemotherapy.

These recommendations were originally formulated for individuals aged 70 and over, [143] and were extended by the American Society of Clinical Oncology to individuals aged 65 and older [144]. Though these recommendations appear to increase the cost of treatment the opposite may well be true. Recent studies of cost-effectiveness demonstrated that the prophylactic use of filgrastim reduces the overall cost of treatment when the risk of neutropenic infection after the first course of treatment is 20% or higher [145]. This threshold is lower than the risk of neutropenic infections in older lymphoma patients receiving CHOP [33-39, 81, 82]. Furthermore, the duration of hospitalization for neutropenic infection is 30% longer in persons aged 65 and over, which implies a higher cost of managing this complication and a higher cost-effectiveness for its prevention [38]. Last but not least, prolonged hospitalization is a risk factor for deconditioning in older individuals, which may involve decreased treatment tolerance, prolonged and costly rehabilitation as well as the need of costly home care and home assistance.

The study of the cost of anemia is more complex, but it appears reasonable to assume that the management of this complication should not substantially affect the total cost of management for the following reasons:

- A recent study demonstrated that the cost of a monthly treatment with erythropoietin is comparable to the cost of two monthly blood transfusions (145).
- Among cancer patients the cost of fatigue is substantial (146).
- Fatigue may reduce the working capacity of as many as 50% of the cancer patients and 25% of their caregivers. Fatigue may precipitate

functional dependence in older individuals (15-18,86), with two costly consequences. First the patient may become incapacitated to provide important money saving functions, such as caregiving for an older spouse or for the grandchildren. Second, the patient himself/herself may need a home caregiver as well as costly rehabilitation.

5. CONCLUSIONS

Aging appears associated with a progressive reduction in hemopoietic reserve due to exhaustion of pluripotent stem cells, increased circulation of catabolic cytokines, and possibly alterations in the microenvironment and in the production of hemopoietic growth factors. In many respects hemopoiesis may reflect general age-related changes.
Whereas hemopoiesis is adequate to maintain the homeostasis of the peripheral blood, it may fail in presence of hemopoietic stress. This event is documented by increased incidence and prevalence of anemia with aging and increased risk of mielodepression following cytotoxic chemotherapy.

In older individuals anemia is associated with increased risk of death, cardiovascular diseases, pharmacologic complications, dementia and functional dependence.

Filgrastim, pegfilgrastim, erythropoietin α and darbepoietin α are effective in older individuals, may prevent complications of cytotoxic chemotherapy, such as neutropenic infections and fatigue, and may lead to cost savings.

The current ASCO guidelines recommend that prophylactic filgrastim or pegfilgrastim be used in patients aged 65 and older who receive moderately toxic chemotherapy and that the hemoglobin of these patients be maintained at 12 gm/dl or higher.

REFERENCES

1. Carreca I; Barbagallo M; Balducci L;Rothstein G: Hemopoiesis cancer and aging, J Natl Cancer Inst, in press
2. Cohen HJ; Harris T; Pieper CF: Coagulation and activation of inflammatory pathways in the development of functional decline and mortality in the elderly. Am J Med, 2003, 114,180-187
3. Rothstein G: Disordered hematopoiesis and myelodysplasia in the elderly. J Am Ger Soc, 2003, 52, 3suppl, 2, 22-26
4. Balducci L; Ershler WB; Krantz S: Anemia in the elderly. Crit Rev Oncol Hematol, 2003, in press

5. Cova and Balducci Cancer Chemotherapy in Balducci L; Ershler WB;Lyman GH: Comprehensive Geriatric Oncology, 2nd edition. Harwood Academic Publishers, Amsterdam, 2003
6. Repetto L; Carreca I; Maraninch D et al: Use of growth factors in the elderly patients with cancer: a report from the second international Society for Geriatric Oncology (SIOG) 2001 meeting. Crit Rev Oncol Hematol, 2003, 45, 123-128
7. Ratain MJ; Schilsky RL; Choi KE et al: Adaptive control of etoposide administration: impact of interpatient pharmacodynamic variability. Clin Pharmacol Ther, 1989, 45, 226-233
8. Silber JH; Fridman M; Di Paola RS et al: First-cycle blood counts and subsequent neutropenia, dose reduction or delay in early stage breast cancer therapy. J Clin Oncol, 1998, 16, 2392-2400
9. Extermann M; Chen A; Cantor AB et al: Predictors of toxicity from chemotherapy in older patients. Eur J Cancer, 2002, 38, 1466-1473
10. Schijvers D, Highley M, DeBruyn E et al. Role of red blood cell in pharmakinetics of chemotherapeutic agents. Anticancer Drugs, 1999, 10, 147-53
11. Izaks GJ, Westendorp RGJ, Knook DL. The definition of anemia in older persons. JAMA. 1999; 281(18): 1714–7
12. Kikuchi M; Inagaki T; Shinagawa N: Five-year survival of older people with anemia: variation with hemoglobin concentration. J Am Ger Soc, 2001, 49, 1226-1228
13. Chaves PH, Volpato S, Fried L. Challenging the World Health Organization criteria for anemia in older women. J Amer Geriatr Soc 2001;S3:A10
14. Anía BJ, Suman VJ, Fairbanks VF, Rademacher DM, Melton JL. Incidence of anemia in older people: an epidemiologic study in a well defined population. J Am Geriatr Soc 1997; 45:825–831
15. Lunney JR; Lynn J; Foley DJ et al: Patterns of functional decline at the end of life. JAMA, 2003, 14, 289, 2387-2392
16. Ferrucci et al, in press
17. Chaves PH; Ashar B; Guralnick JM et al: Looking at the relationship between hemoglobin concentration and prevalent mobility difficulty in older women. Should the criteria currently used to define anemia re-evaluated? J Am Ger Soc, 2002, 50, 257-264
18. Respini D; Jacobsen PB; Thors C et al: Issues of fatigue in the elderly. Crit Rev Hematol Oncol, 2003
19. Albright JW, Makinodan T: Decline in the growth potential of spleen-colonizing bone marrow stem cells of long-lived aging mice. J Exp Med, 1976, 144, 1204-1213
20. Van Zant G: Stem cells and genetics in the study of development, aging and longevity. Results and problems in Cell Differentiation. Vol 29, Springer-Verlag Berlin Heidelberg, 2000, 203-235
21. Lipschitz DA: Age-related decline in hemopoietic reserve capacity. Sem Oncol, 1995, 22 (Suppl 1), 3-6.
22. Baraldi-Junkins CA; Beck AC; Rothstein G: Hematopoiesis and cytokines. Relevance to cancer and aging. Hematol/Oncol Clin N America, 2000, 14, 45-61
23. Moscinski L: The aging bone marrow. In: Balducci L; Lyman GH; Ershler WB: Comprehensive geriatric Oncology. Harwood Academic Publishers, London, 1998, 1998, 414-423

24. Green J: Management of Infectious Complications. In: Balducci L; Lyman GH;Ershler WB: Comprehensive Geriatric Oncology. Harwood Academic Publishers, London, 1998, 733-41
25. Bagnara GP; Bonsi L; Strippoli P et al: Hemopoiesis in healthy old people and centenarian; well maintained responsiveness of CD34+ cells to hemopoietic growth factors and remodeling of cytokine network. J Gerontol A Biol Scie Med Scie, 2000, 55, B61-70
26. Marley SB; Lewis JL; Davidson RJ et al: Evidence for a continuous decline in hemopoietic cell function from birth: application to evaluating bone marrow failure in children. Br J Haematol, 1999, 106, 162-166
27. Chatta C.S; Price TH; Allen RC et al: Effects of "in vivo" recombinant methionyl human granulocyte colony-stimulating factor on the immune response and peripheral blood colony-forming cells in healthy young and elderly adult volunteers. Blood, 1994, 84, 2923-2929
28. Armitage JO; Potter JF: Aggressive chemotherapy for diffuse histiocytic lymphoma in the elderly. J Am Ger Soc 32:269-273, 1984
29. Kim YJ; Rubenstein EB; Rolston KV et al: Colony-stimulating factors (CSFs) may reduce complications and death in solid tumor patients with fever and neutropenia. Proc ASCO, 2000, 19, 612a, abstr 2411
30. Crivellari D; Bonetti M; Castiglione-Gertsch M et al: Burdens and benefits of Adjuvant Cyclophosphamide, Methotrexate and Fluorouracil and Tamoxifen for Elderly Patients with Breast cancer: The international Breast cancer Study Group Trial vii. J Clin Oncol, 2000, 18, 7, 1412-1422
31. Gomez H; Mas L; Casanova L et al: Elderly patients with aggressive non-Hodgkin's lymphoma treated with CHOP chemotherapy plus granulocyte-macrophage colony-stimulating factor: Identification of two age subgroups with differing hematologic toxicity. J Clin Oncol 16:2352-2358, 1998
32. Dees EC, O'Reilly S, Goodman SN, Sartorius S, Levin MA, Jones RJ, Donehower RC, Fetting JH: A prospective pharmacologic evaluation of age-related toxicity and adjuvant chemotherapy in women with breast cancer. Cancer Invest, 2000, 18(6): 521-9
33. Gaynor ER, Fisher RI: Chemotherapy of intermediate-grade non-Hodgkin's lymphoma: "more" or "less" better? Oncology (Huntingt) 1995, Dec 9 (12): 1273-9
34. Zinzani PG; Storti S; Zaccaria A et al: Elderly aggressive histology Non-Hodgkin's Lymphoma: First Line VNCOP-B Regimen: expereince on 350 patients.Blood, 1999, 94, 33-38
35. Sonneveld P; de Ridder M; van der Lelie H et al: Comparison of doxorubicin and mitoxantrone in the treatment of elderly patients with advanced diffuse non-Hodgkin's lymphoma using CHOP vs. CNOP chemotherapy. J Clin Oncol 13:2530-2539, 1995
36. Tirelli U; Errante D; Van Glabbeke M et al: CHOP is the standard regimen in patients ≥ 70 years of age with intermediate and high grade Non-Hodgkin's lymphoma: results of a randomized study of the European organization for the Research and Treatment of Cancer Lymphoma Cooperative Study. J Clin Oncol, 1998,16,27-34
37. Bastion Y; Blay J-Y; Divine M et al: Elderly patients with aggressive non-Hodgkin's lymphoma: Disease presentation, response to treatment and survival. A Groupe d'Etude des Lymphomes de l'Adulte Study on 453 patients older than 69 years. J Clin Oncol 15: 2945-2953, 1997

38. Chrischilles E; Delgado DI; Stolshek BS et al: Impact of age and colony stimulating factor use in hospital length of stay for febrile neutropenia in CHOP treated non-Hodgkin's lymphoma patients. Cancer Control, 2002, 9, 203-211
39. Osby E; Hagberg H; Kvaloy S et al: CHOP is superior to CNOP in elderly patients with aggressive lymphoma while outcome is unaffected by filgrastim treatment: results of a Nordic Lymphoma Group randomized trial. Blood, 2003, 101, 3840-3848
40. Balducci L: Epidemiology of anemia in the elderly: information on diagnostic evaluation. J Am Ger Soc, 2003, 51 (3 suppl), S2-9
41. Kirkeby OJ; Fossum S; Risoe C: Anemia in elderly patients. Incidence and causes of low hemoglobin concentration in a city general practice. Scand J Prim Health Care, 1991, 9, 167-17
42. Joosten E, Pelemans W, Hiele M, Noyen J, Verhaeghe R, Boogaerts MA. Prevalence and causes of anaemia in a geriatric hospitalised population. Gerontology 1992; 38:111–117
43. Anía BJ, Suman VJ, Fairbanks VF, Melton JL. Prevalence of anemia in medical practice: Community versus referral patients. Mayo Clin Proc 1994; 69:730–735
44. Inelmen IM; D'Alessio M; Gatto MR et al: Descriptive analysis of the prevalence of anemia in a randomly selected sample of elderly people living at home: some results of an Italian multicentric study. Aging, 1994, 6, 81-89
45. Rothstein G. Hematopoiesis in the aged: a model of hematopoietic dysregular. Bood, 1993, Nov. 1; 82(9): 2601-4
46. Kumagai T; Morimoto K; Saitoh H et al: Age-related changes in myelopoietic response to lipopolysaccaride in senescence-accelerated mice. Mech Ageing Dev, 2000, 112, 153-157
47. Cai NS, Li DD, Cheung HT et al: The expression of granulocyte/macrophase colony-stimulating factor in activated mouse lymphocytes declines with age. Cell Immunol, 1990, 130:31
48. Matsuo T; Kario K; Kodoma K et al: An inappropriate erythropoietic response to iron deficiency anemia in the elderly. Clin Lab Hematol, 1995, 17, 317-321
49. Kario K; Matsuo T; Kodama K et al: Reduced erythropoietin secretion in senile anemia. Am J Hematol, 1992, 41, 252-257
50. Goodnough LT; Price TH; Parvin CA: The endogenous erythropoietin response and the erythropoietic response to blood loss anemia: the effects of age and gender. J Lab Clin Med, 1995, 126, 57-64
51. Nilsson-Ehle H; Jagenburg R; Landahl S et al: Haematological abnormalities and reference intervals in the elderly. A cross-sectional comparative study of three urban Swedish population samples aged 70, 75 and 81 years. Acta Med Scand, 1988,224, 595-604
52. Biaggioni I; Robertson D; Krantz S et al: The anemia of primary autonomic failure and its reversal with recombinant erythropoietin. Ann Int Med, 1994, 121, 181-186
53. Duthie E: Physiology of aging: relevance to symptom perceptions and treatment tolerance. In: Balducci L; Lyman GH; Ershler WB Comprehensive Geriatric Oncology. Harwood Academic Publishers, London, 1998, 247-262
54. Tasaki T.; Ohto H; Noguchi M et al: Iron and erythropoietin measurements in autologous blood donors with anemia: implications for management. Transfusion. 1994, 34, 337-343

55. Carpenter MA; Kendall RG; O'Brien AE et al: Reduced erythropoietin response to anaemia in elderly patients with normocytic anaemia. Eur J Haematol, 1992, 49, 119-121
56. Cohen HJ: In search of the underlying mechanisms of frailty. J Gerontol MS, 2001, 55a, 706-708
57. Currie MS; Rao KMK; Blazer DG et al: Age and functional correlation of markers of inflammation and coagulation in the elderly: functional implications of elevated cross-linked fibin degradation products (D-Dimers). J Amer Ger Soc, 1994, 42, 738-742
58. Pieper CF; Rao KMK; Currie MS et al: Age, functional status, and racial differences in plasma D-Dimer levels in community dwelling elders. J Gerontol Med Sc, 1999, 55 A, M649-657
59. Harris TB; Ferrucci L; Tracy RP et al: Associations of elevated interleukin 6 and C-reactive protein levels and with mortality in the elderly. Am J med, 1999, 106, 506-512
60. Taaffe DR: Harris TB; Ferrucci L et al: Cross-sectional and Prospective relationshis of interleukin 6 and C-Reactive protein with physical performance in elderly persons: Mac Arthur study of successful aging. J Gerontol MS, 2000, 55A, M709-715
61. Hamermann D; Berman JW; Albers GW et al: Emerging evidence for inflammation in conditions frequently affecting older adults: report of a symposium. J Am Ger Soci, 1999, 47, 995-999
62. Ershler WB: Biological interactions of aging and anemia: a focus on cytokines. J Am Ger Soc, 2003, 51, (3 Suppl), S18-21
63. Martin F: Frailty and the somatopause. Growth Hormone IGF Res, 1999, 9, 3-10
64. Burgess W Liu Q; Zhou J et al: The immune-endocrine loop during aging: role of growth hormone and insuline-like growth factor1. Neuroimmunomodulation, 1999,6, 56-68
65. Morra L; Moccia F; Mazzarello GP et al: Defective burst-promoting activity of T lymphocytes from anemic and non-anemic elderly people. Ann Hematol, 1994, 68, 67-71
66. Hyrota Y; Okamura S; Kimura N et al: Hematopoiesis in the aged as studied by "in vitro" colony assay . Eur J Haematol, 1988, 40, 83-90
67. Joosten E; Van Hove L; Lesaffre E et al: Serum erythropoietin levels in elderly inpatients with anemia of chronic disorders and iron deficiency anemia. J Am Ger Soc, 1993, 41, 1301-1304
68. Nafziger J; Pailla K; Luciani L et al: Decreased erythropoietin responsiveness to iron deficiency anemia in the elderly. Am J Hematol, 1993, 43, 172-176
69. Chatta DS; Dale DC: Aging and haemopoiesis. Implications for treatment with haemopoietic growth factors. Drugs Aging, 1996, 9, 37-47
70. Smith JW 2nd: Tolerability and side-effect profile of rhIL-11. Oncology (Huntingt) 2000; Sept; 14 (2 Suppl 8):41-7
71. Harker LA; Roskos LK; Marzec UM; Carter RA; Cherry JK; Sundell B;Cheung EN; Terry D; Sheridan W: Effects of megakaryocyte growth and development factor on platelet production, platelet life span and platelet function in healthy human volunteers. Book, 2000, Vol 95 No. 8 (April 15): 2514-22
72. Cascinu S; Del Ferro E; Fedeli A et al: Recombinant human erythropoietin treatment in elderly cancer patients with cisplatin-associated anemia. Oncology, 1995, 52, 422-426

73. Fields KK, Vesole DH, Rowlings PA, horowitz MM, Elfenbein GJ: Bone marrow transplant in the older patient. In: Balducci L; Lyman GH;Ershler WB: Coprehensive Geriatric Oncology. Harwood Academic Publishers, London, 1998, 471-80
74. Ballester OF, Vesole D, Corrado C. Multiple myeloma In: Balducci L; Lyman GH;Ershler WB: Comprehensive Geriatric Oncology. Harwood Academic Publishers, London, 1998, 595-609
75. Begg CB; Carbone P: Clinical trials and drug toxicity in the elderly. The experience of the Eastern Cooperative Oncology Group. Cancer, 1983, 52, 1986-1992
76. Gelman RS; Taylor SG: Cyclophosphamide, Methotrexate and 5Fluorouracil chemotherapy in women more than 65 years old with advanced breast cancer. The elimination of age trends in toxicity by using doses based on creatinine clearance. J Clin Oncol, 1984, 2, 1406-1414
77. Christman K; Muss HB; Case D et al: Chemotherapy of metastatic breast cancer in the Elderly. JAMA, 1992, 268, 57-62
78. Giovannozzi-Bannon S; Rademaker A; Lai G et al: treatment tolerance of Elderly cancer patients entered onto phase II clinical trials. An Illinois Cancer center Study. J Clin Oncol, 1994, 12, 2447-2452
79. Ibrahim N; Frye DK; Buzdar AU et al: Doxorubicin based combination chemotherapy in elderly patients with metastatic breast cancer. Tolerance and outcome. Arch Intern med, 1996, 156, 882-888
80. Ibrahim NK; Buzdar AU; Asmar l et al: Doxorubicin based adjuvant chemotherapy in elderly breast cancer patients: The M D Anderson Experience with long term follow-up. Ann Oncol, 2000, 11, 1-5.
81. Morrison VA; Picozzi V; Scotti S et al: The impact of age on delivered dose-intensity and hospitalizations for febrile neutropenia in patients with intermediate –grade non-Hodgkin's Lymphoma receiving initial CHOP chemotherapy: a risk factor analysis. Clin Lymphoma, 2001, 2, 47-56
82. Jacobson JO; Grossbard M; Shulman LN et al CHOP chemotherapy with preemptive granulocyte colony - stimulating factor in elderly patients with aggressive non-Hodgkin's lymphoma: a dose-intensity analysis. Clin Lymphoma 2000, 1, 211-217
83. Doorduijn JK; van derr Holt B; van der hem KG et al: Randomized trials of granulocyte-Colony Stimulating Factor (G-CSF) added to CHOP in elderly patients with aggressive non-Hodgkin's lymphoma. Blood, 2000,96 (11), 133a
84. Rowe JM: Treatment of acute myelogenous leukemia in older adults. Leukemia, 2000, 14, 480-487
85. Lancet JE; Willman CL; Bennett JM: Acute Myelogenous Leukemia and aging: Clinical Interactions. Hematol/Oncol Clinics N America, 2000, 16, 251-268
86. Liao S, Ferrell BA: Fatigue in an older population. JAGS, 2000, 48:426-30
87. Dixon DO, Neilan B, Jones SE, Lipschitz DA, Miller TP, Grozea PN, Wilson HE: Effect of age on therapuetic outcome in advanced diffuse hisiocytic lymphoma: the Southwest Oncology Group experience. Clin Oncol, 1986, Vol. 4, 295-305
88. Meyer RM; Browman GP; Samosh ML et al: Randomized phase II comparison of standard CHOP with weekly CHOP in elderly patients with Non-Hodgkin's Lymphoma. J Clin Oncol, 1995, 13, 2386-2393
89. Wunderlich A; Kloess M; Reiser M et al: Practicability and acute haematological toxicity of 2- and 3- weekly CHOP and CHOEP chemotherapy for aggressive non-Hodgkin's lymphoma: results from the NHL-B trial of the german High Grade Non-Hodgkin's Lymphoma study group. Ann Oncol, 2003, 14, 881-893

90. Valagussa P; BonadonnaG: breast cancer. Cancer Chemother Biol Resp Modif, 2002,20, 493-517
91. Wood WC, Budman DR, Korzun AH, Cooper MR, Younger J, Hart RA, Ellerton JA, Norton L, Ferree CR et al: Dose and dose intensity of adjuvant chemotherapy for Stage II positive breast carcinoma. N Engl J Med, 1994, May 5; 330(18):1253-9
92. Citron ML; Berry DA; Cirrincione C et al: Randomized trial of dose-dense versus conventionally scheduled and sequential versus concurrent combination chemotherapy as postoperative adjuvant treatment of node-positive primary breast cancer: first report of Intergroup Trial C9741? Cancer and leukemia group trial 9741. J Clin Oncol, 2003, 21, 1431-1439
93. Meyer RJ; Davis RB; Schiffer CH et al: Intensive postremission chemotherapy in adult with acute myeloid leukemia. N Engl J Med, 1994, 31, 896-903
94. Bloomfield CD; Lawrence D; Byrd JC et al: Frequency of prolonged remission duration after high-dose cytarabine intensification in acute myeloid leukemia varies with cytogenetics subtype. Cancer Res, 1998, 58, 4173-4179
95. Berman E; Heller G; Santorsa J et al: Results of a randomized trial comparing idarubicin and cytosine arabinoside with daunorubicin and cytosine arabinoside in adult patients with newly diagnosed acute myelogenous leukemia. Blood, 1991, 77, 1666-1674
96. Volger WR; Velez-Garcia E; Weiner RS et al: A phase III trial comparing idarubicin and daunorubicin in combination with cytarabine in acute myelogenous leukemia: a Southeastern Cancer Study Group. J Clin Oncol, 1992, 10, 1103-1111
97. Wiernik PH; Banks PLC; Case DC et al: Cytarabine plus idarubicin or daunorubicin as induction and consolidation therapy for previously untreated adult patients with acute myeloid leukemia. Blood, 1992, 79, 313-319
98. Berman E; Arlin ZA; Gaynar J et al: Comparative trial of cytarabine and thioguanine in combination with amsacrine or daunorubicin in patients with untreated acute non-lymphocytic leukemia: results of the L16M protocol. Leukemia, 1989, 3, 115-121
99. Gurney H: Dose calculations of anticancer drugs: a review of the current practice and introduction of an alternative. J Clin Onc, 1996, Vol. 14:2590-2611
100. Kerr KG: The prophylaxis of bacterial infections in neutropenic patients. J. Antimicrob Chemother, 1999 Nov; 44(5): 587-91
101. Yamada M; Wong FL; Suzuki G: Longitudinal trends of hemoglobin levels in a Japanese population-RERF Adult health Study Subject. Eur J Haematol, 2003, 70, 129-135
102. Salive ME; Cornoni-Huntley J; Guralnik JM et al: Anemia and hemoglobin levels in older persons: relationship with age, gender and health status. J Am Ger Soc, 1992, 40, 489-496
103. Glaspy J; Bukowski R; Steinberg C et al: Impact of therapy with epoietin alfa on clinical outcomes in patients with non-myeloid malignancies during cancer chemotherapy in community oncology practices. J Clin Oncol, 1997,5, 1218-1234
104. Demetri GD; Kris M; Wade J et al: Quality of life benefits in chemotherapy patients treated with epoietin alfa is independent from disease response and tumor type. Result of a prospective community oncology study. The procrit study group. J Clin Oncol, 1998, 16, 3412-3420
105. Gabrilove JL; Einhorn LH; Livingston RB et al: Once weekly dosing of epoietin alfa is similar to three-times weekly dosing in increasing hemoglobin and quality of life. Proc Am Soc Clin Oncol, 1999, 18, 574A.
106. Littlewood TJ; Bajetta E; Nortier JW, et al. Effects of epoetin alfa on hematologic parameters and quality of life in cancer patients receiving nonplatinum chemotherapy: results of a randomized, double-blind, placebo-controlled trial. J Clin Oncol 2001;19(11):2865–2874

107. Cleeland CS; Demetri GD; Glaspy J et al: Identifying hemoglobin levels for optimal Quality of Life. Results of an incremental analysis. Proc Am Soc Clin Oncol, 1999, 16, Astr 2215

108. Anía BJ; Suman VJ,;Fairbanks VF; Melton JL. Prevalence of anemia in medical practice: Community versus referral patients. Mayo Clin Proc 1994; 69:730–735

109. Inelmen EM; Alessio MD; Gatto MRA et al. Descriptive analysis of the prevalence of anemia in a randomly selected sample of elderly people at home: some results of an Italian multicentric study. Aging Clin Exp Res 1994; 6:81–89

110. Smith DL. Anemia in the elderly. Am Fam Physician 2000; 62(7): 1565–1572

111. Mansouri A; Lipschitz DA. Anemia in the elderly patient. Anemia 1992; 76(3): 619–630

112. Zauber PN; Zauber AG. Hematologic data of healthy very old people. JAMA 1987; 257(16): 2181–2184

113. Balducci L; Hardy CL; Lyman GH. Hematopoietic growth factors in the older cancer patient. Curr Opin Hematol 2001;8(3): 170–187

114. Tong EM; Nissenson AR. Erythropoietin and anemia. Semin Nephrol 2001; 21(2): 190–203

115. Krantz SB: Pathogenesis and treatment of the anemia of chronic disease. Am J Med Sci, 1994,307, 353-359

116. Chiari MM, Bagnoli R, De Luca P, Monti M, Rampoldi E, Cunietti E. Influence of acute inflammation on iron and nutritional status indexes in older inpatients. J Am Geriatr Soc 1995; 43:767–771

117. Murphy PT, Hutchinson RM. Identification and treatment of anaemia in older patients. Drugs Aging 1994; 4(2): 113–127

118. Carmel R. Prevalence of undiagnosed pernicious anemia in the elderly. Arch Intern Med 1996; 156(10): 1097–1100

119. Sumner AE, Chin MM, Abrahm JL, et al. Elevated methylmalonic acid and total homocysteine levels show high prevalence of vitamin B_{12} deficiency after gastric surgery. Ann Intern Med 1996; 124:469–76

120. Norman EJ, Morrison JA. Screening elderly populations for cobalamin (vitamin B12) deficiency using the urinary methylmalonic acid assay by gas chromatography mass spectrometry. Am J Med 1993; 94(6): 589–594

121. Gagnon DR, Zhang TJ, Brand FN, Kannel WB. Hematocrit and the risk of cardiovascular disease–the Framingham study: a 34-year follow-up. Am Heart Journal. 1994; 27:674–82

122. Rieger PT: Assessment and epidemiologic issues related to fatigue. Cancer, 2001, S6, 1733-1736

123. Metivier F, Marchais SJ, Guerin AP, Pannier B, London GM. Pathophysiology of anaemia: focus on the heart and blood vessels. Nephrol Dial Transplant 2000; 15(3):14–8

124. Levin A, Singer J, et al. Prevalent left ventricular hypertrophy in the predialysis population: identifying opportunities for intervention. Am J Kidney Dis 1996; 27:347–54

125. Silverberg DS, Wexler D, Blum M, et al. The use of subcutaneous erythropoietin and intravenous iron for the treatment of the anemia of severe, resistant congestive heart failure improves cardiac and renal function and functional cardiac class, and markedly reduces hospitalizations. J Am Coll Cardiol. 2000; 35:1737–44

126. WU WC; Rathore SS; Wang Y et al: Blood transfusions in Elderly patients with Acute Myocardial Infarction, New England Journal of medicine, 2001, 345, 1230-1236
127. Beard CM, Kokmen E, O'Brien P, Anía BJ, Melton LJ. Risk of Alzheimer's disease among elderly patients with anemia: population-based investigations in Olmsted County, Minnesota. Ann Epidemiol. 1997; 7:219–24
128. Nissenson AR. Epoetin and cognitive function. Am J Kidney Dis. 1992; 20(1): 21–4
129. Pickett JL, Theberge DC, Brown WS, Schweitzer SU, Nissenson AR. Normalizing hematocrit in dialysis patients improves brain function. Am J Kidney Dis 1999; 33(6): 1122–30
130. Marcantonio ER; Flacker JM; Michaels M et al: Delirium is independently associated with poor functional recovery after hip fracture. J Am Ger Soc, 2000, 48, 618-624
131. John V; Mashru S; Lichtman S: Pharmacological factors influencing anticancer drug selection in the elderly. Drugs Aging. 2003, 20, 737-759
132. Shank WA, Balducci L: Recombinant hemopoetic growth factors: comparative hemopoietic response in younger and older subjects. J Am Geriatr Soc, 1992, 40:151
133. Price TH; Chatta GS; Dale DC: Effect of recombinant granulocyte colony-stimulating factor on neutrophil kinetics in normal young and elderly humans. Blood, 1996, 88,335-340
134. Zagonel V; Babare R; Merola MC et al: Cost-benefit of granulocyte colony-stimulating factor administration in older patients with Non-Hodgkin's lympghoma treated with combination chemotherapy. Ann Oncol, 1994, 5, suppl 2 127-132
135. Bertini M; Freilone R; Vitolo U et al: The treatment of elderly patients with aggressive non-Hodgkins lymphomas: Feasibiity and efficacy of an intensive multi-drug regimen. Leukemia Lymphoma 22:483-493 1996
136. Heil D; Hoelzer D; Sanz MA et al: A randomized double blind placebo controlled phase III study of filgrastim in remission induction and consolidation therapy for patients with "de novo" acute myeloid leukemia. The International Acute leukemia Study Group, Blood, 1997, 90, 4710-4718
137. Witz F; Sadoun A; Perrin MC: A placebo-controlled study of recombinant human granulocyte macrophage colony-stimulating factor administered during an induction treatment for "de novo" acute myelogenous leukemia in older patients. Blood, 1998, 15, 2722-2730
138. Stone RM; Berg DT; George SL et al: Granulocyte-macrophage Colony stimulating facotr after initial chemotherapy for elderly patients with primary acute myelogenous leukemia. N Engl J Med, 1995, 332, 1671-1677
139. Dombret H; Chastang C; Fenaux P et al: A controlled study of recombinant Human granulocyte Colony-Stimulating factor in elderly patients after treatment for acute myelogenous leukemia. N Engl J Med, 1995, 332, 1678-1683
140. Murphy ST; Parfrey PS: Erythropoietin therapy in chronic uremia: the impact of norm of hematocrit. Curr Opin Nephrol Hypertens, 1999, Sept 8; 573-8
141. Del Mastro L; Venturini M; Lionetto R et al: Randomized phase III trial evaluating the role of erythropoietin in the prevention of chemotherapy-induced anemia. J Clin Oncol, 1997, 15, 2715-2721
142. Brines ML, Ghezzi P, Keenan S, Agnello D, de Lanerolle NC, Cerami O, Cerami A: Erythropoietin crosses the blood-brain barrier to protect against experimental brain injury. Proc Natl Acad Sci USA, 2000, Sept 12:97(19): 10526-31
143. Balducci L; Yates G. General Guidelines for the management of Older patients with Cancer. Oncology (Huntingt), 2000, 14, 221-227
144. Lyman GH; Kuderer N, Balducci L. Cost-Benefit analysis of Granulocyte-Colony stimulating factor in the management of elderly cancer patients. Curr Opin Hematol, 2002, 9, 207-214

145. Cremieux PY; Barrett B; Anderson K: Cost of outpatient blood transfusions in cancer patients. J Clin Oncol, 2000, 2755-2761
146. Curt GA, et al. Impact of cancer-related fatigue on the lives of patient. ASCO Proceeding, 1999, p 573a, 2214
147. Ozer H, Artmitage JO, Bennett CL, Crawford J, Demetri GD et al. 2000 update of recommendations for the use of hematopoietic colony-stimulating factors: evidence-based, clinical practice guidelines. J Clin Oncol, 2003, in press

Chapter 7

CLINICAL AND BIOCHEMICAL EVALUATION CHANGES OVER AGING

Angela Abbatecola, B. Gwen Windham, Stefania Bandinelli, Fulvio Lauretani, Giuseppe Paolisso, Luigi Ferrucci

Angela Abbatecola, Research Scientist, Department of Geriatric Medicine and Metabolic Diseases, II University of Naples, Naples, Italy. B. Gwen Windham, Staff Clinician, Longitudinal Studies Section, Clinical Research Branch, National Institute on Aging, Baltimore, MD, USA. Stefania Bandinelli, Director of Clinical Rehabilitation, Department of Geriatrics, Italian National Institute of Research and Care on Aging (INRCA), Florence, Italy. Fulvio Laurentani, Research Scientist, INRCA, University of Florence, Department of Geriatrics, Firenze, Italy. Giuseppe Paolisso, Professor of Geriatrics, Department of Geriatric Medicine and Metabolic Diseases, II University of Naples, Naples, Italy. Luigi Ferrucci, Director, Baltimore Longitudinal Study on Aging, Longitudinal Studies Section, Clinical Research Branch, National Institute on Aging, Baltimore, MD, USA.

Aging is associated with susceptibility and reduced ability to respond to internal and external stressors. A reduction of functional reserve occurs in many physiological systems and determines increased vulnerability to diseases and high risk of functional dependence. While these modifications can be observed in most persons, particularly in the context of longitudinal studies, they are characterized by extreme variability across individuals and only modest synchronism with chronological aging. As a result, the degree of susceptibility to stressors and exhaustion of functional reserve is dispersed over a wide spectrum in persons of the same age, and the amount of dispersion becomes even greater when we consider older age groups.

By convention, geriatricians define "frail" as those individuals that are at the extreme edge of the severity spectrum in this process. Because of this conventional attitude, frailty is often used as an exchangeable term for disability, comorbidity and poor health status, and it is also considered as an irreversible condition leading to adverse health outcomes. On the contrary, it is important to conceptualize "frailty" as a continuous, other than a discrete process, where several stages or degrees of severity can be defined as they become useful in research and clinical practice, and that below a certain degree of severity it can be reversed with appropriate interventions.

The aging process is probably associated with the development of some unavoidable degree of "frailty" which in the literature is often referred to as "normal aging". Even the healthiest octogenarian is more sensitive to the effects of stressors than the healthiest teenager. Diseases and behavioral risk factors contribute to frailty in ways cannot be completely explained by traditional biomedical expectations. The effect of environment on frailty is complex. An environment that is too challenging causes a rapid exhaustion of functional reserves and leads to an overt instability of the biological homeostasis. On the other hand, an environment that is not at all challenging, leads to a progressive "atrophy" of the homeostatic mechanisms and makes the individual more susceptible to future stressors.

Clinicians who care for older patients face several times daily the complex implications and questions posed by the age-associated frailty. For example, it is clearly difficult to prescribe a pharmacological treatment, make decisions about rehabilitation, give advice to patients about the risk/benefits of a specific surgical procedure or establish the prognosis of diseases, without having information regarding the degree of functional reserve and ability to respond to stress. On the other hand, there is still much disagreement and discussion of the criteria that should be used for the operational definition of frailty, and most have no idea as to how to grade its severity.

There is some consensus that the basic clinical features of the frailty syndrome should include the following domains: a) mobility, such as lower extremity performance and gait abnormalities; b) muscle weakness; c) poor exercise tolerance; d) unstable balance; e) factors related to body composition, such as malnutrition, and sarcopenia (loss of lean body mass), and weight loss. Validity of these factors as critical elements of the frailty syndrome is provided by studies showing that in older, non-disabled persons, individual components are associated with the classical geriatric syndromes (e.g. falls, symptomatic depression, urinary incontinence and functional impairment) and are strong and independent risk factors of disability and death.

In 1999, Walston and Fried [1] developed an interpretive framework that combines the elements of the "body composition" and "mobility" domains of the frailty syndrome into a pathophysiologic pathway where sarcopenia and poor muscle strength, by limiting mobility and physical activity, reduce total energy expenditure and nutritional intake, which, in turn, lead to weight loss and further aggravate sarcopenia. Using data from the Cardiovascular Health Study the elements of the pathway were as follows: 1) unexplained weight loss; 2) poor grip strength; 3) self-reported exhaustion; 4) slow walking speed; and 5) low physical activity. After adjusting for significant confounders, participants with 3 or more of these characteristics were at significantly increased risk of disability, hospitalization and death. The work of Walston and Fried [1] demonstrates that aggregating measures in the domains of physical function and body composition are an effective initial basis for developing screening criteria for an intrinsic vulnerability that have predictive validity. However, without understanding the pathophysiologic pathway that leads to frailty as a syndrome that justifies the aggregation of the domains proposed by Waltson and Fried [1], we lack the critical information to envision any serious attempts to apply the concept of frailty into clinical practice. In this chapter we explore some of the biological mechanisms that tend to become dysregulated with aging and may contribute to the pathophysiology of the frailty syndrome. Some of this information concerns biological markers of frailty that can be already measured. So the possible use of these measures in current clinical practice are pointed out in the various sections of this chapter. As our understanding of the pathophysiology, clinical presentation, and consequences of the frailty syndrome improves, many additional uses of the measures will emerge, and will help identify new potential targets for intervention.

1. HUMAN AGING

Gradual physiological changes that often parallel the aging process contribute to the conventional view of "normal" aging. Normal aging implies a progressive decline of the physiological reserve and the ability to compensate, but it is compatible with autonomy over the entire life span. In frail, older persons the decline in functional reserve is accelerated and compensatory mechanisms start failing with consequent negative health outcomes as the functional reserves are depleted.

A better understanding of physiologic changes that proceed and accompany frailty and, over time, lead to disability is needed if we want to capture this pathological process in an early stage, and develop targeted interventions that will delay or postpone the onset of disability. Unfortunately, we have very little information on this topic and, worse yet, what is known is sparse and difficult to reconnect to an overall paradigm. This chapter attempts to address this problem. We will focus on body composition changes, chronic inflammation, oxidative stress and hormonal changes that often occur in older persons and are accelerated over the aging process. Additionally, in the final part of our discussion, we provide our view on how this information can be used in clinical practice to provide better care to frail older persons.

2. OVERVIEW OF BIOCHEMICAL MARKERS AND AGING (OR FRAILTY)

Many efforts have been made to identify biochemical markers of aging in both normal and frail older individuals [2,3]. Traditionally, clinical chemistry results obtained from laboratory testing are compared with the corresponding reference values in order to determine whether such values fall within the central 95% area under the Gaussian symmetric bell-shaped curve, or the "normal range". Reference values calculated using this method are reported, for example, in the recommendations of the Expert Panel on Theory of Reference Values of the International Federation of Clinical Chemistry and the published guidelines of the National Committee for Clinical Laboratory Standards [4]. In spite of this generalized trend, several lines of research indicate that a purely statistical approach to the identification of "normal" values can be misleading, and methods based on predictive validity in relation to health outcomes should be explored. This is particularly evident for reference values in geriatric patients. Tietz et al. [5] obtained data from 236 individuals, ages 60 to 90 years, 22 individuals, ages 90 to 99 years, and 69, 100 years of age or older. As shown in Table 1 (Tietz et al), plasma levels of dehydroepiandrosterone (DHEA) and DHEA sulphate (DHEAS) were lower in individuals over the age of 90 compared to those of young adults. Other sex hormones, estradiol, estrone and testosterone were found to be much lower in persons over the age of 90 than those of young adults. Interestingly, insulin levels tended to increase in adults aging from 60 to 90 years of age, while a decline in insulin levels was observed in persons over the age of 90.* (Table 1)

The need for biological markers of pathology in the evaluation of older persons is justified by the peculiar relationship that exists between diseases and health status in old age. Because aging is associated with an increment in the global susceptibility to diseases, multiple morbidities are very common. Analogously, diseases that are not clinically overt are often associated with pathological processes that already affect the health status but have not reached the severity threshold that makes them identifiable as "diseases". Thus, the global burden of comorbidity can be captured only indirectly, using functional or biological markers.

---

* Note that age-adjusted "normal" values for most of these hormones are lacking and the values prepared in the literature are highly variable from author to author.

Table 1. Laboratory ranges (95th percentile) and mean values of some hormones in young adults, 60- to 90-year olds, and > 90 years of age

		Young adults		60-90		>90	
Analyte	Sex	Range	Mean	Range	Mean	Range	Mean
DHEA, mg/L	M + F	1.60-8.00				0.17-1.69	0.79
DHEAS, mg/L	M	1800-4500				40-750	287
	F	1200-3150				20-600	231
Estradiol, ng/L	F	Follicular:30-100				<5-20	6
		Luteal:70-300					
Estrone, ng/L	F	Follicular: 30-100					
		Luteal: 60-160				<5-58	29
Insulin (mU/L)	M+F	6-23	11.8	6.6-36.7	16.4	2.4-19.0	7.20
Testosterone total (mg/L)	M	3.50-10.30				2.15-6.71	3.40

As reported by Tietz et al. (5)

Impaired glucose, protein and lipid metabolism in older individuals is common. Aging is associated with impaired glucose handling, mainly due to a decline in insulin activity [6-8]. There is strong evidence that increased resistance to insulin activity is one of the main components of diminished homeostatic glucose regulation in older persons. Insulin-mediated glucose uptake, measured using a glucose clamp technique combined with H^3-glucose infusion, was shown to progressively decline over aging [9]. The response to insulin resistance is increased insulin production. When the ability to compensate for insulin resistance by increasing insulin production is exhausted, the glucose homeostasis becomes dysregulated, and type 2 Diabetes Mellitus occurs. Therefore, insulin resistance along with the reduced ability to secrete insulin, as seen during glucose tolerance test administration in elderly subjects, also contributes to impaired glucose homeostasis [10,11]. However, the dysregulation in the glucose metabolism due to peripheral insulin resistance is important long before diabetes can be diagnosed and cannot be overlooked in the clinical evaluation of older persons.

Total body protein, lean body mass and the rates of protein synthesis decline with increasing age. More importantly, such changes are components of an impaired homeostatic phenomenon, which is not always balanced with adequate dietary protein intake. Furthermore, an altered state of hepatic protein synthesis with reduced fibrinogen and other protein carriers, such as thyroxine-binding protein and iron-binding protein may result in an altered coagulatory state, reduced thyroxine plasma concentrations and an anemic state. In addition, reduced plasma concentrations of albumin have been correlated with a higher degree of oxidative stress.

Lipid and lipoprotein concentrations vary over an individual's lifespan [12]. In particular, total cholesterol and triglyceride levels tend to increase up until 50 years of age and then a gradual decline starts to occur. Interestingly, a positive correlation exists between total cholesterol and/or triglyceride levels with the incidence of cardiovascular disease up to the age of 50 years. However, the ability of total cholesterol to predict coronary heart disease in very old individuals remains controversial. Raiha et al [13] reported that an elevated level of total cholesterol was not a cardiovascular risk in older persons, but predicted survival for non-cardiovascular disease mortality, while Manolio et al [14] did not find any correlation between total cholesterol and all-cause mortality in older subjects [13]. Interestingly, studies have reported that persistently low cholesterol levels increased the risk of mortality in males aged 71 to 93 [15]. Low total cholesterol levels have also been associated with all-cause mortality in elderly Italian men and women, thus underscoring the potential importance of low levels of cholesterol as a warning sign of rapidly declining health [16].

Such discrepancies can be explained by one of the major differences between middle-aged and older populations, which is the presence of an increased prevalence of poorer health of older individuals. In fact, older frail persons with low total cholesterol levels are more likely to have a decreased survival rate than older persons with little or no disease in the presence of chronically low cholesterol values [17]. Interestingly, after adjusting for frailty markers in a large sample of older persons, elevated total cholesterol levels predicted an increased risk for death from CHD, and the risk of death from CHD decreased as cholesterol levels declined [18]. These authors also emphasized the finding that frailty markers were consistently associated with low cholesterol levels, thus confirming similar previous reports. Only further investigations aimed at evaluating controlled clinical trials with lipid-lowering therapy in non-frail older persons can shed light on the risks or the benefits of such treatment.

Regarding lipoproteins, high-density lipoprotein cholesterol (HDL-C) is a considered a protective factor for CHD [19]. In particular, HDL-C levels have been associated with good health status, while reduced HDL-C values are recognized as risk factors for CHD in both middle-aged and older persons. Furthermore, it has been shown that reduced HDL-C also predicts non-CHD/stroke mortality in older persons [20]. Thus, low HDL-C may also be considered a valid biomarker for chronic disease and poor health status in old age.

Ueno et al [3] have recently described biomarkers of aging in women. In particular, these authors suggest that five variables should be considered specific biomarkers for aging in women: forced expiratory volume in 1.0 s (FEV_1), systolic blood pressure (SBP), glucose (GLU, mg/dl), ratio of albumin to globulin (A/G) and mean corpuscular hemoglobin (MCH, pg). Such multiple physiological variables reflect the function of diverse vital functions, in particular, pulmonary function, blood pressure, glucose handling, protein metabolism and hematological functioning. Biological age scores (BAS) were calculated using the parameters mentioned above. Ueno et al [3] concluded that the rate at which women age is relatively slow up until 65 years of age. Then after 65 years of age their rates of aging rapidly increase. Therefore, the biological processes aimed at maintaining a stable homeostasis correctly function up to age 65; after 65, false signaling of such a complex system occurs causing it to lose its effectiveness. This observation is of extreme importance as altered biomarkers are highly correlated with mortality [21] and the frailty syndrome is commonly observed in persons over the age of 65.

The aggregation of variables in global indices based on their predictive role for specific outcomes is very appealing for clinical use, but adds very little to our understanding of the global burden of disease in old age. Recently, authors have also suggested that the involvement in multiple physiological systems that is characteristic of older patients with comorbidity should be interpreted in the context of the "frailty syndrome". According to current views of frailty, homeostasis is disrupted when the ability of individuals to respond to internal and external changes declines below the threshold of effective compensation. When this occurs, abnormal concentrations of specific biomarkers of frailty become detectable in the biological fluids, and structural changes take place in cells and tissues. Unfortunately, serum biomarkers are not currently used to identify frailty, which still remains a clinical diagnosis based on medical history, symptoms, and signs. Clinically, the frailty syndrome is characterized by an excessive reduction in lean body mass, in walking performance and in endurance, associated with a perception of exhaustion and fatigue [22]. Several lines of evidence, however, show that this syndrome is often paralleled by important changes in physiological systems accompanied by changes in serum levels of biomarkers.

3. FRAILTY AND THE NEUROMUSCULAR SYSTEM

There is growing evidence that the core target of the frailty syndrome is motor organization, specifically the muscular and nervous systems. Disease, disuse and aging trigger a mechanism that impoverishes the redundancy of muscular and nervous backup systems, leading to a measurable decline of motor performance. Once the process is activated, its consequences follow a common pathway leading to a more generalized loss of motor functioning. There is good evidence that measures that are related to mobility and motor performance are interpretable as proxy markers of frailty. However, the "diagnosis" of frailty, as a syndrome, hides an array of different pathologic processes that may involve the integrity and functionality of selected physiological subsystems implicated in motor performance [2]. Some of these subsystems include: bone, joints, muscles, peripheral nerves, metabolic efficiency, aerobic capacity and energy production. Clinically, the best criteria for screening of frailty are tests of mobility, gait, balance, manual dexterity, activities of daily living (ADLs) [23], instrumental activities of daily living (IADL) (24) and the Barthel Index [25]. However, it is conceivable that specific biomarkers could be measured in order to identify the involvement of each one of these physiological systems in the early stages of the disablement process.

Lower extremity performance in non-disabled persons is an excellent predictor of poor quality of life, deterioration of health status, incident disability, health care utilization, nursing home admission and death. Thus, physical performance measures have been considered "vital signs" of functional decline in older persons [26]. In particular, gait speed and the short performance battery, developed in the context of the EPESE study, have been identified as quantitative estimates of future risk for functional decline and hospitalization [26] Observational studies provide good evidence that performance-based measures of mobility are valid proxy measures of frailty and global susceptibility to adverse health outcomes.

In older persons, poor muscle strength and poor physical performance often coexist. Midlife handgrip muscle strength has been recognized as an important factor that predicts old age functional ability [27]. Observational studies have consistently shown that chronic conditions such as coronary heart disease, diabetes and pulmonary obstructive disease are associated with lower muscle strength. These findings suggest that a core mechanism exists that is responsible for changes in body composition and disease susceptibility in old age and ultimately to the age-associated changes in functional capacity. Possible links between diseases in old age and "frailty" are: nutritional depletion, inflammation, reduced physical activity or inactivity. These mechanisms are, in turn, risk factors for mortality. Thus, in persons afflicted with chronic illness, reduced muscle strength could be considered an important marker of disease severity. Indeed, handgrip muscle strength has also been associated with overall mortality, independently of poor nutritional status, inflammation and physical inactivity [28]. These findings suggest that muscle strength has a direct effect on mortality or increases the risk of mortality through a mechanism that is still unclear.

4. BODY COMPOSITION CHANGES

The two main components of body composition are fat mass and lean (fat-free) mass. Fat-free mass consists of body cell mass, extracellular fluid and the extracellular solids such as collagen and bone mineral [29]. The body cell mass may be further subdivided into the fat-free portion of cells within muscle, viscera and the immune system. The body cell mass is functionally the most important compartment in determining energy production and expenditure, protein needs, and metabolic response to stress (acute phase response).

There are substantial changes in body composition that accompany the aging process [30]. In particular, the fat mass increases and accumulates preferentially in the abdominal area, while a parallel decline in muscle mass and bone density occurs. Interestingly, the changes in body composition that begin to manifest during adulthood may be partially explained by an imbalance of energy intake and expenditure. In older adults, however, these changes are extremely accelerated compared to younger cohorts, and cannot be explained simply as an imbalance between energy intake and expenditure.

In most older persons, fat mass constitutes a greater percentage of total weight than individuals at younger ages. A population-based study in which anthropometric parameters were measured over the entire life span (age range: 20-103 yrs.) demonstrated that the accumulation of abdominal fat with age occurs primarily during middle age [31] but is different for men and women. In particular, the greatest change of waist circumference seems to occur in men between 20 and 55 years of age, while in women, the waist circumference tends to increase progressively across the entire life span.

Many studies have shown that increased visceral fat is a risk factor for age-related diseases such as hypertension, type 2 diabetes, cardiovascular disease and some types of cancer [20,32]. Adipose tissue has also been correlated with oxidative stress, reduced glucose uptake, and reduced insulin clearance. Understanding how changes in body composition and, in particular, fat distribution, affect the risk for many disease states and mortality is one of the most important research questions that should be addressed in future studies.

The simplest clinical indicator of visceral fat is the waist circumference. A number of studies have shown that waist circumference is an independent risk factor for cardiovascular disease in adults, including those 65 years and older. On the contrary, the relationship between body mass index (BMI), cardiovascular disease and all-cause mortality is controversial. The highest mortality rates have been found in older persons with very low BMI, while in middle-aged persons, BMI was positively associated with mortality [33]. These data suggest that the relationship between body composition and health-related outcomes in older persons cannot be evaluated simply in conventional terms of body fat, but rather fat distribution and type of fat accumulated, both providing essential information for assessing such risk.

The notion that aging is associated with gradual reduction of lean body mass is also generic. In fact, selected tissues seem to be more affected by aging than others. In particular, the decline in non-fat mass is largely attributed to sarcopenia. Sarcopenia has been increasingly used to describe the age-related decline in both muscle mass and muscle strength. However, despite the term "sarcopenia", the precise criteria that define such a state have still not been agreed upon.

Changes in body composition that parallel the aging process are strongly associated with a decline in physical function and mortality risk. The underlying mechanisms responsible for the excess age-associated decline of muscle mass and function compared to other sections of lean body mass are still unknown. Several hypotheses have been proposed, which include: i) intrinsic biochemical and physical changes leading to muscle atrophy [34]; ii) reduced neuronal stimulation due to reduction in the number of α-motorneurons or their activity [35]; iii) oxidative damage of mitochondrial DNA with accumulations of mutations that reduce the efficiency of the metabolic pathways aimed at energy production [36,37]; iv) influence of external factors such as malnutrition, sedentary life-style and disease typically observed in older persons (38); v) loss of endogenous hormone production [39,40]; and vi) dysregulation of catabolic cytokines [41,42]. Over the aging process, both changes in the contractile efficiency of muscle fibers and changes in tissue quality, such as an increase in connective tissue and pericellular fat infiltration, may also contribute to altered muscle function.

There are many methods that simultaneously measure body fat and fat-free components of body composition. Some important measures are as follows: 1) skin-fold measurements are obtained using hand-held calipers, which exert a standardized pressure at various body locations. The sum of these measurements is used to derive body fat percentage. The caliper method is based on the idea that the thickness of subcutaneous fat reflects a constant proportion of the total body fat and that the sites selected for measurements represent the average thickness of the subcutaneous fat [43,44].

Also, the mean arm circumference with triceps skin-fold thickness is used to calculate muscle area and thus, derive fat-free mass; 2) hydrodensitometry or underwater weighing is another instrumental method that measures whole body density by determining body volume. This technique is based on the two-compartment model (fat and fat-free mass). The densities of bone and muscle are higher than water. Body fat percentage is then calculated from body density using standard equations (sirk or brozek); 3) bioelectrical impedance analysis (BIA) is measured utilizing a safe electrical signal that passes through the body. Impedance is greatest in fat tissue (10-20% water), while fat-free mass (70-75% water) allows the signal to pass much more easily. The measurement obtained is entered into a formula along with height, weight, and gender to determine lean and fat mass. However, in order to obtain correct evaluations from the BIA it is necessary that the body is within normal hydration ranges.

Newer more sophisticated methods for the assessment of body composition include the Dual Energy X-ray Absorptiometer (DEXA), computed tomography (CT), magnetic resonance imaging (MRI) and air displacement plethysmography . DEXA is a relatively new method that uses three compartments (total body mineral, fat-free mass, and fat mass). DEXA consists of a dual energy beam (two low dose x-ray sources) that scans bone and soft tissue simultaneously. DEXA is currently considered the "gold standard" measure because of the high degree of precision in a single measurement and the ability to provide the exact location of fat tissue distribution. CT scanning produces cross-sectional scans of the body. As the beam rotates data is collected, stored and applied to algorithms to build images that describe body composition. MRI utilizes a magnetic field that "excites" water and fat molecules, producing a measurable signal, which is then measured and analyzed. Whole body air displacement plethysmography (trade name BOD POD) is a new technique that is similar to the underwater method, but uses air displacement instead of water. It is based on Boyle's law, which states that volume and pressure are inversely related. All the methods described above are summarized in Table 2 (shown on page 154), with information on their reliability, advantages and disadvantages.

It is interesting to speculate on the consequences of sarcopenia that are not directly related to poor muscle strength. A number of physiological functions that take place within muscle tissues have a critical effect on human metabolism: muscles are a reservoir of body proteins and energy that can be utilized in periods of extreme stress or malnutrition; amino-acids can be mobilized during acute infections and are used as building blocks for antibodies; hormones are produced and catabolized in muscle tissue. Thus, age-related muscle mass reduction may explain the lower metabolic adaptation and immunological response to disease. Indeed, poor muscle strength is a strong predictor of mortality, independent of any other known risk factors for poor muscle strength. The rate of decline varies among individuals and is influenced by factors that modulate the balance between catabolic and anabolic processes. There are several possible mechanisms that may be involved in the genesis of sarcopenia (Fig. 1). The most important of these mechanisms are prolonged pro-inflammatory state, change in hormone secretion signaling activity, and unopposed oxidative stress. However, recent data suggest that these three pathophysiological mechanisms are highly interconnected and should be interpreted as components of a unique process leading to frailty and disability in old age [45].

Figure 1. Possible factors involved in the genesis of sarcopenia

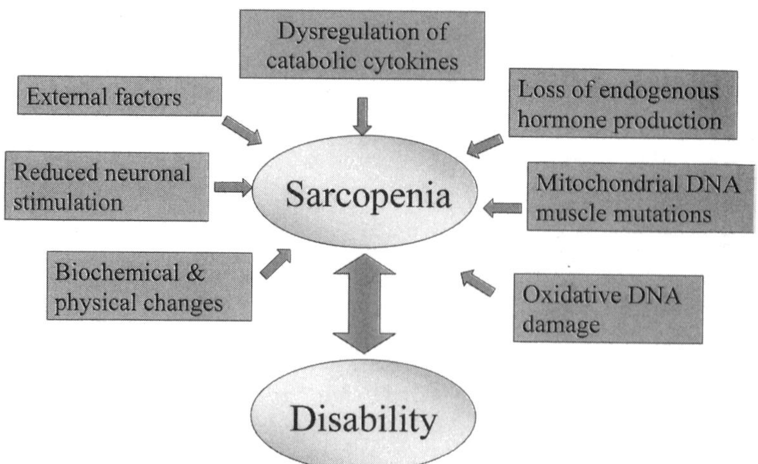

5. INFLAMMATION

Increased circulating and tissue levels of inflammatory markers have been observed in older persons, especially those who are frail and/or affected by comorbidity. Normally, cytokines or other biomarkers of inflammation initiate and regulate the acute phase inflammatory response during an infection, a trauma or any other type of stress. However, studies have suggested that a primary dysregulation of the mechanisms that initiate, modulate and shut off an inflammatory response often occurs with aging [46,47]. Such a dysregulation is mainly testimonied by high plasma levels of pro-inflammatory cytokines such as tumor necrosis factor-α (TNF-α), Interleukin-6 (IL-6) (48-50), (Interleukin-1) IL-1 and acute phase proteins in older persons [46]. In extreme situations, such as diseases that cause prolonged hypercatabolic states, severe muscle "wasting" may develop over a short period. However, a certain degree of muscle "decline" has been attributed to the reduced capacity of skeletal muscles to synthesize new proteins in the aging process [29]. An imbalance between muscle protein synthesis and degradation occurs, ultimately leading to reduced muscle mass, protein content and strength. Such imbalance has been linked to pro-inflammatory cytokines capable of inducing proteolysis or inhibiting protein synthesis. TNF-α induces muscle proteolysis and plays a significant role in muscle wasting (cachexia). TNF-α and IL-6 can also inhibit protein synthesis, either directly or by interfering with IGF-1 signaling [51].

Elevated plasma levels of each of the pro-inflammatory cytokines mentioned above have also been observed in many age-related diseases, such as anemia, osteoporosis, sarcopenia, atherosclerosis, cancer, type 2 DM, impaired cognitive functioning, and Alzheimer's disease. This further supports the theory that a core mechanism contributes to overall age-associated changes in functional capacity.

6. HORMONES

Anabolic agents shift the anabolic/catabolic balance of protein metabolism toward the synthesis of new proteins, which is needed to replace the proteins that are continuously catabolized, therefore maintaining muscle integrity and volume. Hypertrophy requires the proliferation of muscle nuclei (hyperplasia) in order to maintain the nuclear/cytoplasmic ratio (52). Hormonal factors shown to be related to muscle hypertrophy are: Insulin-like Growth Factor-1 (IGF-1), Growth Hormone (GH), testosterone and dehydroepiandrosterone. High IGF-1 concentrations are associated with characteristics that are opposite to those typical of aging, including decreased body fat content, increased muscle mass and improved metabolic homeostasis of glucose and lipids. At the muscular level, IGF-1 stimulates protein synthesis and satellite cell differentiation, thus, playing a crucial role in the maintenance of muscle mass and function. Many studies have provided insight into the signaling pathways by which IGF-1 affects muscle anatomy and function [53-55]. Circulating IGF-1 concentrations decrease with advancing age. The age-associated decline in IGF-1 plasma concentrations is influenced by reduced GH levels, and also by nutritional status, insulin and inflammatory cytokines. Specifically, the biologic activity of IGF-1 on muscle strength can be inhibited by IL-6 [55], suggesting that the detrimental effect of inflammation on muscle functioning may be mediated by IGF-1. Furthermore, studies provide evidence that the higher concentrations of pro-inflammatory cytokines found in older persons directly interferes with the IGF-1 gene protein expression and receptor sensibility in muscles [55,56]. High IL-6 and low IGF-1 plasma concentrations are considered risk factors for poor muscle strength, poor lower extremity performance and disability.

The aging process is associated with the loss of many anabolic signals to muscle function. Recent studies have shown that age is not only accompanied by a decline in anabolic activity, but an increase in catabolic signals as well. In fact, impairment of the anabolic IGF-1 signaling pathway may have several negative effects:

1) Reduced physical activity that is often observed in advanced age causes decreased stretch-activation stimulation of different muscle isoforms of IGF-1;
2) An age-related decline of GH influences IGF-1 muscle response;
3) The progressive loss of appetite with reduced food intake can result in malnutrition and eventual "wasting";
4) Loss of motoneurons that are essential for skeletal muscle functioning leads to atrophy and increased proteolysis.

There is evidence that the age-associated decline in GH levels in combination with lower IGF-1 levels also contributes to the development of sarcopenia [57,58]. The reduced pituitary secretion of GH is probably due to age-related changes in the GH-releasing hormone (GHRH). Unfortunately, treatment with GH has demonstrated many adverse effects, such as peripheral edema, arthralgias, glucose intolerance and type 2 diabetes [40]. Investigations have demonstrated that therapy with GHRH (somatorelin) in older persons is capable of restoring the age-related decline of the GH response [59]. More studies attempting to verify whether such pharmacological approaches can restore muscle functioning as well as the metabolic homeostasis in elderly persons while minimizing side effects are underway.

Testosterone affects muscle mass and muscle strength both directly and indirectly. It has been reported that testosterone increases protein synthesis and intramuscular mRNA concentrations of IGF-1 and decreases inhibitory IGF binding protein 4 concentrations [60]. Due to evidence that testosterone levels decline with advancing age, a negative impact on muscle function is not surprising. Older men with low circulating levels of testosterone tend to have lower muscle strength than men of the same age with normal testosterone, and studies utilizing supplemental therapy with testosterone have shown an increase in muscle mass and strength in elderly males. Testosterone has also been linked to body composition changes such as an increase in muscle mass and a decrease in fat mass [61]. The widespread use of testosterone replacement remains controversial due to safety concerns and inconsistent reports regarding clinically important outcome measures.

The production and the circulating levels of adrenal sex hormone precursors, dehydroepiandrosterone (DHEA) and DHEA sulphate (DHEAS), decline significantly with aging [62]. DHEAS serum levels have been correlated with parameters of body composition. Some clinical trials have shown that supplementation with DHEA resulted in increased muscle strength and decreased body fat [63]. However, more recently these findings were not confirmed in a large randomised controlled trial performed in men 60 to 80 years old. The mechanism by which DHEA acts on muscle function is probably related to the peripheral conversion to testosterone and dihydrotestosterone, but a direct effect of DHEAS cannot be excluded since specific receptors have been identified in muscle tissue.

Estrogen levels also decline with aging. Although estrogen has a direct anabolic effect on muscle cells in vitro, several authors believe that the effect of estrogen on muscle is mediated by their conversion to testosterone [64]. Interestingly, both estrogen and testosterone are capable of inhibiting IL-6 production, suggesting that an age-related decline of such hormones would play a pivotal role in catabolic signaling on muscle tissue. However, the available information regarding the effects of supplemental therapy of estrogen on muscle function is limited and the results are inconclusive. While some studies have concluded that estrogen therapy in postmenopausal women does not significantly affect muscle mass or strength [65,66], others suggest that estrogen therapy has a positive effect on body composition. For example, Sorensen et al [67] demonstrated that estrogen replacement therapy was significantly associated with an increase in lean body mass and also a decrease in total body fat.

As previously mentioned, advancing age is associated with impaired glucose handling mainly due to a reduction of insulin peripheral activity. Since insulin plays a pivotal role for muscle contraction by increasing glucose uptake and promoting intracellular glucose metabolism, it is plausible that age-related insulin resistance (IR) may be an important cause of poor muscle strength in old age. Furthermore, a reduction of insulin peripheral activity may reduce the muscle tissue anabolic rate leading to a relative catabolic state and in turn, facilitating sarcopenia. The contraction of Type I fibers is especially dependent on glucose entry and metabolism compared to contraction of Type IIa (fast twitch, oxidative, glycolytic) or IIb (fast twitch, glycolytic) fibers [68]. Type I fibers are more responsive to insulin, and are more representative of the muscle in older persons [69].

Over the aging process, changes in both the contractile efficiency of muscle fibers and changes in tissue quality, such as an increase in connective tissue and pericellular fat infiltration, may contribute to altered muscle function [70]. Moreover, insulin resistance (IR) could be further worsened by the occurrence of pericellular fat accumulation both directly and through the increased production of pro-inflammatory cytokines, such as IL-6 and TNF-α. Furthermore, a recent study demonstrated that a decline in aged skeletal muscle force might also be due to a reduction of L-type calcium channels, resulting in excitation-contraction uncoupling and less Ca^{2+} release by the sarcoplasmic reticulum (SR) [71]. Insulin has a stimulatory effect on intracellular calcium uptake [71]; thus, an age-related state of IR may negatively affect muscle contraction via this mechanism. It is well known that IGF-1 actively stimulates insulin receptors. Since IGF-1 levels decline throughout aging, the decline in muscle strength that is associated with aging may be mediated by decreasing plasma IGF-1 levels that contribute to IR. Studies will be needed in order to verify if the impact of IR on specific muscle tissue and functioning in aged individuals exists.

Certain changes typically occur in muscles of older adults. The quantity of muscle declines, although this varies between individuals, but the composition of the muscle changes with aging as well. Increased infiltration of fat deposited in skeletal muscle tissue may affect muscular function. Much of the existing data on the association between intramyocellular lipid (IML) content has been obtained directly from muscle tissue biopsies. However, the use of muscle attenuation through computed tomography (CT) scanning, as a measure of IML, has been validated [72]. In 45 men and women, the muscle fiber lipid content determined histologically with oil red staining was correlated with muscle attenuation. Thus, the use of CT-derived muscle attenuation should be considered a non-invasive method of measuring IML. In fact, Visser et al [73] demonstrated that increased skeletal muscle fat infiltration measured by CT scanning was associated with poorer lower extremity performance independently of total body fat and muscle area in older men and women.

7. OXIDATIVE STRESS

The accumulation of lipofuscina [74] and increased cross-linking of collagen [75] were the first observations reported on the effect of the aging process at the cellular level. At that time it was unknown that these modifications are, at least in part, related to oxidative stress. More recently, researchers have focused on the progressive changes that occur in the DNA structure and the underlying causes and potential consequences of these mutations. For example, a number of studies suggest that excess and unopposed oxidative stress is the main cause of increasing mitochondrial DNA (mtDNA) mutations with aging and in several age-related diseases. Accordingly, oxidative stress characterized by an uncontrolled production of free radicals is considered a major factor in the aging process. In aerobic biological systems, free radicals are primarily derived from oxygen and are produced by splitting a covalent bond into atoms or molecules with an unpaired electron, therefore forming highly reactive oxygen species (ROS). In normal physiological conditions, the intra-mitochondrial environment is characterized by a substantial equilibrium between the production of ROS and the activity of anti-oxidant mechanisms, such as glutathione peroxidase (GSH-Px) and superoxide dismutase (SOD). Several lines of research suggest that the endogenous production of ROS increases with age and, in parallel, the activity (but not the tissue concentration) of anti-oxidants declines, therefore increasing the risk of damage due to oxidative stress, especially at the level of the mtDNA. In addition to its effect on mtDNA, oxidative stress also adversely impacts other vulnerable targets, including lipid and protein components of membranes. Free radicals can cause lipid oxidation with a consequent reduction in transmembrane transportation. Age-related overproduction of ROS may also lead to the activation of apoptosis. Therefore, the accumulation of oxidatively damaged mtDNA, together with enhanced apoptosis act synergistically to cause the general decline of biochemical and physiological function of tissues over the aging process. The underlying mechanisms by which these events accompany the aging process remain to be identified and merit further investigation.

Studies suggest that the degree of unopposed oxidative stress is predictive of mortality. In particular, the production of free radicals in the heart, kidney and liver is inversely proportional to the maximum lifespan [76] and rate of mitochondrial oxygen radical generation is negatively associated with animal longevity. In animal models, caloric restriction, which decreases the rate of aging, also decreases mitochondrial oxygen radical production and oxidative damage to mtDNA.

The mitochondrial DNA/oxidative stress hypothesis can explain certain age-related disease states such as Parkinson's disease, Alzheimer's disease and skeletal muscle myopathies. Recently, epidemiological studies have suggested that dietary anti-oxidants may have a significant impact on age-related disease states [77,78]. This remains unproven in clinical trials. The clinical implications of oxidative stress are complex, and intervention studies are needed to further clarify the role of dietary and supplemental antioxidants in the prevention of age-associated frailty.

8. SUCCESSFUL AGING

The possibility of reaching the extreme end of the human lifespan results from the continuous adaptation of the body to respond to negative insults over the aging process. Healthy centenarians are a very selective group of persons representing one of the best living models of "successful aging". Many studies have focused on centenarians' anthropometric, endocrine and metabolic characteristics in order to formulate a clearer clinical picture of successful aging. They report that the average fat free mass (FFM) of healthy centenarians is similar to that of other aged subjects but lower than middle-aged adult subjects [79]. However, most healthy centenarians do not undergo the usual anthropometric derangement found in elderly persons. For example, the waist/hip ratio has been found to be lower in healthy centenarians than in other aged individuals. Regarding endocrine factors, total plasma IGF-1 concentrations were similar in both healthy centenarians and aged subjects, but the molar ratio IGF-1/IGF binding protein-3, an expression of free plasma IGF-1 concentration, was observed to be significantly elevated in healthy centenarians compared to elderly subjects [80]. This ratio is negatively correlated with body mass index, body fat content, plasma triglycerides, and FFA and LDL concentrations [80].

While serum markers may be useful for helping identify successful aging, caution should be used since the interpretation may be different in younger adults than in older persons. For example, in older persons, the ability of total cholesterol to predict age-related diseases such as coronary heart disease (CHD) has been challenged. In middle-aged adults, total cholesterol levels have been shown to have a direct association with CHD and mortality, but such a relationship in individuals over the age of 65 remains controversial. In older persons, a J or U-shaped association has been reported, suggesting that extremely high or low concentrations have an increased risk of death [81,82]; total cholesterol levels have also been shown to have a positive association, an inverse association, and no association with mortality in older persons.

Up to now, most studies have considered the association of total cholesterol on CHD in subjects under the age of 85 years. Interestingly, a recent study reporting data on fractionated lipoprotein levels among persons over the age of 85 years, concluded that low HDL cholesterol, but not high LDL cholesterol, is a risk factor for mortality from CHD and stroke in persons over the age of 85 [83]. Lipoprotein (a) [Lp(a)], a genetically controlled cholesterol-rich lipoprotein, has been hypothesized as an independent risk factor for premature CHD, stroke, and peripheral artery disease in elderly persons [84,85]. This observation may be due to the presence of Lp(a) in atherosclerotic plaques and its ability to stimulate smooth muscle proliferation [86].

The physiological and pathological roles of Lp(a) probably change with aging. Support for this comes from a study by Baggio et al [87], which reported no significant differences in Lp(a) serum concentrations among healthy centenarians, persons <65 and >65 years of age, even though Lp(a) has been proposed as an independent risk factor for cardiovascular disease. Centenarians with high Lp (a) levels had significantly higher IL-6 levels, thus characterizing the paradox of successful aging. Such data questions the idea that Lp(a) is under strict genetic control and suggests that environmental factors may play a significant role in older adults, including subclinical inflammatory states. Thus, a continuous remodeling of lipid metabolism may occur with aging and may be critical for successful aging. The deleterious reshaping of serum lipids and lipoproteins in young, adult and elderly individuals are considered risk factors for age-related diseases, while their biological significance in healthy centenarians remains unknown. Thus, only future investigations highlighting age-related changes in lipid physiology of healthy centenarians on mortality rates will resolve such discrepancies.

Healthy centenarians have a lower degree of oxidative stress. In fact, it has been shown that healthy centenarians have greater plasma antioxidant defenses than aged individuals. According to the remodeling theory on aging, the body continuously and correctly adapts to deleterious changes over time. As previously mentioned, an age-related up-regulation of the inflammatory response takes place over the aging process. In both sick and healthy elderly individuals, peripheral blood markers of inflammation (albumin, cholesterol, IL-6 and CRP) have been associated with increased risk for mortality. Interestingly, the age-related increase of serum IL-6 levels has been seen in both elderly and centenarian individuals [49,87]. IL-6 dysregulation has been suggested to play a role in the pathogenesis of a variety of age-related diseases, such as diabetes and atherosclerosis [88]. Indeed, healthy centenarians have elevated pro-inflammatory cytokine concentrations, but do not have the same high incidence of most age-related disease states in other elderly persons. Thus, in healthy centenarians such abnormal cytokine levels may reflect a state of subclinical inflammation. The reason why healthy centenarians adapt correctly to such insults remains unknown.

Whether healthy centenarians have some protective genetic factors that can protect against deleterious changes or facilitate the remodeling process remain unknown. Future investigations will be needed in order to provide the necessary answers.

Tables 3 and 4 summarize some of the clinical and biochemical evaluations described in the text above, and that can be used to assess the degree of "successfulness: of the aging process. Note that these are only examples. An exhaustive list would be very large, and out of the scope of this chapter.

Table 2.

Table 2. Diverse Techniques for Body Composition Evaluations

Method	Reliability	Advantages	Disadvantages
Hydrodensitometry	++	Traditional reference method for body composition research	High cost; long test duration (15-60'); difficult for persons who dislike, can't be submersed in water, or have difficulty expelling air from their lungs; reading errors if air remains in lungs; reading may vary due to body hydration.
Skin-fold Measurements	++	Low cost; test duration: 10-20'	Precision depends on the skill of the technician; accuracy depends on sites measured; difficulty in grasping skin-fold of obese; multiple readings are required for accuracy.
BIA	++++	Test duration: 10'; Moderate cost; low to moderate technician skill.	Electrolyte gel can be uncomfortable; accuracy depends on minimal variability caused by body hydration level; measures derived by the equation used.
DEXA	+++++	Test duration: 10-20';subjects only have to lie still; measures fat distribution throughout the body in a single scan; no need to account for air mass in the lungs.	Very high cost.
MRI	++++	Very useful for high quality images for body fat distribution.	Very high cost; requires a highly skilled technician.
CT	++++	Very useful for ratio intra-abdominal fat to extra-abdominal fat.	Very high cost; exposure to radiation
BOD POD	++++	Brief test duration: 20 sec;	Very high cost; limited in availability; requires further testing in order to verify test accuracy in measuring body composition.

Table 3.

Table 3. Summary of diverse techniques described in the text in older persons

Test	Purpose	Clinical Situation	Specific Examples
Glucose Clamp	To assess insulin action and secretion	Impaired glucose handling	Measurement of insulin-mediated glucose uptake and glucose stimulated insulin secretion (11)
Isometric Muscle strength (upper limb)	To assess handgrip muscle strength	Sarcopenia, predictor of disability and mortality	Handheld dynamometer (27)
Isometric Muscle strength (lower limb)	To assess lower extremity muscle strength	Sarcopenia	Hip Flexion, Knee Extension, Ankle dorsal flexion, Hip abduction
Balance	To assess static balance	Screening for falls	FICSIT balance score (89)
ADL	To assess self-care, mobility and incontinence	Disability screening	Katz (ADL) (23) Barthel Index (25)
IADL	To assess the ability to shop, cook, perform household activities and finances	Disability screening	Lawton (IADL) (24)
Physical performance tests	Quantitatively assess gait, balance, and risk of falls	Valid proxy for frailty and global susceptibility to adverse health outcomes	Tinetti performance oriented mobility (90) assessment Short physical performance battery (91)

Table 4. Summary of some laboratory tests utilized in older people

Test	Values	Clinical Importance
Fasting glucose (mg/dl)	≥126	Diabetes mellitus
OGTT 2 hr glucose (mg/dl)	≥200	Diabetes mellitus
Fasting glucose (mg/dl) +	<110 + <140	Normal glucose homeostasis
OGTT 2 hr glucose (mg/dl)	110-125 + <140	Impaired fasting glucose (IFG)
	<110 + 140-199	Impaired glucose tolerance (IGT)
	110-125 + 140-199	Combined IFG + IGT
Total cholesterol (mg/dl)		
	>200	Hypercholestolemia with increased cardiovascular risk
	<50	Frailty marker
HDL	≤ 35	Risk of atherosclerosis
	≥160	Risk of atherosclerosis
LDL		
Albumin (g/dl)	<3.5	Malnutrition
C-reactive protein	>0.5mg/dl	Inflammatory state
Hemoglobin	men: <12g/dl	Anemic state
	women: <13g/dl	Anemic state
Red blood cells	men: <4.3 x 10^6	Anemia, hemorrhage, hemolysis
	women: <4.0 x 106	
	men: >5.5 x 10^6/μl	Polycythemia
	women: >5.1 x 106/μl	
White blood cells	neutrophils: >7500/μl	Infection, inflammatory state, neoplasms, metabolic disease states
	eosinphils: >500/μl	allergies, neoplasms,
	monocytes: >1000/μl	infection, sarcoidosis
	lymphocytosis: >4000/μl	mieloproliferative disorders
	neutrophils:<1500/μl	neutropenia: altered production, excessiva destruction
	lymphocytes: <1000/μl	lymphopenia: altered immune response

8. CONCLUSIONS

It is widely recognized that the assessment of diseases status performed according to the traditional dichotomy "no disease vs. disease" is insufficient to understand the complexity of problems that influence health and well being in older persons. This concept was recognized long ago by geriatricians and implemented in the paradigm of "Comprehensive Geriatric Assessment". Accordingly, many researchers and clinicians have proposed that the direct assessment of physical and cognitive function provides the essential information that is needed to design effective interventions in frail older persons. However, this approach has never been completely translated into clinical practice and many geriatricians claim that the administration of any available medical treatment is still conditioned to a previous diagnosis of specific diseases and hypotheses about specific pathophysiological pathways. Furthermore, significant changes in health status may occur and be amenable to effective treatment long before any clear effect on physical and cognitive function is detected.

We propose that the concept of frailty – a condition that involves impairment in multiple physiological systems and is characterized by exhaustion of functional reserve, massive use of compensatory strategies and high risk of homeostatic breakdown – can be used by clinicians to gain a better understanding of the global burden of disease and reduced physical function in older persons and their interaction with the "pure" effect of aging. Unfortunately, there is still no agreement on the criteria that should be used in order to identify frail older persons. However, there is general consensus that comorbidity, disease susceptibility and risk of developing multiple health outcomes are commonly associated with the detection of abnormal circulating levels of several biomarkers and changes in body composition. Thus, composite measures of mobility, body composition, strength, circulating hormones and biomarkers of inflammation may help clinicians understand the severity of health status deterioration in their patients over and beyond the information provided by the simple diagnosis of diseases. Aggregate measures of these outcomes should be developed in future studies and are likely to replace the current criteria for the definition of frailty, both in research projects and in clinical practice.

REFERENCES

1) Walston J, Fried LP: Frailty and the older man. Med Clin North Am, 1999 Sep;83(5):1173-94
2) Ferrucci L, Cavazzini C, Corsi A, Bartali B, Russo CR, Lauretani F, Ferrucci L. Cavazzini C, Corsi AM, Bartali B, Russo CR, Lauretani F, Bandinelli S, Bandinelli S, Guralnik JM: Biomarkers of frailty in older persons. J Endocrinol Invest, 2002;25;10-5
3) Ueno L, Yamashita Y, Moritani T, Nakamura E: Biomarkers of aging in women and the rate of longitudinal changes. J Physiol Anthropol, 2003; 22: 37-46
4) NCCLS: How to define, determine, and utilize reference intervals in the clinical laboratory; proposed guideline. NCCLS document C28P (ISBN 1-56238-143-1), NCCLS, 940 West Valley Road, Suite 1400, Wayne, Penn 19087, USA, 1992
5) Tietz NW, Shuey DF, Wekstein DR: Laboratory values in fit aging individuals--sexagenarians through centenarians. Clin Chem, 1992 Jun;38(6):1167-85
6) Fink RI, Kolterman OG, Griffin J, Olegsky JM: Mechanism of insulin resistance in ageing. J Clin Invest, 1983; 71: 1523-35
7) Rowe JW, Minaker KL, Pallotta JA, Flier JS: Characterization of the insulin resistance in aging. J Clin Invest, 1983; 71: 1581-7
8) Gumbiner B, Thorburn AW, Ditzler TM, Bulacan F, Henry RR: Role of impaired intracellular glucose metabolism in the insulin resistance of aging. Metabolism, 1992;41:1115-21

9) Ferrannini E, Vichi S, Beck-Nielsen H, Laakso M, Paolisso G, Smith U: European Group for the study of Insulin Resistance (EGIR). Insulin action and age. Diabetes, 1996; 45:947-53
10) Kosaka K, Kuzuya T, Hagura R, Yoshinaga H: Insulin response to oral glucose load is consistently decreased in established non-insulin-dependent diabetes mellitus: the usefulness of decreased early insulin response as a predictor of non-insulin-dependent diabetes mellitus. Diabet Med, 1996:S109-19
11) Defronzo 79: Glucose intolerance and aging: evidence for tissue insensitivity to insulin. Diabetes, 1979 Dec;28(12):1095-101
12) Lipid Research Clinics Program Epidemiology Committee: Plasma lipid distributions in selected North American populations: the Lipid Research Program Prevalence Study. Circulation 1979;60: 427-439
13) Raiha I, Marniemi J, Puukka P, Toikka T, Ehnholm C, Sourander L: Effect of serum lipids, lipoproteins, and apolipoproteins on vascular and nonvascular mortality in the elderly. Arterioscler Thromb Vasc Biol, 1997 Jul;17(7):1224-32
14) Manolio TA, Ettinger WH, Tracy RP, Kuller LH, Borhani NO, Lynch JC et al: Epidemiology of low cholesterol levels in older adults. The Cardiovascular Health Study, Circulation 1993; 87: 728-37
15) Schatz IJ, Masaki K, Yano K Chen R, Rodriguez BL, Curb JD: Cholesterol and all-cause mortality in elderly people from the Honolulu Heart Program: a cohort study, Lancet. 2001 Aug 4;358(9279):351-5
16) Brescianinni S, Maggi S, Farchi G, Mariotti S, Di Carlo A, Baldereschi M, Inzitari S: Low total cholesterol and increased risk of dying: Are low levels clinical warning signs in the elderly? Results from the Italian Longitudinal Study on Aging. JAGS, 2003; 51: 991-6
17) Pekkanen J, Nissinen A, Vartiainen E, Salonen JT, Punsar S, Karvonen MJ: Changes in serum cholesterol level and mortality: a 30 year follow up. Am J Epidemiol, 1994; 139: 155-65
18) Corti MC, Guralnik J, Salive M, Harris T, Ferrucci L, Glynn R, Havlik R: Clarifying the direct relation between total cholesterol levels and death from coronary heart disease in older persons. Annuals of Internal Medicine, 1997; 126: 753-760
19) Schaefer EJ, Moussa PB, Wilson PW, McGee D, Dallal G, Castelli WP: Plasma lipoproteins in healthy octogenarians: lack of reduced high density lipoprotein cholesterol levels: results from the Framingham Heart Study. Metabolism, 1989 Apr;38(4):293-6
20) Volpato S, Leveille S, Corti MC, Harris T, Guralnik J: The value of serum albumin and high-density lipoprotein cholesterol in defining mortality risk in older persons with low serum cholesterol. JAGS, 2001; 49: 1142-1147
21) Masoro EJ: Physiological system markers of aging. Exp Gerontol, 1988;23(4-5):391-7
22) Fried LP, Tangen CM, Walston J, Newman AB, Hirsch C, Gottdiener J, Seeman T, Tracy R, Kop WJ, Burke G, McBurnie MA: Cardiovascular Health Study Collaborative Research Group. Frailty in older adults: evidence for a phenotype. J Gerontol A Biol Sci Med Sci, 2001;56(3):M146-56
23) Katz S, Akpom CA: 12 Index of ADL. Med Care May, 14 (5 suppl):116-8; 1976
24) Lawton MP, Brody EM: Assessment of older people:self-maintaining and instrumental activities of daily living. Gerontologist, 1969; 9: 179-186
25) Wade DT, Colin C: The Barthel ADL Index – a standard measure of physical disability. Int Disabil Studies, 1988; 10: 64-67
26) Studenski S, Perera S, Wallace D, Chandler JM, Duncan PW, Rooney E, Fox M, Guralnik JM: Physical performance measures in the clinical setting. J Am Geriatr Soc, 2003;51(3):314-22

27) Rantanen T, Guralnik JM, Foley D, Masaki K, Leveille S, Curb JD, White L: Midlife hand grip strength as a predictor of old age disability. JAMA, 1999; 10;281(6):558-60
28) Rantanen T, Volpato S, Ferrucci L, Heikkinen E, Fried LP, Guralnik JM: Handgrip strength and cause-specific and total mortality in older disabled women: exploring the mechanism. J Am Geriatr Soc, 2003 May;51(5):636-41
29) Roubenoff R: The Pathophysiology of Wasting in the Elderly. J Nutr, 1999;129:256S-259S
30) Williamson DF: Descriptive epidemiology of body weight and weight changes in 17,000 adults. Int J. Obes, 1988; 12:391-401
31) Bartali B, Benvenuti E, Corsi AM, Bandinelli S, Russo CR, Di Iorio A, Lauretani F, Ferrucci L: Changes in anthropometric measures in men and women across the life-span: findings from the InCHIANTI study. Soz Praventivmed, 2002; 47(5): 336-48
32) Elahi D, Dyke MM, Andres R: Aging, fat, metabolism and obesity. In Masoro EJ (ed): Handbook of Physiology. Section 11: Aging. Oxford University Press, New York, 1995:47
33) Visscher TL, Seidell JC, Molarius A, van der Kuip D, Hofman A, Witteman JC: A comparison of body mass index, waist-hip ratio and waist circumference as predictors of all-cause mortality among the elderly: the Rotterdam study. Int J Obes Relat Metab Disord, 2001;25(11):1730-5
34) Carmeli E, Coleman R, Reznick AZ. The biochemistry of aging muscle. Exp. Gerontol, 37:477-89, 2002
35) Zeynep E, Faisal Beg M, Burke D, De Luca C: Effects of aging on motor-unit control properties. Am Physiol Soc, 2081-91,1999
36) Mecocci P, Fano G, Fulle S, MacGarey U, Shinobu L, Polidori MC, Cherubini A Vecchiet J, Senin U, Beal MF: Age-dependent increases in oxidative damage to DNA, lipids and proteins in human skeletal muscle. Free Radic Biol Med, 26:303-8, 1999
37) McKenzie D, Bua E, McKiernan S, Cao Z, Aiken JM, Wanagat J: Mitochondrial DNA deletion mutations: a causal role in sarcopenia. Eur J Biochem, 269:2010-5, 2002
38) Baumgartner R, Koehler K, Romero L, Garry P: Serum albumin is associated with skeletal muscle in elderly men and women. Am J Clin Nutr, 64:552-8,1996.Frisancho AR. Triceps skinfold and upper arm muscle norms for assessment of nutritional status. Am J Clin Nutr. 1974; 27:1052-8.
39) Kamel H, Maas D, Duthie E: Role of hormones in the pathogenesis and management of sarcopenia. Drugs Aging, 2002; 19: 869-877
40) Blackman MR, Sorkin JD, Munzer T, Bellantoni MF, Busby-Whitehead J, Stevens TE, Jayme J, O'Connor KG, Christmas C, Tobin JD, Stewart KJ, Cottrell E, St Clair C, Pabst KM, Harman S: Growth hormone and sex steroid administration in healthy aged women and men: a randomized controlled trial. JAMA, 2002 Nov 13;288(18):2282-92
41) Iovino M, Monteleone P, Steardo L: Repetitive growth hormone-releasing hormone administration restores the attenuated growth hormone (GH) response to GH-releasing hormone testing in normal aging. J Clin Endocrinol Metab, 1989;69(4):910-3
42) Roubenoff R: Inflammatory and hormonal mediators of cachexia. J Nutr, 1997;127:1014S-1016S
43) Roubenoff R: Catabolism of aging: is it an inflammatory process? Curr Opin Clin Nutr Metab Care, 2003;6(3):295-9
44) Frisancho AR: Triceps skinfold and upper arm muscle norms for assessment of nutritional status. Am J Clin Nutr 1974; 27:1052-8

45) Ferrucci L, Guralnik J: Inflammation, hormones, and body composition at a crossroad. Am J Med, 2003 Oct 15;115(6):501-2
46) Heymfield SB, McManus C, Smith et al: Anthropometric measurement of muscle mass: revised for equations for calculating bone free arm muscle area. Am J Clin Nutr, 1982; 36: 680-690
47) Brunnsgard H, Pederson M, Pederson BK: Aging and proinflammatory cytokines. Curr Opin Hematol 8: 131-136, 2001
48) Franceschi C, Bonafè M, Valensin S et al: Inflamm-aging: An evoluzinary perspective on immunosenescence. Ann NY Acad Sci, 908: 244-254, 2000
49) Ershler WB: Interleukin-6: a cytokine for gerontologists. J Am Geriat Soc, 41:176-181, 1993
50) Fagiolo U, Cossarizza A, Scala E, et al: Increased cytokine production in mononuclear cells of healthy elderly people. Eur J Immunol, 23: 2375-2378,1993
51) Albright JW, Albright JF: Soluble receptors and other substances that regulate proinflammatory cytokines in young and aging humans. J Geronto A Biol Sci Med Sci, 55: 20-25, 2000
52) Frost RA, Lang CH: Regulation of insulin-like growth factor-1 in skeletal muscle and muscle cells. Minevra Endocrinol, 2003;28(1):53-73
53) Barton-Davis ER, Shoturma DI, Sweeney HL: Contribution of satellite cells to IGF-I induced hypertrophy of skeletal muscle. Acta Physiol Scand, 1999;167(4):301-5
54) Cappola AR, Bandeen-Roche K, Wand GS, Volpato S, Fried LP: Association of IGF-I levels with muscle strength and mobility in older women. J Clin Endocrinol Metab, 2001;86(9):4139-46
55) Cappola A, Qian-Li X, Ferrucci L, Guralnik JM, Volpato S, Fried LP: Insulin-like Growth Factor I and Interleukin-6 Contribute Synergistically to Disability and Mortality in Older Women. JCEM, 88: 2019-25, 2003
56) Barbieri M, Ferrucci L, Ragno E, Corsi A, Bandinelli S, Bonafe M, Olivieri F, Giovagnetti S, Franceschi C, Guralnik JM, Paolisso G: Chronic inflammation and the effect of IGF-I on muscle strength and power in older persons. Am J Physiol Endocrinol Metab, 2003;284(3):E481-7
57) Ferrucci L, Penninx BW, Volpato S, Harris TB, Bandeen-Roche K, Balfour J, Leveille SG, Fried LP, Md JM: Change in muscle strength explains accelerated decline of physical function in older women with high interleukin-6 serum levels. J Am Geriatr Soc, 2002;50(12):1947-54
58) Rudman D: Growth hormone, body composition and aging. J Am Geriatr Soc, 1985; 33: 800-1
59) Kelijam M: Age-related alterations of growth hormone/insulin-like-growth-factor J axis. J Am Geriatr Soc, 1991; 39: 295-307
60) Baumgartner RN, Waters DL, Gallagher D, Morley JE, Garry PJ: Predictors of skeletal muscle mass in elderly men and women. Mech Ageing Dev. 1999;107(2):123-36
61) Mooradian AD, Morley JE, Korenman SG: Biological actions of androgens. Endocr Rev, 1987; 8: 1-28
62) Baulieu EE, Thomas G, Legrain S, Lahlou N, Roger M, Debuire B, Faucounau V, Girard L, Hervy MP, Latour F, Leaud MC, Mokrane A, Pitti-Ferrandi H, Trivalle C, de Lacharriere O, Nouveau S, Rakoto-Arison B, Souberbielle JC, Raison J, Le Bouc Y, Raynaud A, Girerd X, Forette F: Dehydroepiandrosterone (DHEA), DHEA sulfate, and aging: contribution of the DHEAge Study to a sociobiomedical issue. Proc Natl Acad Sci U S A, 2000;97(8):4279-84
63) Tummala S, Svec F: Correlation between the administered dose of DHEA and serum levels of DHEA and DHEA-S in human volunteers: analysis of published data. Clin Biochem, 1999;32(5):355-61

64) Grinspoon S, Corcoran C, Miller K, Biller BM, Askari H, Wang E, Hubbard J, Anderson EJ, Basgoz N, Heller HM, Klibanski A: Body composition and endocrine function in women with acquired immunodeficiency syndrome. J Clin Endocrinol Metab 1997;82: 1332-7
65) Haarbo J, Marslew U, Gotfredsen A, Christiansen C: Postmenopausal hormone replacement therapy prevents central distribution of body fat after menopause. Metabolism, 1991;40(12):1323-6
66) Gower BA, Nyman L: Associations among oral estrogen use, free testosterone concentration, and lean body mass among postmenopausal women. J Clin Endocrinol Metab, 2000;85(12):4476-80
67) Sorensen MB, Rosenfalck AM, Hojgaard L, Ottesen B: Obesity and sarcopenia after menopause are reversed by sex hormone replacement therapy. Obes Res, 2001; 9: 622-6
68) Song XM, Ryder JW, Kawano Y, Chibalin AV, Krook A, Zierath JR: Muscle fiber type specificity in insulin signal transduction. Am J Physiol, 277:R1690-6, 1999
69) Staron R, Hagerman F, Hikida R, Murrey T, Hostler D, Crilll M, Ragg K, Toma K: Fiber type composition of the vastus lateralis muscle of young men and women. Journal of histochemistry & cytochemistry, 48:623-629, 2000. Lexell J, Henriksson-Larsen K, Wilblad B, Siostrom M: Distribution of aging studied in whole muscle cross-sections. Muscle Nerve, 6:588-595,1983
70) Madsen OR, Lauridsen UB, Hartkopp A, Sorensen OH: Muscle strength and soft tissue composition as measured by dual energy x-ray absorptiometry in women aged 18-87 years. Eur J Appl Physiol Occup Physiol, 76: 239-45, 1997
71) Paolisso G, Gambardella A, Balbi V, Galzeranno D, Verza M, Varricchio M, D'Onofrio F : Effects of magnesium and nifedipine infusions on insulin action. Substrate oxidation and blood pressure in aged hypertensive patients. Am J Hypertens, 920-26,1993
72) Goodpaster BH, Kelley DE, Thaete FL, He J, Ross R: Skeletal muscle attenuation determined by computed tomography is associated with skeletal muscle lipid content. Appl Physiol, 2000;89(1):104-10
73) Visser M, Deeg DJ, Lips P, Harris TB, Bouter LM: Skeletal muscle mass and muscle strength in relation to lower-extremity performance in older men and women. J Am Geriatr Soc, 2000;48(4):381-6
74) Strehler BL: Time, cells and aging. Academic Press, New York, 1981
75) Kohn RR: Aging of animals: possible mechanisms. In Kohn RR, ed, Principles of mammalian aging, Prentice-Hall, Englewood Cliffs, NJ, 1978
76) Sohal RS, Svensson I, Sohal BH, Brunk UT: Superoxide anion radical production in different animal species. Mech Ageing Dev, 1989;49(2):129-35
77) Gilgun-Sherki Y, Melamed E, Offen D: Antioxidant treatment in Alzheimer's disease: current state. J Mol Neurosci, 2003;21(1):1-12
78) Paolini M, Sapone A, Canistro D, Chieco P, Valgimigli L: Antioxidant vitamins for prevention of cardiovascular disease. Lancet, 2003 ;362(9387):920
79) Paolisso G, Gambardella A, Balbi V, Ammendola S, D'Amore A, Varricchio M: Body composition, body fat distribution, and resting metabolic rate in healthy centenarians. Am J Clin Nutr, 1995;62(4):746-50
80) Paolisso G, Ammendola S, Del Buono A, Gambardella A, Riondino M, Tagliamonte MR, Rizzo MR, Carella C, Varricchio M: Serum levels of insulin-like growth factor-I (IGF-I) and IGF-binding protein-3 in healthy centenarians: relationship with plasma leptin and lipid concentrations, insulin action, and cognitive function. J Clin Endocrinol Metab, 1997;82(7):2204-9
81) Frank JW, Reed DM, Grove JS, Benfante R: Will lowering population levels of serum cholesterol affect total mortality? Expectations from the Honolulu Heart Program. J Clin Epidemiol, 1992;45(4):333-46

82) Stemmermann GN, Chyou PH, Kagan A, Nomura AM, Yano K: Serum cholesterol and mortality among Japanese-American men. The Honolulu (Hawaii) Heart Program. Arch Intern Med, 1991;151(5):969-72
83) Weverling-Rijnsburger AW, Jonkers IJ, van Exel E, Gussekloo J, Westendorp RG: High-density vs low-density lipoprotein cholesterol as the risk factor for coronary artery disease and stroke in old age. Arch Intern Med, 2003 14;163(13):1549-54
84) Maher V, Brown BG: Lipoprotein (a) and coronary heart disease. Curr Opin Lipidol, 1995; 6: 229-235
85) Dahlen G: Lp(a) lipoprotein in cardiovascular disease. Atherosclerosis, 1994; 108: 111-26
86) Sansoni P, Cossarizza A, Brianti V, Fagnoni F, Snelli G, Monti D, Marcato A, Passeri G, Ortolani C, Forti E, et al: Lymphocyte subsets and natural killer cell activity in healthy old people and centenarians. Blood, 1993;82(9):2767-73
87) Baggio G, Donazzan S, Monti D, Mari D, Martini S, Gabelli C, Dalla Vestra M, Previato L, Guido M, Pigozzo S, Cortella I, Crepaldi G, Franceschi C: Lipoprotein(a) and lipoprotein profile in healthy centenarians: a reappraisal of vascular risk factors. FASEB J, 1998;12(6):433-7
88) Pickup JC, Mattock MB, Chusney GD, et al: NIDDM as a disease of the innate immune system: association of acute-phase reactants and interleukin-6 with metabolic syndrome X. Diabetologia, 1997; 40:1286-1292
89) Judge JO, Schechtman K, Cress E: The relationship between physical performance measures and independence in instrumental activities of daily living. The FICSIT Group. Frailty and Injury: Cooperative Studies of Intervention Trials. J Am Geriatr Soc, 1996;44(11):1332-41
90) Tinetti ME: Performance oriented assessment of mobility problems in elderly patients. J Am Geriatr Soc, 1986;34: 119-126
91) Guralnik JM, Simonsick EM, Ferrucci L, Glynn RJ, Berkman LF, Blazer DG, Scherr PA, Wallace RB: A short physical performance battery assessing lower extremity function: association with self-reported disability and prediction of mortality and nursing home admission. J Gerontol, 1994;49(2):M85-94

Chapter 8

BIOLOGICAL SCREENING AND IMPACT IN ELDERLY CANCER PATIENTS

Anne-Chantal Braud and Martine Extermann

Martine Extermann, H. Lee Moffitt Cancer Center and Research Institute, Tampa, Florida, Professor of Oncology and Medicine, University of South Florida College of Medicine, Tampa, Florida. Anne Chantal Braud, Institut Paoli-Calmettes, Marseille, France.

Aging is a universal phenomenon but the aging of human beings involves a number of special mechanisms. Some may be useful in assessing elderly cancer patients before starting chemotherapy. Oncologists will be interested if biological tests may predict response, toxicity or survival of elderly patients. There is still a lot of uncertainty in the prediction of life expectancy in individuals, even if the concept of "biological age" has been created. This concept has been largely used subjectively especially when a patient look younger or older than he is. In a contrast a number of attempts were made in this connection to establish batteries of biomarkers able to predict age, survival, functional status. It is noteworthy that there are any reliable biomarkers for mental function or functional state despite the fact that earlier decline are often noted in elderly patients regardless of their pathology In elderly cancer patients, these laboratory tests might be useful indicators to predict life expectancy, functional status, risk of acute toxicity and to improve follow up during treatment. We will discuss all these aspects in cancer patients and in specific diseases as soon as feasible We will state all the aspect of biology in elderly cancer patients, test available, value and impact in helping medical decision making.

1. BIOLOGY AND THE RELATIONSHIP BETWEEN CANCER AND AGING

Although several hypotheses have been postulated, the cellular and molecular mechanisms regulating the physiological process of ageing and senescence have not been fully elucidated. Ageing cannot be considered to be directly responsible for the carcinogenic process but the susceptibility of older cells to environmental carcinogens may facilitate some molecular changes involved in carcinogenesis. Some of the mechanism of both geriatric and oncologic interest are the production of reactive oxygen species and free radicals, telomere length, control of tumor suppressor genes No clinically usable test is presently available along those lines.

In the same way there is a well-characterized remodeling of immune function with advancing age [1,2]. However, the consequences are not fully established even if it is apparent that healthy older individuals are more susceptible to reactivation of tuberculosis or herpes zoster. A clear change in T-cell function with age can be measured in vitro. There is an accumulation of T cells that have cell surface characteristics of memory cells while naïve T cells decrease. Distinct studies suggest that T cells acting as "primitive" natural killer cells (NK cells) with phenotype intermediate between T and NK cells increase with ageing. B cell immunity is poorly modified but some data suggest that ageing is associated with reduce level of specific gamma globulin and increased level of polyvalent B cells. The concentration of antibodies specific for foreign antigens declines and can be partially explained by a decrease in the number of specific antibody forming cells and impaired T-lymphocyte help as the response of T lymphocyte help [3]. Link between immune system and cancer is not yet clearly established but might partly explain changes observed in term of immunity, increased incidence of cancer in old people.

Normal human cells especially leukocytes might be responsible for changes in the pattern of cytokine secretion, increased level of interleukin 4 and interferon gamma, and regulation of cancer growth. All these mechanisms might be involved in specific and most often slow tumoral growth observed in old patients.

These immune changes play an important role when physician discuss specific treatment for example immunotherapy, bone marrow transplantation or management of infections and other side effects. However, prognostic value of such parameter is unknown, screening tests are unknown since they have never been investigated. They might help physicians to identify elderly patients with high risk of infection due to lymphopenia or low level of immunoglobulin as well as inadequate response to immunotherapy.

2. THE RELATIONSHIP BETWEEN BIOLOGY AND SURVIVAL

Biological markers of ageing and risk of death are still poorly known. Frailty was associated with increased level of interleukine-6 and D-dimer. Cohen et al recently reported these parameters in 4162 participants aged 65 years or older. More than 1763 people with informative blood samples, both high levels of interleukine-6 or D-dimer alone or in combination were associated with poorer functional status. Levels of interleukine-6 and D-dimer were not correlated (p:0.44). Both were significantly associated with mortality. In the sample 20% of patients died of cancer, 23.8% died of myocardial infarction and 23% of other circulatory conditions. In the high IL6 and d-dimer group, one third dead from myocardial infarction, while activity of daily living, instrumental activity of daily living, and decline of function were significantly correlated with these two parameters [4]. This correlation between inflammatory markers and the risk of coronary disease as well as with adverse outcome had been largely demonstrated but is still poorly investigated in cancer patients. Its value and impact on treatment are unexplored. Cytokine of inflammation have various pejorative effects on the neuroendocrine system, skeletal muscle, bone and central nervous system perhaps via increase production of oxygen free radicals and distinct mechanism. The activation of the coagulation system interact with immunocytes [5], cell migration, vascular remodeling as well as endothelial cell activation that could partly explain it pejorative value in elderly cancer patients [6].

On another side, anaemia and haemoglobin levels was correlated not only with functional decline but also mortality [7]. An analysis from Optime study, based on older patients with cardiac heart failure, median age 65, hemoglobin level less than 11.6g/dl was a co-morbid condition, a significant predictor of death and rehospitalization after the adjustment for a variety of baseline co-factors (p:0.015).

3. THE RELATIONSHIP BETWEEN BIOLOGY AND FUNCTIONAL STATUS

Frailty and increased vulnerability are associated with various biological changes in elderly patients. However, the major question in elderly cancer patients is to predict the frailty or the loss of autonomy rather than to determine biological pattern of these advanced and most often poorly reversible states.

Most oncologists search clinical and biological predictive parameters. Anaemia and blood cell counts are correlated with increased functional dependence in elderly patients [8,9] and recommendations for the level of haemoglobin is largely higher than in younger cancer patients since NCNN and ASCO recommended to maintain haemoglobin level higher than 12g/dl. Anaemia is correlated with dementia [10], iatrogenic complications, and dependence. Lymphopenia at diagnosis is currently associated with malnutrition and frailty [11]. Lymphopenic patients (<1000/mm3) had functional disability, cognitive impairment as measured by the mini mental status test and poor prognostic. As a result, lymphopenia may be considered as a significant marker of vulnerability in elderly patients.

In a recent study Cohen et al suggest that activation of inflammatory pathway is predictive of loss of autonomy [4]. In elderly patients with no baseline impairment, high level of interleukine-6 or D-dimer are significantly associated with loss of autonomy in basal activities (ADL) Only changes in ADL and IADL were associated with IL-6 and d-dimer level (RR: 2.00), without any evidence of interaction between interleukine-6 and d-dimer levels (interaction 0.44). A trend of correlation is observed when baseline ADL or Instrumental Activity Daily Living (IADL) are abnormal. Same predictive value has been reported for CRP and acute patient's status for example or 3 and 7 year survival [12]. These results might be interesting in elderly cancer patients but are still poorly used. One of the limitation concerning the use of these parameters in elderly cancer patients is the well-established link between cancer and inflammation especially d-dimer. Surrogate increase of d-dimer might be a useful indicator but remains poorly used and investigated.

4. THE RELATIONSHIP BETWEEN BIOLOGY AND TOXICITY OF TREATMENT

Initial assessment is supposed to predict as soon as feasible toxicity and outcome of treatment. Clinical assessment gives some insights but only predicts partially toxicity and tolerance of treatment. Some authors tried to identify biological parameters to help the assessment of the risk of toxicity before starting the treatment of cancer. Freyer found that albumin was correlated with grade III or grade IV toxicities [13]. Other suggested that pre-albumin, another marker of metabolism and inflammation, might be a better predictor of toxicity of chemotherapy in patients with cancer.

Nevertheless, serum albumin can be easily and routinely measured in most clinics. Low levels of serum albumin indicate chronic problems. However, it is important to eliminate malnutrition as a cause of low serum albumin. Patients with low serum albumin can still have chemotherapy but should be closely monitored for complications. Extermann et al. demonstrated a straight correlation between albumin level and tolerance of chemotherapy. Low level of albumin was significantly correlated with non-hematological grade III or IV toxicity (p:0.007) while grade IV hematological toxicity was correlated with initial red blood cell count [14].

Beside albumin and red blood cell counts, creatinine clearance helps dose adjustment in elderly patients. These parameters are fully necessary to predict the risk of toxicity or dose adaptation of treatment. Clearance of creatinine must be used rather than creatinine because of physiological sarcopenia in elderly [15]. It is to note that some drugs such as cisplatin or capecitabine may have major toxicity in elderly due to renal failure. Mucositis and haematological toxicity rather than cutaneous toxicity of capecitabine in elderly patients have been largely correlated with creatinine clearance [16], whereas vinorelbine or docetaxel toxicity have never been associated with renal function. Specific pharmacokinetic studies will help us to investigate dose adjustment of some drugs in elderly patients.

Significance of early fall in lymphocytes count during chemotherapy is unknown in elderly since it is predictive of increased risk of febrile neutropenia in younger cancer patients [17].

5. ARE BIOCHEMICAL MARKERS INDICATORS OF AGING OR CANCER?

Biochemical markers indicating poor prognosis in patients with prostate cancer for example (eg, increased CRP, increased IL-6, decreased pre-albumin) were independent of age. This observation raised the question of whether these factors were markers of ageing or of cancer. Clinicians are most often faced with two issues: assessment of cancer and assessment of ageing and it is most often very difficult to identify biological parameters of these two distinct mechanisms: some elderly patients have normal levels of certain biochemical parameters, which support the belief that disease, not ageing, is the main cause of the change in such markers.

6. CONCLUSIONS

As a result, a single biochemical parameter could not give an overall assessment of the patient, but might be significant for a specific clinical problem such as malnutrition or organ malfunction. The question concerning assessment of frailty or future disability remains unsolved and further research is needed. Simple assessments of clinical diagnosis or biochemical markers or a combination of both are probably more suitable. However screening test such as CRP, albumin, and haemoglobin could be used for initial general screening as these were based on evidence of predicting toxicities.

ADDENDUM

As this chapter was in press, we deplored the accidental death of Anne-Chantal Braud. Her dynamism and input will be missed by the geriatric oncology community.

REFERENCES

1. Ginaldi L; De Martinis M; D'Ostilio A; Marini L; Loreto MF; Corsi MP; Quaglino D: The immune system in the elderly: I. specific humoral immunity. Immunol Res. 1999;20(2):101-8
2. Burns EA, Leventhal EA. Aging, immunity, and cancer. Cancer Control. 2000. Nov-Dec; 7(6):513-22
3. Issa JP. Age-related epigenetic changes and the immune system. Clin Immunol. 2003 Oct; 109(1):103-8
4. Cohen HJ; Harris T; Pieper CF: Coagulation and activation of inflammatory pathways in the development of functional decline and mortality in the elderly. Am J Med. 2003;114:180-187
5. Opal SM: Phylogenetic and functional relationships between coagulation and the innate immune response. Crit Care Med. 2000 Sep;28(9 Suppl):S77-80
6. Malek AM; Alper SL; Izumo S: Hemodynamic shear stress and its role in atherosclerosis. JAMA. 1999 Dec 1;282(21):2035-42
7. Chaves PH; Ashar B; Guralnik JM; Fried LP: Looking at the relationship between hemoglobin concentration and prevalent mobility difficulty in older women: should the criteria currently used to define anemia in older people be reevaluated? J Am Geriatr Soc. 2002 Jul;50(7):1257-64
8. Siena S; Secondino S; Giannetta L; Carminati O; Pedrazzoli P: Optimising management of neutropenia and anaemia in cancer chemotherapy-advances in cytokine therapy. Crit Rev Oncol Hematol. 2003 Oct 15;48(Suppl):S39-47
9. Evans WJ. Physical function in men and women with cancer. Effects of anemia and conditioning. Oncology (Huntingt). 2002 Sep;16(9 Suppl 10:109-15
10. Milward EA; Grayson DA; Creasey H; Janu MR; Brooks WS; Broe GA: Evidence for association of anaemia with vascular dementia. Neuroreport. 1999 Aug 2;10(11):2377-81
11. Jazwinski SM: Biological aging research today: potential, peeves, and problems. Exp Gerontol. 2002 Oct-Nov;37(10-11):1141-6
12. Reuben DB; Cheh AI; Harris TB et al: Peripheral blood markers of inflammation predict mortality and functional decline in high-functioning community-dwelling older persons. J Am Geriatr Soc. 2002;50:638-644
13. Freyer G; Tranchand B; Ligneau B; Ardiet C; Souquet PJ; Court-Fortune I; Riou R; Rebattu P; Boissel JP; Trillet-Lenoir V; Girard P: Population pharmacokinetics of doxorubicin, etoposide and ifosfamide in small cell lung cancer patients: results of a multicentre study. Br J Clin Pharmacol. 2000 Oct;50(4):315-24
14. Extermann M; Yoder J; Overcash J; Wallace K; Vranas P; Braud AC; Luciani A; Carbonel A; Cantor AB: Influence of concomitant medications metabolized by cytochrome P-450 on toxicity from chemotherapy. 8th International Conference on Geriatric Oncology, Rome, Italy, Nov 21-22, 2003
15. Newman AB; Yanex D; Harris T et al. Weight change in old age and its association with mortality. J Am Geriatr Soc. 2001;49:1309-1318
16. Poole C; Gardiner J; Twelves C; Johnston P; Harper P; Cassidy J; Monkhouse J; Banken L; Weidekamm E; Reigner B: Effect of renal impairment on the pharmacokinetics and

tolerability of capecitabine (Xeloda) in cancer patients. Cancer Chemother Pharmacol. 2002 Mar;49(3):225-34

17. Blay JY; Chauvin F; Le Cesne A; Anglaret B; Bouhour D; Lasset C; Freyer G; Philip T; Biron P: Early lymphopenia after cytotoxic chemotherapy as a risk factor for febrile neutropenia. J Clin Oncol. 1996 Feb;14(2):636-43

Chapter 9

BIOLOGICAL BASIS OF THE ASSOCIATION OF CANCER AND AGING COMORBIDITY

Martine Extermann

Program Leader, Senior Adult Oncology Program, H. Lee Moffitt Cancer Center and Research Institute, Tampa, Florida, Associate Professor of Oncology and Medicine, University of South Florida College of Medicine, Tampa, Florida.

Age is the single most important risk factor for the development of cancer. A 20 year-old person has some 1/10,000 risk of developing a cancer per year. At 50, the risk is about 1/1000, and at 80, it is about 1% per year. The mechanisms for this effect are hotly debated: time to accumulate mutations and epigenetic modifications, oxidative damage, modifications of the immune system, decreased cell repair mechanisms, all have been hypothesized. One of the aspects of aging, however, is an increased prevalence of comorbidity in general. Cancer patients aged 70 and above have on average 3 comorbidities [1]. This comorbidity may affect cancer risk, detection, evolution, and treatment. The increased comorbidity is also associated with a parallel polymedication. At the H. Lee Moffitt Cancer Center, older cancer patients take on average six concomitant drugs [2]. In this chapter, we will focus on the way comorbidity interacts with cancer risk and evolution, trying to understand the underlying biological mechanisms.

1. GENERAL COMORBIDITY INTERACTIONS

Some studies attempted identifying whether there was an interaction between comorbidity and cancer prognosis. Many found that comorbidity modifies the treatment of older cancer patients [3]. However, do comorbidities impact the outcome of the cancer itself? A study by Satariano and Ragland shows an equivalent rate of breast cancer deaths at three years in patient subgroups with various levels of comorbidity. The rate of non-cancer deaths increased 16 times across groups [4]. Another study by Newschaffer et al. was showing a non-significant trend compatible with either no or a low level of interaction [5].

On the other hand, a randomized study by Frasci et al. showed that older metastatic lung cancer patients with severe comorbidity had a worse tolerance to chemotherapy and poorer survival than those without. This was independent from ECOG performance status [6].

Can we gain more insight from observing specific diseases? In this chapter, we will focus on two syndromes that have been generating quite a lot of interest in the last few years: 1) diabetes and the metabolic syndrome; 2) inflammatory diseases and anti-inflammatory drugs.

1.1. Diabetes and Metabolic Syndrome

The relationship between diabetes and cancer is the focus of a lot of attention. This interest is often expanded to include the metabolic syndrome. Two parallel definitions of the latter exist. The Guidelines from the National Cholesterol Education Program (Adult Treatment Panel [ATP] III) [7] require the presence of any three of the following:

- Abdominal obesity, defined as a waist circumference in men >102 cm (40 in) and in women >88 cm (35 in)*
- Triglycerides >150 mg/dL (1.7 mmol/L)
- HDL cholesterol <40 mg/dL (1 mmol/L) in men and <50 mg/dL (1.3 mmol/L) in women
- Blood pressure > 130/85 mmHg
- Fasting glucose > 110 mg/dL (6.1 mmol/L)

* Some men can develop multiple metabolic risk factors when waist circumference is only marginally increased [94 to 102 cm (37 to 39 in)] as such patients may have a genetic contribution to insulin resistance.

The World Health Organization [8] uses as a definition:
Either hyperinsulinemia (defined as the upper quartile of the nondiabetic population) or a fasting plasma glucose > 110 mg/dL (6.1 mmol/L) plus at least two of the following:

- Abdominal obesity, defined as a waist-to-hip ratio >0.90, a body mass index >30 kg/m2, or a waist girth >94 cm (37 in)
- Dyslipidemia, defined as serum triglyceride >150 mg/dL (1.7 mmol/L) or HDL cholesterol <35 mg/dL (0.9 mmol/L)
- Blood pressure > 140/90 mmHg or the administration of antihypertensive drugs.

The association of diabetes mellitus and cancer has been most studied in the case of colorectal cancer. Diabetic patients have an increased incidence of colorectal cancer [9-11]. A recent study highlights that diabetes is also associated with a shorter disease-free survival (Figure 1) [12]. Another study focused on patients undergoing hepatic colorectal cancer metastasis resection [13]. Diabetic patients had a higher peri-operative mortality (8% versus 2%, $p<0.02$) but no difference in long-term survival.

In a study by Weiss et al., no significant impact on breast cancer was found from diabetes, thyroid disease, gallbladder disease, colorectal polyps, high blood pressure, high cholesterol or surgery for endometriosis in women less than 55 years. There was some evidence of increased breast cancer risk in women with ovarian cysts who did not receive oophorectomy (RR=1.94(1.0-3.9)) [14]. There was also a non-significant increase following diagnosis of other cancers.

Figure 1. Disease-free survival for patients with colon cancer by diabetes mellitus status. (Reprinted with permission from Meyerhardt, J.A. et al. JCO; 21:433-440 2003)

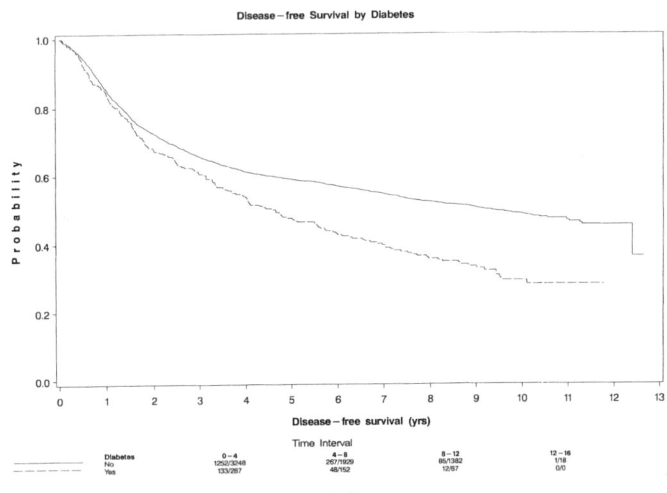

An Italian series found an increased risk of Hodgkin's disease in patients with diabetes (OR 2.1) [15]. This study found also an increased risk of Hodgkin's disease in patients with a history of infectious mononucleosis (4.0), herpes zoster (2.9), pyelonephritis (3.3), tuberculosis (2.3), chronic bacterial diseases (1.4), rheumatoid arthritis (2.4), and psoriasis (2.7). For NHL, the odds ratio were 2.9 for infectious mononucleosis, 1.8 for herpes zoster, 4.9 for pyelonephritis, 1.8 for tuberculosis, 1.9 for malaria, 1.7 for chronic bacterial diseases, 1.7 for rheumatoid arthritis, and 2.5 for psoriasis. Interestingly, most of these associations were showing an age-related trend, with the association being stronger in elderly patients.

Since the metabolic syndrome was defined relatively recently, few studies are available on its impact on cancer. A study linked obesity in colon cancer patients with an increase in overall mortality and a borderline significant increase in disease recurrence [16]. A case control study of probants undergoing colonoscopy studied the association of colon cancer and adenomatous polyps with diabetes, hypertension, cardiovascular diseases and hypercholesterolemia [7]. They found a significant association, with the strongest effects being familial diabetes and hypertension. In stratified analyses, familial diabetes, hypertension and strokes were significantly associated with adenomatous polyps in the subgroups of probants that were older and/or had symptoms at the time of colonoscopy. Only diabetes was possibly associated with colon cancer. An increase of the strength of the association with age was also found in another study [8]. In that study, the association of diabetes with colon cancer was only observed in patients 60 years and older. A Japanese case control study showed that not only diabetes, but also glucose intolerance was associated with an increased risk of colorectal adenomas [17].

The main postulated mechanism for the association of diabetes and the metabolic syndrome with cancer is insulin-resistance. Several studies provide support to this hypothesis [18]. Since aging is associated with an increased insulin resistance, this mechanism could be one of the pathways by which the risk of cancer increases with age. Insulin resistance has been associated with hyperinsulinemia, increased growth factors, including IGF-1, activation of the NF-κB anti-apoptotic pathway via activation of the IκB kinase β, and activation of peroxysome proliferators-activated receptors [18].

Conversely, there is evidence that patients treated for cancer are at increased risk of metabolic syndrome later in life. In a study, 16% of long term childhood cancer survivors, average age 12.6 years, had a metabolic syndrome, versus none of the controls [19]. These children had a decreased spontaneous growth hormone secretion, which may contribute to this syndrome.

1.2 Inflammatory and autoimmune Disease

Even in the absence of overt diseases, aging is associated with an increase in several inflammatory markers, such as IL-6, C-reactive protein, and sedimentation rate [20]. Non-specific markers of auto-immunity, such as antinuclear antibodies, tend also to increase with age. But does this lead to cancer? Some insight may come from studies with inflammatory and autoimmune diseases, as well as their treatment.

A study analyzed the association of osteoarthritis and rheumatoid arthritis with NHL. They found no impact of osteoarthritis, and an increased risk with rheumatoid arthritis [21]. A study examined the association with cancer of finger and hand joint and temporo-mandibular joint prostheses [22]. It found no association, except for an association with NHL in the subgroup that received finger and hand joint replacement for rheumatoid arthritis. The Italian study mentioned above found a significant association of rheumatoid arthritis with both NHL and Hodgkin's [15]. A particular presentation of rheumatoid arthritis, Felty's syndrome, shows a strong association with large granular lymphocytosis and leukemia. Rheumatoid arthritis is present in 30% of LGL syndromes, and there is a strong association with HLA-DRB1*04 [23]. A Scottish study on patients with rheumatoid arthritis and 5 other rheumatoid conditions found more detailed results [24]. There was an increased risk of death from lung cancer: SMR 1.4 (1.2-1.5) in males, 1.6 (1.5-1.8) in females. There was also an increased risk of death from hematologic malignancies: M 1.8 (1.4-2.3), F: 2.0 (1.7-2.3). There was however a decreased risk of death from GI tract malignancies: M 0.82 (0.7-1.0), F 0.8 (0.7-0.9).

A Finn study did compare the incidence of cancer in patients with celiac disease to that of the general population. They did not find any difference [25].

A well-known association between an autoimmune disease and cancer is Sjögren's disease and lymphoma [26]. New intriguing data have been published. A study observed many analogies between Sjögren's derived lymphomas and those arising from hepatitis C-related cryoglobulinemia [27]. A direct link with HCV infection remains yet to be demonstrated. Another study noted that seronegative Sjögren patients did not develop systemic complications, over 10 years, whereas those positive for Ro/La antibodies had a 49.7 relative risk of developing an NHL [28]. In the study by Ioannidis et al., patients with a low C4 level or palpable purpura at presentation were at high risk of developing lymphoproliferative disorders [26].

Several studies addressed the association of systemic lupus erythematosus (SLE) and cancer. In an English clinical database of 276 SLE patients, there was no increased risk of malignancy compared to expected: standardized incidence rate 1.16 (95% CI 0.55-2.13) [29]. The increase of Hodgkin's disease was trending toward significance: SIR 17.82 (95% CI 0.45-99.23). Another study analyzed a Swedish population registry. Again, they found no overall increased rate of cancer [30]. Males had a standardized morbidity rate of 2.24 (95% CI: 0.6-5.7), and females had 1.02 (CI 0.4-2.1). However, some tumors were significantly more frequent: NHL: 11.63 (1.4-42), lung cancer 5.55 (1.3-18.7), and prostate cancer 6.41 (1.3-18.7). A Danish registry study found again an increased incidence of NHL (RR 5.2, CI 2.2-10.3) [31]. They also found an increased incidence of lung cancer (RR

1.9), liver cancer (RR 8.0), and vagina/vulva cancers (RR 5.7). A Canadian study reviewed a clinical cohort of 297 SLE patients and found an increased risk of cancer (SIR 1.59 (1.05-2.32) [32]. The specific sites at risk were cervical cancer: SIR 8.15 (1.63-23.81), and hematopoietic malignancies: SIR 4.9 (1.57-11.4), notably NHL. Another Canadian study found however no increased risk of cancer (SIR 1.08, CI 0.70-1.62), except for hematologic malignancies, mostly NHL (SIR 4.1) [33]. An American study examined patients from the Chicago Lupus Cohort, which focused on women with SLE [34]. It found an increased incidence of malignancies. The SIR was 2.0 (CI 1.4-3.9) overall. Lung cancer was the only individual cancer significantly increased (3.1, 1.3-3.9). In Caucasian women, breast cancer was the only significantly increased cancer: 2.9 (1.4-6.4).

The general conclusions that can be drawn from this overview is that whereas the evidence points toward an increase in hematologic malignancies in patients with auto-immune diseases, the evidence is conflicting concerning solid tumors.

A key physiopathological question is whether it is the immune disease itself that increases the risk of malignancy or its treatment. A study of 128 SLE patients found that those exposed to IV cyclophosphamide were at higher risk of cervical dysplasia ($p<0.04$) [35]. In the study by Cibere et al., the increased risks of malignancy were independent from the use of cytotoxic agents [32]. A prospective 3-year study in rheumatoid arthritis patients treated with methotrexate found a significant increase in the risk of Hodgkin's disease (SMR 7.4, 3.0-15.3), but no difference with the general population for NHL (SMR 1.07, 0.6-1.7) [36]. These numbers are very similar to those mentioned in larger rheumatoid arthritis studies. Of note however is that 3/8 patients treated with methotrexate withdrawal underwent a remission. Another study found that EBV-associated lymphomas represented only a very small fraction of NHL associated with rheumatoid arthritis [37]. A large study showed that patients with inflammatory bowel disease treated with azathioprine did not present an increased risk of cancer, compared to their counterparts who did not receive it [38]. The role of TNF-alpha inhibitors is ambiguous. A case reports study describes the early appearance of squamous cell carcinomas of the skin within a few months after starting etanercept therapy for rheumatoid arthritis, even if it postulated that prolonged TNF-alpha inhibition may have antitumoral effect [39]. A revue of the FDA database of patients treated with etanercept or infliximab showed 26 cases of lymphoproliferative disorders, 81% of them lymphomas [40]. The median time between the start of treatment and the development of the lymphoma was again very short (median 8 weeks). In two instances, regression was observed on discontinuation of the treatment. The present available evidence does not allow definitive conclusions, but seems to indicate that increased risks of cancer, if any, appear linked more strongly to the auto-immune disease than to its treatment. A possible exception is anti-TNF-alpha treatments.

There is epidemiological evidence that allergies and immune-related diagnoses might reduce the risk of glioma and meningioma. In three large cohorts of Swedish patients, Schwartzbaum et al. found decreased ratios of gliomas in most cases: 0.45 (95% CI 0.19-1.07), 0.45 (0.11-1.92) (high-grade gliomas only, no reduced risk of low-grade gliomas), and 0.46 (0.14-1.49) [41]. In an American case control study 40 patients with a history of allergies were less likely than controls to have gliomas (OR 0.67, 95% CI 0.38-0.62), but not meningiomas or acoustic neuromas [42]. Patients with autoimmune diseases, including diabetes, were less likely to have gliomas (OR 0.49, 95% CI 0.35-0.69), or meningiomas (OR 0.59, 95% CI 0.38-0.92).

1.3. NSAIDS and Statins

Interestingly, the two groups of syndromes mentioned above share common treatments within each category. Inflammatory diseases are often treated with NSAIDS, and diabetics and patients with the metabolic syndrome often take statins. These two categories of medications have been analyzed for their role in cancer prevention.

The tumor in which the role of NSAIDS is the most studied is colorectal cancer. There is large epidemiological evidence that the regular use of aspirin, other NSAIDS, including COX2 inhibitors, and aminosalicylates are associated with an about 50% decreased incidence of colon cancer [43-45]. Several randomized studies have been published. They often use the occurrence of adenomas as a surrogate end-point, given the orderly progression of colorectal neoplasms. An American intergroup study randomized 635 colorectal cancer patients to 325mg of aspirin a day or placebo [46]. Patients underwent at least one colonoscopy at a median of 12.8 months after randomization. Adenomas were found in 17% of the aspirin group and 27% of the control group (p=0.004). The mean number of adenomas was also decreased. The time to detection of first adenoma was increased in the aspirin group (hazard ratio 0.64, 95% CI 0.43-0.94, p=0.022). This study targeted patients with a low risk of cancer recurrence, and patients with familial adenomatous polyposis or inflammatory bowel disease were excluded. A second study by the same group, again in patients without familial risk syndromes, did randomize 1121 patients with colorectal adenomas to placebo, aspirin 81mg/day, or 325mg/day [47]. On control colonoscopy at least 1 year after randomization, the incidence of adenomas was 47% in the control group, 38% in the 81mg group, and 45% in the 325mg group. The relative risks were 0.81 (0.69-0.96), and 0.96 (0.81-1.13) compared to placebo respectively. Another study in patients with colorectal adenomas randomized 272 patients to lysine acetylsalicylate 160 or

300mg/day or placebo [48]. After 1 year, the incidence of adenoma was 30% in the aspirin group and 41% in the placebo group (RR 0.73, 0.52-1.04, p=0.08). On stepwise regression, treatment with aspirin had a significant impact (p=0.01). One study attempted to reduce already present polyps in patients with familial adenomatous polyposis (FAP) [49]. Patients were randomized to celecoxib, 100 or 400 mg twice daily, or placebo. The patients receiving 400mg of celecoxib had a 28% reduction in the number of polyps (p=0.003), and a 30.7% reduction in the sum of polyp diameters (p=0.001), compared to a reduction of 4.5 and 4.9% respectively in the placebo group. In the group receiving 100mg of celecoxib, the reductions were 11.9% (p=0.33), and 14.6% (p=0.09). The same authors also looked at the decrease of duodenal polyps in these patients [50]. They found a 14.5% decrease after 6 months of celecoxib 400mg bid, compared with 1.4% for placebo. Again, the results obtained with 100mg bid of celecoxib were intermediate. A third study addressed patients with FAP [51]. They were randomized to sulindac 75 or 100 mg twice daily or placebo. After 4 years of treatment, adenomas developed in 43% of the treated subjects, versus 55% of the placebo group (p=0.54).

The impact of NSAIDS use on the incidence of breast cancer was also analyzed. A meta-analysis of 14 studies found an 18% risk reduction, comparable for aspirin and other NSAIDS [52]. A recent study on the Women's Health Initiative cohort, focusing on 80,741 post-menopausal women between ages of 50 and 79, found a 21% reduction for 5-9 years of regular NSAIDS, and a 28% reduction for 10 or more years [53]. The effect was more pronounced for ibuprofen: 49%, than for aspirin: 21%.

A recently published meta-analysis reviews the effect of NSAIDS on other solid tumors [43]. In addition to breast cancer, reviewed above, a decreased risk was found for cancer of the esophagus, stomach, ovary, prostate, and lung. No significant effect was found for pancreas, kidney, and bladder cancer (Table 1).

By contrast, in a recent article, Cerhan et al., using the SEER data, showed an association between the use of NSAIDS and an increased incidence of lymphoma [21]. The incidence of NHL was increased about twofold in patients taking aspirin, other NSAIDS, or both. The authors corrected for a history of osteoarthritis or rheumatoid arthritis. Although rheumatoid arthritis was associated with an increased risk of NHL, the association of aspirin with NHL was independent of arthritis history. These data are highly consistent with studies of rheumatoid arthritis patients, found to have a decreased risk of colon cancer and an increased risk of NHL [21]. Other series, however, did not find a similar association, and a case control study found a protective effect of NSAIDS on NHL [21].

Table 1. Overall relative risks and 95% confidence interval according to cancer site and type of exposure. (Reproduced with permission from González-Pérez et al.)

Overall relative risks and 95% confidence interval according to cancer site and type of exposure

	N†	NSAIDs RR (95%CI)	N	Aspirin RR (95%CI)	N	NA-NSAIDs RR (95%CI)
Esophagus	4	0.65 (0.46–0.92)	4	0.51 (0.38–0.69)		
Stomach	3	0.54 (0.39–0.75)	5	0.73 (0.63–0.84)	2	0.91 (0.66–1.25)
Pancreas	2	1.09 (0.59–2.01)	3	0.69 (0.40–1.20)		
Breast	9	0.77* (0.66–0.88)	11	0.77 (0.69–0.86)	5	0.86 (0.73–1.00)
Ovary	6	0.74 (0.61–0.90)	6	0.91 (0.79–1.06)		
Prostate	4	0.64* (0.34–1.21)	7	0.92 (0.81 – 1.05)	2	0.84 (0.68–1.05)
Kidney			6	1.23* (0.86–1.75)		
Bladder	3	0.91 (0.71–1.18)	3	0.91 (0.73–1.13)		
Lung	3	0.65* (0.34–1.22)	5	0.84* (0.66–1.07)		

*$p < 0.05$ (Heterogeneity test); †Number of studies.

What are the mechanisms by which NSAIDS prevent solid tumors and might induce NHL? The evidence points to both cyclooxygenase dependent and independent pathways [54]. In vitro, apoptosis is the dominant anti-proliferative effect of each class of NSAIDS. Cell cycle arrest further contributes to this effect [55, 56]. COX 2 is known to enhance VEGF secretion. It is also an inducer of the NF-κB pathway [21]. In at least one animal model, COX 2 can induce Her2 expression in mouse mammary tumor [57]. Recent evidence suggests an interaction between NSAIDS and angiotensin II pathway inhibitors, via their impact on the insulin-like growth factor-1 receptor [58]. Human studies are still rare. A study of the impact of rofecoxib 25mg daily on subsequently resected colorectal liver metastases measured apoptosis index, proliferation index, and microvessel density [59]. It showed a 29% reduction in microvessel density (p=0.15), but little difference in apoptosis and proliferative index compared to placebo. Another study found that celecoxib was reducing the perioperative increase in VEGF in patients undergoing surgery for breast cancer [60]. An extremely interesting study provides a potential link between NSAIDS and diabetes, suggesting that the metabolic syndrome and inflammatory diseases may not be that independent from each other when it comes to controlling carcinogenesis [61]. Hundal et al. studied 9 type 2 diabetics before and after two weeks of treatment with aspirin, about 7g/day. The treatment reduced plasma glucose by about 25%, total cholesterol and C-reactive protein by some 15%, triglycerides by 50%, and insulin clearance by 30%, despite no change in body weight. The postulated mechanism is inhibition of IKKβ activation, a mechanism independent of COX inhibition by salicylates.

For celecoxib, the effect appears to be dose-dependent, with higher doses needed than for benign antalgia. This was found in both animal models and human studies [62,49,50]. The picture is less clear for aspirin. One study suggests an increased effect with prolonged exposure [53]. Another study, using rectal mucosal PGE2 as a biomarker of effect at 4 weeks found an equal effectiveness of 81 and 650mg per day [63].

Patients with a metabolic syndrome often receive statins. Mortimer and colleagues studied recently a large health plan database [64]. They analyzed the risk of breast cancer in women aged 35 and older taking statins. In women less than 50 years, there was no difference with the controls (1.4% versus 1.2%). However, women aged 50 and older were less likely to develop breast cancer than controls (1.0% versus 2.6%). Interestingly, women on both hormone replacement therapy and statins had the same risk as those taking statins alone, whereas controls without concomitant statins were at increased risk. A prospective cohort study observed older women (mean age 77 years) treated with statins in community centers [65]. The age-adjusted incidence of breast cancer over an average of 6.8 years was 3.1/1000 for women on statins, 1.4 for women using other lipid-lowering agents, and 5.0 among non-users. The relative risk of breast cancer among statin users was 0.28 (95% CI 0.14-0.99), compared to non-users. These results are supported by a Dutch case-control trial showing that statins users were 20% less likely to develop cancers [66]. On the other hand, a meta-analysis of five randomized trials of statins for cardiovascular diseases prevention did not show a difference in the risk of cancer over a five-year follow-up period [65]. Two other case-control studies did not find a protective effect of statins against breast cancer [68, 69]. A Canadian retrospective cohort did not show a benefit either, even in women older than 55 years of age or on hormone replacement therapy [70].

Interesting laboratory results are appearing in hematologic malignancies as well. Simvastatin induces apoptosis of B-CLL cell lines by activation of caspase 9 [71]. Statins also trigger tumor-specific apoptosis in AML cell lines, cerivastatin being the most effective [72]. Further exploration is needed before we fully understand the impact of statins on cancer.

2. CONCLUSIONS

Comorbidity and its treatment appear to be an important influence on the behavior of cancer in older patients. Rather than a blanket effect, this may be attached to groups of syndromes with common pathophysiological mechanisms. In addition to paying attention to the impact of cancer treatment on comorbidity, or on the impact of comorbidity on the ability to deliver cancer treatment, we will have in the future to pay attention on the direct impact of comorbidity on the behavior of the cancer in elderly patients.

REFERENCES

1. Extermann M, Overcash J, Lyman GH, Parr J, Balducci L: Comorbidity and functional status are independent in older cancer patients. Journal of Clinical Oncology 16:1582-7, 1998

2. Extermann M, Yoder J, Overcash J, Wallace K, Vranas P, Braud AC, Luciani A, Carbonel A, Cantor AB: Influence of concomitant medications metabolized by cytochrome P-450 on toxicity from chemotherapy. 8th International Conference on Geriatric Oncology, Rome, Italy, Nov 21-22, 2003

3. Greenfield S, Blanco DM, Elashoff RM, Ganz PA: Patterns of care related to age of breast cancer patients. JAMA 1987 May 22-29;257(20):2766-70

4. Satariano WA, Ragland DR: The effect of comorbidity on 3-year survival of women with primary breast cancer. Ann Intern Med. 1994 Jan 15;120(2):104-10

5. Newschaffer CJ, Bush TL, Penberthy LE, Bellantoni M, Helzlsour K, Diener-West M Does comorbid disease interact with cancer? An epidemiologic analysis of mortality in a cohort of elderly breast cancer patients. J Gerontol A Biol Sci Med Sci. 1998 Sep;53(5):M372-8

6. Frasci G, Lorusso V, Panza N, Comella P, Nicolella G, Bianco A, De Cataldis G, Iannelli A, Bilancia D, Belli M, Massidda B, Piantedosi F, Comella G, De Lena M: Gemcitabine plus vinorelbine versus vinorelbine alone in elderly patients with advanced non-small-cell lung cancer. J Clin Oncol. 2000 Jul;18(13):2529-36

7. Expert panel on detection, evaluation, and treatment of high blood cholesterol in adults (Adult Treatment Panel III): Third report of the national cholesterol education program (NCEP). Circulation 2002; 106:3143

8. Alberti KG, Zimmet PZ: Definition, diagnosis and classification of diabetes mellitus and its complications. Part 1: diagnosis and classification of diabetes mellitus provisional report of a WHO consultation. Diabet Med 1998 Jul;15(7):539-53

9. Brauer PM, McKeown-Eyssen GE, Jazmaji V et al: Familial aggregation of diabetes and hypertension in a case-control study of colorectal neoplasia. Am J Epidemiol 156:702-713, 2002

10. Le Marchand L, Wilkens LR, Kolonel LN et al : Assocaitions of sedentary lifestyle, obesity, smoking, alcohol use and diabetes with the risk of colorectal cancer. Cancer Res 57:4787-94, 1997

11. Hu FB, Manson JE, Liu S, et al : Prospective study of adult onset diabetes mellitus (type 2) and risk of colorectal cancer in women. J Natl Cancer Inst 91:542-7, 1999

12. Meyerhardt JA, Catalano PJ, Haller DG, Mayer RJ, Macdonald JS, Benson AB III, Fuchs CS: Impact of diabetes mellitus on outcomes in patients with colon cancer. J Clin Oncol. 2003 Feb 1;21(3):433-40

13. Little SA, Jarnagin WR, DeMatteo RP, Blumgart LH, Fong Y: Diabetes is associated with increased perioperative mortality but equivalent long-term outcome after hepatic resection for colorectal cancer. J Gastrointest Surg 6:88-94, 2002

14. Weiss HA, Brinton LA, Potischman NA, Brogan D, Coates RJ, Gammon MD, Malone KE, Schoenberg JB: Breast cancer risk in young women and history of selected medical conditions. Int J Epidemiol. 1999 Oct;28(5):816-23

15. Tavani A, La Vecchia C, Franceschi S, Serraino D, Carbone A: Medical history and risk of Hodgkin's and non-Hodgkin's lymphomas. Eur J Cancer Prev 9:59-64, 2000

16. Meyerhardt JA, Catalano PJ, Haller DG et al: Influence of body mass index on outcomes and treatment-related toxicity in patients with colon carcinoma. Cancer 98:484-495, 2003

17. Marugame T, Lee K, Eguchi H, Oda T, Shinchi K, Kono S: Relation of impaired glucose tolerance and diabetes mellitus to colorectal adenomas in Japan. Cancer Causes Control 13:917-921, 2002

18. Komninou D, Ayonote A, Richie JP, Rigas B: Insulin resistance and its contribution to colon carcinogenesis. Exp Biol Med 228:396-405, 2003

19. Talvensaari KK, Lanning M, Tapanainen P, Knip M: Long-term survivors of childhood cancer have an increased risk of manifesting the metabolic syndrome. J Clin Endocrinol Metab, 81:3051-5, 1996

20. Cohen HJ, Harris T, Pieper CF: Coagulation and activation of inflammatory pathways in the development of functional decline and mortality in the elderly. Am J Med. 2003 Feb 15;114(3):180-7

21. Cerhan JR, Anderson KE, Janney CA, Vachon CM, Witzig TE, Habermann TM: Association of aspirin and other non-steroidal anti-inflammatory drug use with incidence of non-Hodgkin lymphoma. Int J Cancer. 2003 Sep 20;106(5):784-8

22. Fryzek JP, Mellemkjaer L, McLaughlin JK, Blot WJ, Olsen JH: Cancer risk among patients with finger and hand joint and temporo-mandibular joint prostheses in Denmark. Int J Cancer 81:723-5, 1999

23. Coakley G, Brooks D, Iqbal M, et al: Major histocompability complex haplotypic associations with Felty's syndrome and large granular lymphocyte syndrome are secondary to allelic association with HLA-DRB1*0401. Rheumatology 39:393-8, 2000

24. Thomas E, Symmons DP, Brewster DH, Black RJ, Macfarlane GJ: National study of cause-specific mortality in rheumatoid arthritis, juvenile chronic arthritis, and other rheumatic conditions: a 20 year follow-up study. J Rheumatol 2003 May;30(5):958-65

25. Collin P, Reunala T, Pukkala E et al: Coeliac disease-associated disorders and survival. Gut 35:1215-8, 1994

26. Ioannidis JP, Vassiliou VA, Moutsopoulos HM: Long-term risk of mortality and lymphoproliferative disease and predictive classification of primary Sjogren's syndrome. Arthritis Rheum. 2002 Mar;46(3):741-7

27. De Re V, De Vita S, Gasparotto D et al: Salivary gland B-cell lymphoproliferative disorders in Sjögren's syndrome present a restricted use of antigen receptor gene segments similar to those used by hepatitis C virus-associated non-Hodgkin's lymphomas. Eur J Immunol 32:903-910, 2002

28. Davidson BKS, Kelly CA, Griffiths ID: Primary Sjögren's syndrome in the North East of England: a long-term follow-up study. Rheumatology 38:245-253, 1999

29. Sultan SM, Ioannou Y, Isenberg DA: Is there an association of malignancy with systemic lupus erythematosus? An analysis of 276 patients under long-term review. Rheumatology (Oxford) 39:1147-52, 2000

30. Nived O, Bengtsson A, Jonsen A, Sturfelt G, Olsson H: Malignancies during follow-up in an epidemiologically defined systemic lupus erythematosus inception cohort in southern Sweden. Lupus. 2001;10(7):500-4

31. Mellemkjaer L, Andersen V, Linet MS et al : Non-Hodgkin's lymphoma and other cancers among a cohort of patients with systemic lupus erythematosus. Arthritis Rheum 40:761-8, 1997

32. Cibere J, Sibley J, Haga M: Systemic lupus erythematosus and the risk of malignancy. Lupus 10:394-400, 2001

33. Abu-Shakra M, Gladman DD, Urowitz MB: Malignancy in systemic lupus erythematosus. Arthritis Rheum 39:1050-4, 1996

34. Ramsey-Goldman R, Mattai SA, Schilling E, et al: Increased risk of malignancy in patients with systemic lupus erythematosus. J. Investig Med 46:217-222, 1998

35. Bateman H, Yacizi Y, Leff L, Peterson M, Paget SA: Increased cervical dysplasia in intravenous cyclophosphamide-treated patients with SLE : a preliminary study. Lupus 9:542-4, 2000

36. Mariette X, Cazals-Hatem D, Warszawski J et al: Lymphomas in rheumatoid arthritis patients treated with methotrexate: a 3-year prospective study in France. Blood 99:3909-15, 2002
37. Kamel OW, Holly EA, van de Rijn M, Lele C, Sah A: A population based, case control study of non-Hodgkin's lymphoma in patients with rheumatoid arthritis. J Rheumatol. 26:1676-80, 1999
38. Fraser AG, Orchard TR, Robinson EM, Jewell DP: Long-term risk of malignancy after treatment of inflammatory bowel disease with azathioprine. Aliment Pharmacol Ther 16:1225-32, 2002
39. Smith KJ, Skelton HG: Rapid onset of cutaneous squamous cell carcinoma in patients with rheumatoid arthritis after starting tumor necorsis factor alpha receptor IgG1-Fc fusion complex therapy. J Am Acad Dermatol 45:953-6, 2001
40. Brown, SL, Greene MH, Gershon SK, Edwards ET, Braun MM: Tumor necrosis factor antagonist therapy and lymphoma development. Arthritis & Rheumatism 46:3151-8, 2002
41. Schwartzenbaum J, Jonsson F, Ahlbom A et al: Cohort studies of association between self-reported allergic conditions, immune-related diagnoses and glioma and meningioma risk. Int J Cancer 106:423-8, 2003
42. Brenner AV, Linet MS, Fine HA et al: History of allergies and autoimmune diseases and risk of brain tumors in adults. Int J Cancer 99:252-9, 2002
43. González-Pérez A, García Rodríguez LA, López-Ridaura R: Effects of non-steroidal anti-inflammatory drugs on cancer sites other than the colon and the rectum: a meta-analysis. BMC Cancer 3:28, 2003
44. Eaden J: Review article: the data supporting a role for aminosalicylates in the chemoprevention of colorectal cancer in patients with inflammatory bowel disease. Aliment Pharmacol Ther 18(suppl 2):15-21, 2003
45. Rahme E, Barkun AN, Toubouti Y, Bardou M: The cyclooxygenase-2-selective inhibitors rofecoxib and celecoxib prevent colorectal neoplasia occurrence and recurrence. Gastroenterology 125:404-412, 2003
46. Sandler RS, Halabi S, Baron JA et al: A randomized trial of aspirin to prevent colorectal adenomas in patients with previous colorectal cancer. N Engl J Med 348:883-890, 2003
47. Baron JA, Cole BF, Sandler RS, et al : A randomized trial of aspirin to prevent colorectal adenomas. N Engl J Med 348:891-899, 2003
48. Benamouzig R, Deyra J, Martin A et al: Daily soluble aspirin and prevention of colorectal adenoma recurrence : one-year results of the APACC trial. Gastroenterology 125:328-336, 2003
49. Steinbach G, Lynch PM, Phillips RK et al: The effect of celecoxib, a cyclooxygenase-2 inhibitor, in familial adenomatous polyposis. N Engl J Med 342:1946-52, 2000
50. Phillips RK, Wallace MH, Lynch PM, et al: A randomized, double blind, placebo controlled study of celecoxib, a selective cyclooxygenase 2 inhibitor, on duodenal polyposis in familial adenomatous polyposis. Gut, 50:857-60, 2002
51. Giardello FM, Yang VW, Hylind LM et al: Primary chemoprevention of familial adenomatous polyposis with sulindac. N Engl J Med 346:1054-9, 2002
52. Khuder SA, Mutgi AB: Breast cancer and NSAID use: a meta-analysis. Br J Cancer. 2001 May 4;84(9):1188-92
53. Harris RE, Chlebowski RT, Jackson RD, Frid DJ, Ascenseo JL, Anderson G, Loar A, Rodabough RJ, White E, McTiernan A: Women's Health Initiative. Breast cancer and nonsteroidal anti-inflammatory drugs: prospective results from the Women's Health Initiative. Cancer Res. 2003 Sep 15;63(18):6096-101
54. Kundu N, Fulton AM: Selective cyclooxygenase (COX)-1 or COX-2 inhibitors control metastatic disease in a murine model of breast cancer. Cancer Res 62:2343-6, 2002
55. Elder DJ, Paraskeva C: Induced apoptosis in the prevention of colorectal cancer by non-steroidal anti-inflammatory drugs. Apoptosis 4:365-372, 1999

56. Rice PL, Kelloff J, Sullivan H et al: Sulindac induces caspase- and proteasome-dependent degradation of beta-catenin protein in human colon cancer cells. Mol Cancer Ther 2:885-892, 2003
57. Howe LR, Subbaramiah K, Patel J et al: Celecoxib, a selective cyclooxygenase 2 inhibitor, protects against human epidermal growth factor receptor 2 (HER2/neu)-induced breast cancer. Cancer res 62:5405-7, 2002
58. Yasumaru M, Tsuji S, Tsujii M et al : Inhibition of angiotensin II activity enhanced the antitumor effect of cyclooxygenase-2 inhibitors via insulin-like growth factor I receptor pathway. Cancer Res 63:6726-6734, 2003
59. Fenwick SW, Toogood GJ, Lodge JP, Hull MA: The effect of the selective cyclooxygenase-2 inhibitor rofecoxib on human colorectal cancer liver metastases. Gastroenterology 125:716-729, 2003
60. O'Donoghue GT, Roche-Nagle G, Connolly EM et al: Selective COX-2 inhibition attenuates the perioperative increase of the tumour enhancing pro-angiogenic cytokine Vegf in human breast cancer patients. J Surg Res 114:243, 2003
61. Hundal RS, Petersen KF, Mayerson AB, Randhawa PS, Inzucchi S, Shoelson SE, Shulman GI: Mechanism by which high-dose aspirin improves glucose metabolism in type 2 diabetes. J Clin Invest. 2002 May;109(10):1321-6
62. Abou-Issa HM, Alshafie GA, Seibert K et al : Dose-response effects ot the COX-2 inhibitor, celecoxib, on the prevention of mammary carcinogenesis. Anticancer res 21:3425-32, 2001
63. Sample D, Wargowich M, Fisher SM et al: A dose-finding study of aspirin for chemoprevention utilizing rectal mucosal prostaglandin E(2) levels as a biomarker. Cancer Epidemiol Biomarkers Prev 11:275-9, 2002
64. Mortimer JE: The protective effects of statins on the incidence of breast cancer in older women. 8th International Conference on Geriatric Oncology, Rome, Italy, Nov 21-22, 2003
65. Cauley JA, Zmuda JM, Lui LY et al: Lipid-lowering drug use and breast cancer in older women: a prospective study. J Womens Health (Larchmt) 12:749-756, 2003
66. Graaf MR, Beiderbeck AB, Egberts ACG et al: The risk of cancer in statin users. Proc Am Soc Clin Oncol 22:846, 2003
67. Bjerre LM, LeLorier J: Do statins cause cancer? A meta-analysis of large randomized clinical trials. Am J Med 110:716-723, 2001
68. Coogan PF, Rosenberg L, Palmer JR et al : Statin use and the risk of breast and prostate cancer. Epidemilogy 13:262-267, 2002
69. Kaye JA, Meier CR, Walker AM, Jick H: Statin use, hyperlipidemia, and the risk of breast cancer. Br J Cancer 86:1436-9, 2002
70. Beck P, Wysowski DK, Downey W, Butler-Jones D: Statin use and the risk of breast cancer. J Clin Epidemiol 56:280-5, 2003
71. Chapman-Shimshoni D, Yuklea M, Radnay J, Shapiro H, Lishner M: Simvastatin induces apoptosis of B-CLL cells by activation of mitochondrial caspase 9. Exp Hematol 2003 Sep;31(9):779-83
72. Wong WW, Tan MM, Xia Z, Dimitroulakos J, Minden MD, Penn LZ: Cerivastatin triggers tumor-specific apoptosis with higher efficacy than lovastatin. Clin Cancer Res. 2001 Jul;7(7):2067-75

Chapter 10

BIOLOGICAL BASIS OF CANCER IN THE OLDER PERSON

Claudia Beghe' and Lodovico Balducci

Claudia Beghe', Associate Professor of Medicine, University of South Florida College of Medicine, Tampa, Florida, Head, Geriatric Section, James A. Haley Veterans Hospital, Tampa, Florida. Lodovico Balducci, Program Leader, Senior Adult Oncology Program, H. Lee Moffitt Cancer Center and Research Institute, Tampa, Florida, Professor of Oncology and Medicine, University of South Florida College of Medicine, Tampa, Florida.

Cancer prevention is the most attractive form of cancer control, as it avoids the complications of cancer and cancer treatment that are particularly burdensome to the older person [1]. Cancer prevention may also reduce cancer-related mortality and thus prolong the life expectancy and the active life expectancy of older individuals. This aspect of cancer prevention is counter-intuitive and should be highlighted. A common tenet holds that cancer prevention is at most marginally effective in older individuals, who have limited life expectancy and high prevalence of disability and functional dependence. The truth is that cancer is the second most common cause of mortality for Americans aged 65 and older and it may become the first during the next decade, as mortality rate from cardiovascular diseases is declining [2-4]. In addition, cancer preferentially affects active and independent older individuals [5-11] with years of active life expectancy in front of them were it not for cancer.

In this chapter the rationale and the effectiveness of primary and secondary cancer prevention in the older person are examined and the practical application of cancer prevention to the geriatric population is explored. Primary prevention includes inhibition of carcinogenesis; secondary prevention involves reduction of cancer-related death through early detection and timely management of cancer.

1. CHEMOPREVENTION

The administration of substances capable to stop or reverse carcinogenesis appears the most promising form of cancer prevention in older individuals. It is more practical than elimination of environmental carcinogens that may have already caused permanent damage to older individuals [12]. As discussed in another session of this book [13], age itself is associated with molecular changes mimicking carcinogenesis, which prime older individuals to the effects of late-stage carcinogens. It is not far fetched to fathom that by blocking the progression of these changes, chemoprevention of cancer may also delay aging. Another appealing feature of chemoprevention is avoidance of invasive intervention necessary for early diagnosis and treatment of cancer [6]. Potential drawbacks of cancer chemoprevention in the elderly include toxicity and cost of treatment, in addition to the fact that limited life expectancy may minimize the benefits.

After reviewing the principles of chemoprevention, we explore the practical application of this strategy to older individuals.

1.1 Principles of Chemoprevention

Two aspects of carcinogenesis suggest that chemoprevention may be effective [14]. First, carcinogenesis is a step-wise time consuming process, during which oncogenes are activated, and anti-proliferative genes are disabled, under the influence of different carcinogens [13-15]. Thus carcinogenesis offers both plenty of time and of targets to chemoprevention. Second, carcinogenesis is a "field process" that may involve all cells exposed to the same carcinogens. Thus chemoprevention may affect the development of multiple neoplasms.

Figure 1 illustrates the possible mechanism of action of chemopreventative agents and Table 1 lists some of the most promising among them. The formation of highly electrophilic DNA adducts, is one of the first step in carcinogenesis. The early stage carcinogens responsible for their formation may be present in nature as procarcinogen, activated by the P450 enzymatic system, and neutralized by type II liver reactions [16], that involve glutathione-S-tranferases (GST); diphosphate-glucuronsyl transferase, quinone reductase and epoxide hydrolase [17]. Chemoprevention

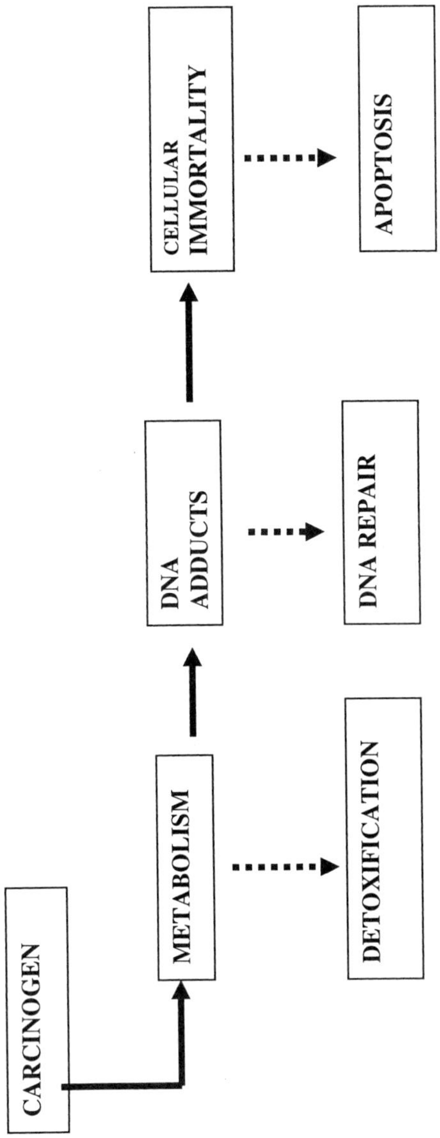

Figure 1: Potential targets of chemoprevention

Fig. 1

Table 1. Promising chemopreventive agents

Mechanism of action	Agent
Inhibition of carcinogen activation	**Inhibition of P-450 enzymes** • Isothiocyanates (cruciferous vegetables) • Diallil sulfide (garlic) • Flavonoids, Isoflavonoids, coumarins (different plants) **Inhibition of electrophilic groups derived from carcinogen activation** • 2-mercaptoethanol • Riboflavin • Ellagic acid and other plant phenols • Epigallocatechin-3-gallate (EGCG) (green tea)
Enhanced carcinogen detoxification	**Inducers of Glutathion-S-transferases (GSTs)** • Diallyl-sulfide and s-allyl-cystein (garlic) • Isothiocyanantes (cruciferous vegetables) • Oltipraz (antischistosomal drug) • N-Acethylcystein (synthetic) **Inducers of quinone transferase** • Resveratrol (Grape and other fruits)
Enhancers of DNA damage repair	• Calorie restriction • Selenium • Epigallocatechin galate
Inhibitors of induced cell proliferation	**Reactive Oxygen Species (ROS) scavengers** • Antioxidants (ascorbic acid, alfa-tocopherol, selenium, polyphenolic compounds from green tea, spices and vegetables) • Calorie restriction **Anti-proliferative and differentiating agents** • Retinoids • DMFO • Hormonal agents (SERMs, aromatase inhibitors, androgen deprivation) **Prostaglandin synthesis-inhibitors** • COX 1 and 2 inhibitors • Corticosteroids
Inducers of apoptosis	• Retinoids • Hormonal agents • COX1 and 2 inhibitors

may inhibit the activation and enhance the elimination of the carcinogen, and in addition may inhibit some metabolic by-products with carcinogenic activity. In the animal model, isothiocyanates and diallyl-sulfate prevent carcinogenesis by acting on the P450 system [18-23] and Oltipraz [24] and N-acetyl-cistein [18], by inducing GSTs.

The formation of DNA adducts is the crossroad of chemical, radiation-induced and light-induced carcinogenesis [25]. These substances may be repaired by DNA repairing enzymes, such as methyl-transferase, base-excision repair and nucleotide-excision repair enzymes [26], whose activity is enhanced by selenium, calorie restriction, and epigallocatechin galate [25]. Carcinogenesis is also subjected to a number of endogenous influences, including reactive oxygen species (ROS), generated as by-products of cellular metabolism [25], hormones, growth factors [27] and eicosenoids [28-31]. The majority of the efforts of chemoprevention have been focused on these late carcinogenetic stages and have involved:

- Antioxidants, such as alpha tocopherol, selenium and ascorbic acid able to scavenge free radicals [25]. Calorie restriction may also play an important role, by reducing the formation of ROS and promoting endogenous antioxidant activities.
- Modulation of steroid receptors that are ligand-activated nuclear transcription factors [32], that may inhibit cell proliferation and promote differentiation and apoptosis.
- Inhibition of polyamine synthesis, that are essential for cell proliferation. This may be accomplished with Dimethylfluoro ornithine (DMFO) [33], which competitively inhibits of the rate-limiting enzyme Ornithine-decarboxylase.
- Inhibition of eicosanoids synthesis by Non-steroidal anti-inflammatory drugs (NSAIDs) [28-31,34.]

Three groups of substances were proven to prevent cancer in humans: hormonal agents, retinoids, and NSAIDS. Of the hormonal agents, the best studied have been the Selective Estrogen receptor Modulators (SERMs) and in particular tamoxifen [35] and raloxifene [36-38] for breast cancer, and the α reductase inhibitor finsteride for prostate cancer (NEJM). The SERMs compete with estrogens for the Estrogen Receptors (ER) [32] and prevent the chain of events triggered by estrogen, that stimulates the proliferation of the neoplastic breast cells. SERMs may also suppress the secretion of Insulin-like Growth Factor-1 (ILF-1) that stimulate the release of Transforming Growth Factor β (TGF-β) from the tumor stroma [39]. Other hormonal agents that may be used for chemoprevention of breast cancer include the aromatase inhibitors [40] that eliminate the production of estrogen in post-menopausal women. Finsteride inhibit the transformation of testosterone into the more active form dihydrotestosterone and was recently proven to reduce the incidence of prostate cancer [41-43].

Synthetic and natural vitamin A derivatives (retinoids) reverse preneoplastic lesions and prevent second primary cancers in the upper airways [44], by inducing differentiation and apoptosis of the preneoplastic cells [45]. Retinoids may also enhance the immune response and inhibit angiogenesis [45, 46]. The activity of different retinoids is determined by the affinity for different Retinoid receptors, of which two broad categories exist [47, 48]. The 4-N-(4-hydroxiphenyl)retinamide (4-HPR, fenretinide) is unique position among the retinoids, as it induces apoptosis of transformed cells *in vitro* without binding to retinoid receptors [48].

Though all NSAIDs may have cancer-preventative activity, selective COX-2 inhibitors are the most appealing substances for this purpose, because they are associated with lower risk of gastrointestinal bleeding and have a more specific action. Unlike COX1, that is a structural enzyme, present in all normal tissues, COX2 is induced in pathological condition, such as infection or neoplasia [49].

1.2 Issues Related to Clinical Studies of Chemoprevention

Clinical trials of chemoprevention need to overcome a number of problems that include adequate sample size, duration, toxicity, and cost [50]. As the risk of cancer is relatively small in the general population, it may take several thousand patients and a prolonged period of time to minimize the type II (beta) error and conclude the study. It took almost 14,000 women and more than five years to demonstrate that tamoxifen reduced by 50% the risk of new breast cancer in the Breast cancer prevention trial BCPT (NSABP-P1) [35].

A clear precondition of chemoprevention is negligible toxicity of the agent. Toxicity is of special concerns to older individuals who are more subject to adverse effects of drugs due to altered pharmacokinetics, reduced functional reserve of organ and systems, and increased risk of drug interactions [1]. Toxicity is a concern with available agents. Even at low doses, cis-retinoic acid is considered too toxic for routine prevention of cancer of the upper digestive and respiratory tract [51]. Tamoxifen increased threefold the risk of endometrial cancer and twofold that of cerebrovascular accidents in women enrolled in the BCTP [35] and caused hot flushes, depression, and sexual disfunction [32, 52].

The cost issue is not well defined, but there is general agreement in the Western society that preventive interventions should not exceed a certain cost. An informal reference point has been the cost of screening mammography for women aged 50-70, that was calculated around $50000.00-60000.00/year of life saved [53] Higher costs are generally considered excessive. Cost estimates should include the cost of the intervention, of the complications and of the many saved from treating the disease.

To some extent two strategies may reduce the sample size and the duration of the study, improve the benefit/risk ratio and limit the cost. These include enrollment in the study of only individuals who are at high risk of disease, and use of intermediary end-points as surrogate of outcomes (phase IIb trials) [53-55]. Unfortunately, regression of premalignant lesions is not always proof that the agent under study may prevent cancer. For example premalignant lesions of the cervix may undergo spontaneous regression in as many as 60% of cases [56]; retinoids cause regression of squamous metaplasia of the bronchus [14], but they may hasten the development of lung cancer in smokers [14]. Also, reversal of a preneoplastic lesion does not necessary mean a correction of the genetic alterations [57]: loss of heterozygosity at chromosome 9p persisted in the oropharyngeal mucosa, despite regression of leukoplakia following treatment with retinoids.

With this background we will examine the results of clinical trials of chemoprevention of concern to elderly patients

1.3 Clinical Trials of Chemoprevention

1.3.1 Breast Cancer

Age is the single most important risk factor for breast cancer [58] and older women appear ideal candidates for chemoprevention. The results of chemoprevention should be compared with result of other preventative strategies such as screening mammography that has reduced by 20-30% the mortality from breast cancer in women aged 50-70 and may reduce the mortality of even older women [59, 60]. The effectiveness of SERMS in chemoprevention is suggested by experimental and clinical studies:

- Treatment with ovariectomy, tamoxifen, raloxifene or exemestane prevented chemically induced breast cancer in rodents [39].
- The incidence of contralateral breast cancer was reduced by 39% in women who had received adjuvant tamoxifen for five years, according to the Oxford meta-analysis [61].

- The Multiple Outcome Raloxifene Evaluation (MORE) [36-38, 62] showed a reduction of approximately 70% in the incidence of hormone-receptor rich breast cancer among women receiving this SERM for the prevention of osteoporosis.
- In the NSABP-B24 study tamoxifen reduced by 43% the incidence of ipsilateral invasive breast cancer and by 30% that of non-invasive breast cancer among women treated with partial mastectomy and radiotherapy for Ductal Carcinoma in situ (DCIS) [63].
- Tamoxifen reduced the incidence of benign breast lesions, including epithelial hyperplasia and cyst of the breast [64].
- Tamoxifen reduced by 45% the incidence of invasive breast cancer and by 50% that of non-invasive breast cancer after 48 months of treatment in the BCPT (NSABP-P1 trial) [21] In this trial 13,300 women with a $\geq$ 1.67 risk of developing breast cancer over 5 years were randomized to receive tamoxifen or placebo [35]. All women aged 60 and older were eligible in terms of breast cancer risk. The reduction in invasive breast cancer was limited to hormone-receptor rich tumors, and was highest for women at higher risk of cancer, that is those with a risk of 5.01 or higher at five years according to the Gail model. The use of tamoxifen resulted in a 19% reduction in bone fractures, but a threefold increase in endometrial cancer and pulmonary embolism and a modest increase (14%) in cataracts. The risk of stroke was also increased in the tamoxifen treated group of women. The risk of complications increased with the age of the patient.

In addition to the NSABP-P1, two other trials explored the chemoprevention of breast cancer with tamoxifen. The Italian trial [65] closed prematurely due to high dropout rate, but eventually showed a statistically significant reduction of breast cancer in women treated with tamoxifen, and the Royal Marsden trial [66], that was negative. It should be said however that this trial involved 2741 women, with a drop out around 20%. This number may be inadequate to establish the effect of tamoxifen.

The weight of evidence indicates that tamoxifen, and possibly raloxifen do prevent breast cancer. The opened question is when chemoprevention of breast cancer is indicated, especially in older women. A decision analysis, based on the BCPT, established that the breast cancer risk threshold for which tamoxifen was beneficial increased with age and was 7% in 5 years for women aged 70 and older [67]. Not unexpectedly, the threshold increased with age, and for women aged 70 corresponded to a 7% risk of breast cancer in 5 years. Possibly this threshold is too low, as it does not take into account the deterioration in quality of life caused from hot flushes and mood changes. An additional concern is that tamoxifen might affect cognition of older women. Paganini Hill el al showed a twofold increase in memory disorder [68] and Chlebowski worsening of MR spectroscopy after myo-inositol [69] in women receiving tamoxifen.

Other chemopreventative strategies are under study including the use of raloxifen, that does not cause endometrial cancer nor memory deterioration [70], the use of aromatase inhibitors, of phyto-estrogen [71], and of COX-2 inhibitors [72].

The benefits of aromatase inhibitors was suggested by the Anastrozol Tamoxifen Alone or in Combination (ATAC) study, showing that the incidence of contralateral breast cancer was lower for women receiving adjuvant anastrozole than for those receiving adjuvant tamoxifen [73] In rodents, the combination of celecoxib and the aromatase inhibitor exemestane was more effective than exemestane alone in the prevention of DMBA-induced breast cancer [72].

1.3.2 Prostate Cancer

As in the case of breast cancer, age is the major risk factor for prostate cancer [74]. Familiarity [75] accounts for 50% of cancers before age 50, but is of limited interest to the older man. Other risk factors include elevated concentration of serum testosterone and of insulin-like growth factor 1 (ILF-1) [76], and inadequate dietary intake of phyto-estrogens (soya) [77], lycopenes (tomato) [78], and selenium [79, 80].

A well-recognized pre-neoplastic lesion, prostatic intra-epithelial neoplasia (PIN) [81, 82] provides a useful surrogate end-point for clinical trials of chemoprevention. PIN involves lesions of different malignant potential from dysplasia to high grade PIN (HGPIN). The most advanced lesions are associated with phenotypic and genotypic changes that are typical of prostatic cancer. The major impediment to the use of PIN as surrogate end-point of chemoprevention studies is the need for serial biopsies.

Androgen deprivation as chemoprevention is supported by clinical and experimental evidence, that include negligible incidence of prostate cancer among castrated experimental animals [83] and humans, association of prostate cancer with high life-long levels of testosterone [76], and regression of HGPIN following castration [84].

The main challenge in chemoprevention of prostate cancer appears then to provide androgen deprivation of the prostate minimizing the systemic effects of androgen deprivation, such as loss of libido and osteoporosis [42, 85]. The 5-α reductase inhibitor finasteride held this promise. In a large study involving 18,882 men aged 55 and older, with a median follow-up of 7 years, finasteride treatment resulted in a 24% decline in the incidence of prostate cancer [43, 85]. This achievement is mitigated by the fact that the incidence of high-grade tumor was 37% in the finasteride group and 22% in the

individuals receiving placebo. Clearly, finasteride cannot be recommended unless the impression that it causes a more aggressive disease is dispelled.

Other agents that may be studied include SERMs [86] and androgen antagonists [87], that prevent the growth of prostate cancer in the experimental model, and COX-2 inhibitors, that appear synergistic with hormonal deprivation [88] and Vitamin E and selenium [89]. These compounds have been selected for the The Selenium and Vitamin E Cancer Prevention Trial (SELECT), because vitamin E seemed to prevent prostate the ATBC (Alpha-Tocopherol, Beta Carotene Cancer Prevention Trial) [90].

1.3.3 Cancer of the Large Bowel

The incidence of this cancer increases with age [91]. Early detection of colorectal cancer through screening asymptomatic individuals reduces the mortality related to this disease [92-94]. To be acceptable chemoprevention needs to prove to be at least as effective and not more costly nor more risky than secondary prevention.

In recent year the NSAIDs and especially the COX-2 inhibitors have shown potential for chemoprevention of cancer of the large bowel. In favor of this hypothesis, the concentration of prostaglandin is higher in many malignant tissues than in normal gastrointestinal mucosa [30, 31], sulindac and celecoxib prevent cancer of the large bowel in experimental animals after carcinogen exposure [30], and both celecoxib [49], and aspirin [30] reduced the number and size of polyps in patients with familial polyposis of the colon. To this evidence it should be added the results of two retrospective studies, showing that regular aspirin intake was associated with reduced risk of death from cancer of the large bowel [30, 95].

Despite these encouraging results, chemoprevention of colorectal cancer with NSAIDs should be considered still hypothetical and should not be instituted in practice until results of randomized trials are available. Due to lesser gastrointestinal toxicity and risk of bleeding COX-2 inhibitors may be preferable to non-specific NSAIDs, but the long-term complications of these compounds, that may include coronary artery disease [96], are not established yet.

1.3.4 Lung Cancer

Cigarette smoking is the most important risk factor for lung cancer. Of interest to this book is the fact that the age at diagnosis of lung cancer has become more and more advanced during the last twenty years, and the mortality from lung cancer has increased approximately 25% among people older than 65, while has decreased to the same extent among those younger than 55 [97, 98]. This trend may be ascribed to smoking cessation, resulting in decreased mortality from cardiovascular diseases and delayed development of lung cancer [97]. Passive smoking, exposure to asbestos and arsenic [97] and cyclic amines in the diet [98, 99] may also play a role in the genesis of lung cancer. Molecular epidemiology of lung cancer reveals potential targets of chemoprevention, as lung cancer is more common in individuals with defective repair of mutagen-induced DNA damage [100-102], enhanced mutagen sensitivity [103, 104], increased activity of hepatic phase I and reduced activity of phase II enzymes [104]. At the moment there is no effective secondary prevention for lung cancer through early detection and chemoprevention may become the most important form of lung cancer control. Unfortunately, none of the trials of chemoprevention of lung cancer have been positive (Table 2). Nonetheless, these trials have taught important lessons to be carried on in future trials. First, it is clear that these trials are feasible, as many thousands of patients were enrolled both in phase IIb and phase III trials, and age did not appear an obstacle to recruitment. Second, the need for prospective trials was emphasized. It was reasonable from epidemiologic and experimental data to expect that β-carotene and retinoids were beneficial. Instead, β-carotene increased incidence and the mortality of lung cancer in the ATBC [90] and the CARET study (that was closed prematurely when the ATBC results emerged) [110]. After the harmful effect of β- carotene had emerged, it was found that affected mainly current smokers, and experiments were designed to clarify its mechanisms [114]. The exposure to a high doses of β-carotene and of smoke in combination, suppressed the expression of the β-receptors for retinoic acid and enhanced that of Activator protein 1 in ferret lungs. Consistent with these results isotretinoin increased the risk of secondary tumor and of recurrence of primary tumors in current smokers [113], in the Lung Inter-group Trial.

Based on these results, future studies of chemoprevention of lung cancer should target ex-smokers, and may include serial examination of sputum cytology for the study of molecular markers, including retinoid acid receptor, DNA-hypermethylation, P53 abnormalities, telomerase, ras abnormalities and loss of heterozygosity [14].

1.3.5 Other Cancers

Though chemoprevention in humans was first demonstrated for cancer of the head and neck [44], this has limited clinical applications, given the chronic toxicity of retinoic acid, even at low doses [44, 115] and the development of resistance to this substance [51].

Two strategies of chemoprevention of bladder cancer are under study and include use of feneretinaide and COX-2 inhibitors. Fenretinide blocks experimental carcinogenesis in experimental systems, and celecoxib appears synergistic with BCG in the treatment of carcinoma *in situ* [116].

Table 2. Randomized clinical trials of chemoprevention of lung cancer

Study	End-point	Agent (s)	Patients	Results
Phase II b				
Heimburger et al (1988) (105)	Reverse of metaplasia	Vitamin B12+ folate	73	Negative
Arnold et al (1992) (106)	Reverse cytology	Etretinate	150	Negative
Lee et al (1994) (107)	Prevention of metaplasia	Isotretinoin	87	Negative
Kurie et al (2000) (108)	Prevention of metaplasia	Fenretinide	68	Negative
Mclarty et al (1995) (109)	Sputum atypia in asbestos workers	Beta-carotene and vitamin A	755	Negative
Phase III, smokers				
ATBC (Alpha-tocopherol-Beta-Carotene) (90)	Prevention lung cancer in smokers	Alpha-tocopherol-Beta carotene	29133	Beta carotene was harmful; alpha-tocopherol may decrease the incidence of prostate cancer
Beta-carotene and Retinol Efficacy Trial (CARET) (Omenn) (110)	Prevention of lung cancer in smokers and asbestos workers	Beta carotene and retinol	18324	Increased incidence of and mortality from lung cancer
Phase III: previous history of lung cancer				
Pastorino (1993) (111)	Prevention second lung cancer	Retinyl palmitate	307	Negative
EUROSCAN (2000) (van Zandijk) (112)	Prevention second lung or head and neck cancer	Nacetyl cysteine, retinyl palmitate	2592	Negative
Lippman et al (2001) (113)	Prevention second lung cancer	isotretinoin	1166	Negative

1.4 Conclusions

Chemoprevention appears promising for older patients. The establishment of reliable surrogate end points and the development of safer agents may render clinical trials of chemoprevention speeder and risk less. Currently, only tamoxifen has been proven capable to prevent a cancer (breast cancer) beyond doubt, but this compound has limited application given the lack of improvement in breast cancer-related mortality and the risk of complications.

2. SECONDARY PREVENTION OF CANCER IN THE ELDERLY

Theoretical basis: Three assumptions support secondary cancer prevention (Figure 2) [6]:

- Cancer presents a preclinical phase, during which symptoms and signs of cancer are absent. In addition to asymptomatic invasive cancer, the pre-clinical phase involves premalignant lesions. Some of these, including carcinoma "in situ" (DCIS) of the breast and adenomatous polyps of the large bowel are recognizable at light microscopy. Other premalignant lesions may be detected only by genomic analysis (example obliteration of the rb (retinoblastoma) gene in normally appearing cells of the colonic mucosa predict the development of adenocarcinoma of the colon [6].
- Cancer may be diagnosed during the pre-clinical phase by screening the asymptomatic population at risk.
- Diagnosis of cancer at early stages is associated with improved cure rates.

The validity of these assumptions is established by randomized clinical trials demonstrating improved outcome for asymptomatic persons undergoing regular cancer screening. Controversy lingers as to which end-points are appropriate in these trials, especially for older individuals. A reduction in cancer-related deaths is considered the definitive proof that screening is effective [6], but this end-point has a number of shortcomings. Several years are required to achieve this goal, while new and more sensitive diagnostic techniques may be developed that render obsolete the results of the studies. Furthermore a number of lives maybe unnecessarily lost among the controls, if screening proves effective. To avoid these difficulties alternative end-points, achievable in a shorter time period, have been proposed, all of which are fraught by serious problems. Comparison of cancer-related survival in lieu of mortality rate between the screened and the control population is fraught by the lead-time bias, implying that screened patients appear to live longer because their cancer has been diagnosed earlier. The demonstration that cancer is diagnosed at an earlier stage in the screened than in the control population is fraught by the so-called lead-time and over-detection biases [6]. Length time bias implies that only indolent tumors are diagnosed at screening, while rapidly dividing tumors "sneak through" screening intervals (Figure 3); over-detection bias *implies* that a number of cancers diagnosed at screening would have never become clinically detectable during a patient's lifetime.

Figure 2. Early detection of precancerous lesions or early cancer may lead to improved surgical cure.

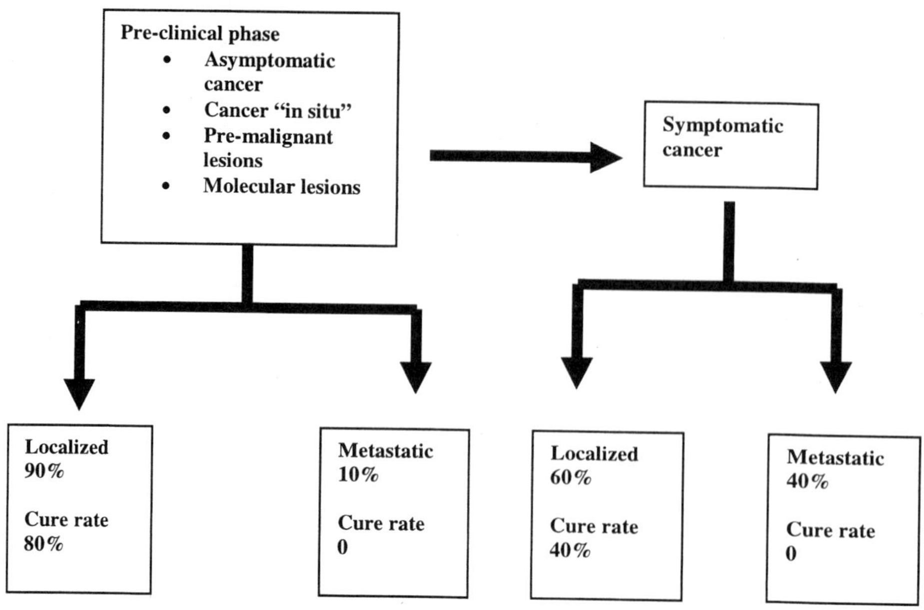

Figure 3: Length time bias. Rapidly growing tumors (black circles) may become symptomatic during screening intervals (arrows). In this example, the rabidly growing tumor reaches a diagnosable size between screening interval. Because of this effect, screening is more likely to diagnose slowly growing tumors, whose prognosis may be better. Thus, screening may give the impression of improving patient's survival from diagnosis simply because it detects prevalently slowly growing, less aggressive tumors.

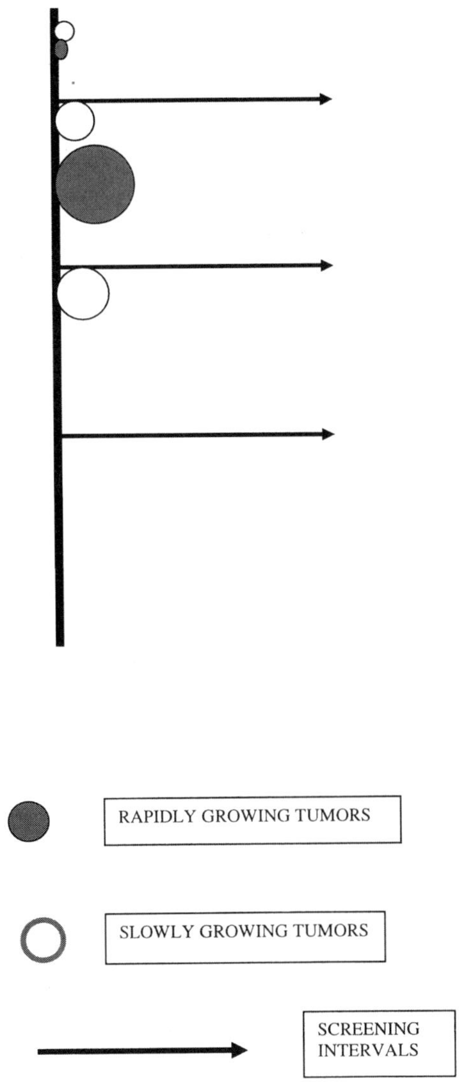

Even a reduction in cancer-related mortality may not represent a satisfactory end-point. First it is not clear whether a reduction in cancer-related mortality is desirable when the overall mortality of the population is not reduced. This issue is of particular concern for older individuals subjected to competitive causes of death by multiple comorbidities and is exemplified by the case of prostate cancer. A Swedish randomized controlled study of radical prostatectomy vs observation in men up to age 75 has demonstrated that surgery reduces the cancer-related mortality but not the overall mortality of these individuals [117]. As an inference, screening older individuals for prostate cancer is unlikely to affect their mortality. Second the effects of screening on quality of life of older individuals should be assessed. Screening may involve a number of complications including discomfort, cost, inconvenience, anxiety and the risk related to diagnostic tests. It is reasonable to fear that these complications may deny the limited benefits of screening on survival [118].

2.1 Effects of Aging on Accuracy and Effectiveness of Cancer Screening

The accuracy of some screening tests may improve with age. As the prevalence of common cancers increases [2, 3] with age, the predictive value positive of diagnostic examinations improves [6, 119]. Also, physiologic changes of aging, such as atrophy of the mammary tissue may allow better appreciation of new lesions suspicious of cancer. At the same time, shorter life expectancy and reduced tolerance of antineoplastic treatment may limit the benefits of cancer screening. Other considerations may also mitigate the value of screening asymptomatic older individuals for cancer. Previous screening examinations may have eliminated all prevalence cases of cancer and have made negligible the diagnostic yield of subsequent examinations [6]. The behavior of some neoplasms, including breast cancer, becomes more indolent in the elderly and less threatening of patient's survival and quality of life [6]. Accordingly, early detection of these neoplasms may not be beneficial.

Clearly, the balance of benefits and risks of cancer screening in the elderly varies from an individual to the other. The estimate of whether this balance is negative or positive may be based on two considerations: individual life expectancy and risk that the cancer may compromise a patient's quality of life, even when it is unlikely to shorten the survival.

Life expectancy may be determined by life table methods [120] (Fig. 4). On the basis of a patient function and comorbidity one may decide whether the patient belongs to the upper intermediate or lower quartile of life expectancy. Seemingly, cancer screening would not be beneficial for persons with a life-expectancy shorter than five years, as the earliest effects of screening on cancer-related deaths are seen five years after the institution of the screening program. As a practical rule, vulnerable and frail patients, that is patients who have increased circulating concentrations of Il-6 and D-Dimer [121], or patients with a score ≥ 4 in the Vulnerable Elderly Survey 13 (VES-13) [122], patients with difficulty in performing tests of physical performance such as the get up and go tests [123], patients with moderate dementia or other geriatric syndromes, such as multiple falls, neglect and abuse, failure to thrive, spontaneous bone fracture, should not undergo cancer screening except for very special circumstances, that increase their risk to develop cancer over the following two three years. These conditions include recent history of cancer of the breast and of the large bowel.

To establish a positive balance between benefits and risks of screening two combined approaches appear reasonable. The influence of cancer on the quality of life of older individual depends both on the nature of the cancer and on the attitude of the person. For example: both breast and prostate cancer are unlikely to cause the death of the patient when they are found in a 85 year old person, but cancer of the breast is much more likely to cause local complications including fungating masses, pain, infections and bleeding than cancer of the prostate. Furthermore, the management of localized breast cancer is associated with a lower risk of surgical complications than that of prostate cancer. On the basis of this consideration it may be sensible to screen 85-year-old women for breast cancer and not to screen 85-year-old men for prostate cancer.

A recent study established that older individuals vary in their willingness to take risk [124]. High-risk takers are more likely to accept cancer treatment even when the predicted benefits are minimal and are more likely to benefit from cancer screening in terms of quality of life.

A number of approaches have been suggested to make cancer screening of older individuals more cost and time effective. For example, Kerlikowske [53] recommended that of women aged 70 and older only those with a bone density in the upper quintile undergo screening mammography, because 9 out of 10 breast cancers occur in this group of women and serial bone density assessment to screen for osteoporosis are recommended in all post-menopausal women. This approach is at present only a theoretical model, but it exemplifies a reasonable attempt to target cancer screening on the older population at highest risk. With this background one may now examine the value of screening older individuals for common neoplasms.

Figure 4. Upper, middle and lower quartiles of life expectancy for women and men at selected ages. Data from the Life Tables of the United States. (Reprinted with permission, JAMA 2001, 285:2750-56, "*Copyright© (2001) American Medical Association*, all rights reserved.")

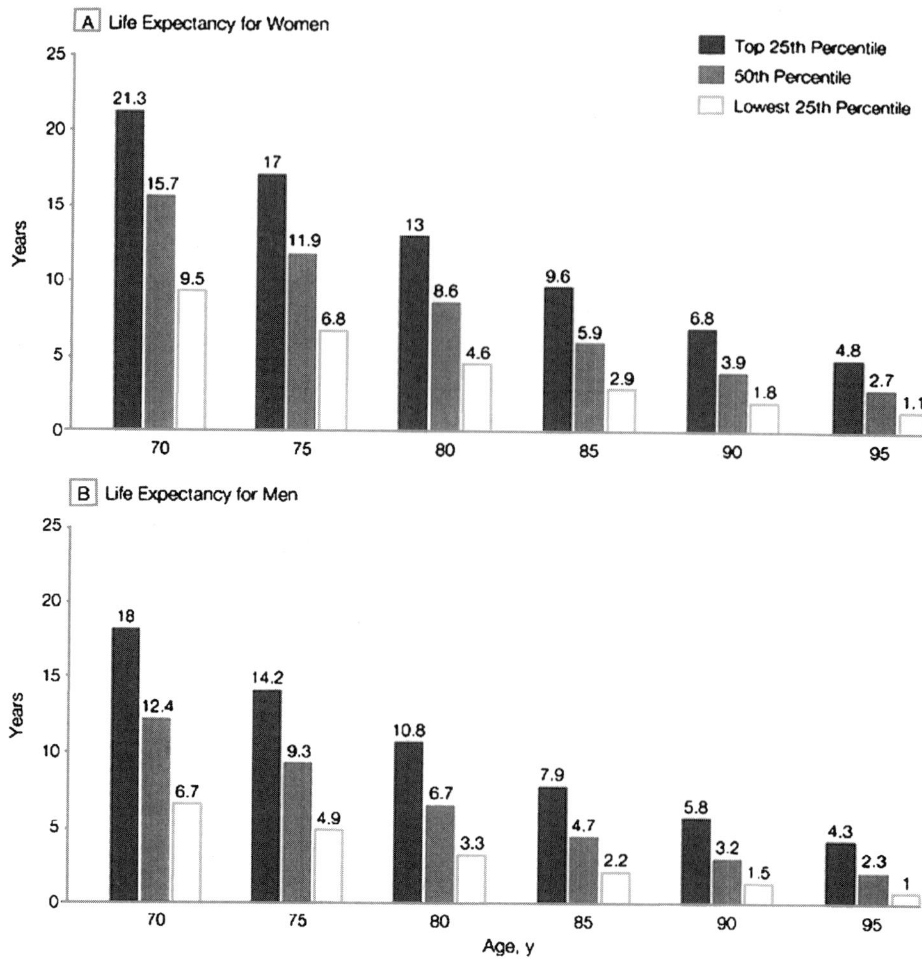

2.2 Approach to Individual Diseases

2.2.1 Breast Cancer

Of the screening examinations promoted for early detection of breast cancer (mammography, clinical examination of the breast and breast self-examination) only screening mammography has proved effective in randomized clinical trials (level 1 evidence) [125-130]. With one exception [126], all these trials, reported a 20-30% reduction in breast cancer mortality in the screened population. Screening mammography has been the object of a recent controversy. A meta-analysis of randomized trials claimed that the six positive trials were fraught by so many biases to make the results unreliable, and only the two negative studies were free of bias [131]. This position has not found general acceptance however, because one of the negative studies, the Malmö trial, turned positive at the last analysis [132], and the other negative study, the Canadian trial, was criticized because it had used "single view" mammography, that appears less sensitive [125, 126]. The unbalanced randomization in the Edinburgh trial, that was positive, would have minimized rather that amplified the effects of mammography [133]. Furthermore, it appears difficult to assume that the degree of bias in the other positive trials would have been responsible for the dramatic results observed [130]. This controversy did not change the recommendations of major organizations, including the United States Preventive Service Task Force (USPSTF), that women aged 50-70 undergo serial screening mammography. The benefits of screening mammography were not conclusively demonstrated for women aged 70+, who had been involved in only two trials [130]. However, some degree of benefit appears likely even for older women, for the following reasons:

- A Dutch study showed in a retrospective analysis that screening mammography reduced breast cancer mortality in women aged 70-75 [134].
- A number of recent analysis of the Surveillance, Epidemiology and End results (SEER) data supported screening mammography for older women by showing that women aged 70 and older undergoing at least two mammographic evaluations after age 70 were two and half fold less likely to die from breast cancer than women who had not undergone mammography after age 70 [59]; that breast cancer patients aged 75 and older presented with earlier stage breast cancer if they had undergone mammography [135], and that mammography appeared beneficial even to older women with moderate degree of comorbidity [60].
- Both total and partial mastectomy may be performed under local anesthesia, with minimal morbidity and negligible mortality. The treatment of early breast cancer may thus improve a patient's quality of

life by eliminating the risk of local complications, even when it does not lead to survival prolongation.

On the basis of these considerations it appears reasonable to recommend that women aged 70 and older undergo some form of screening for breast cancer, if their life expectancy is estimated to be 5 years or longer [130]. A fruitful debate may concern cost-effective screening of older women, rather than the value of screening. To this purpose it is important to remember that in some randomized controlled studies, mammography was performed at interval of 18-36 months [130], without compromise of effectiveness. For older women, bearing tumors that in general are more indolent, intervals longer than one year may reduce the cost, discomfort and inconvenience of screening. The clinical breast examination (CBE), that may be performed at any clinic visit, with minimal inconvenience for the patient, time investment for the provider, and cost for the health care system, may represent a complement or even an alternative to mammography. The Canadian study [125] and the Breast Cancer Detection Demonstration Project (BCDDP) [136] showed that CBE and mammography were equivalent in detecting invasive cancer. Focusing screening efforts on women at high risk of the disease, as proposed in the Kerlikowske model may further improve the cost-effectiveness of breast cancer screening [53].

Any recommendations related to breast cancer screening will evolve with the results of studies employing newer and more accurate imaging techniques such as digital mammography and MRI of the breast.

2.2.2 *Cancer of the Large Bowel*

Of the screening tests proposed for early diagnosis of cancer of the large bowel, serial examinations of voided stools for FOB have proven effective in randomized controlled studies [92-94, 137] involving asymptomatic individuals aged 50-80. Annual examination was more effective than the biennial one [94]. Retrospective studies support the value of serial endoscopic examinations, and of these, full colonoscopy is favored, as it allows visualization of the whole large bowel and removal of adenomatous polyps, a procedure that prevents the development of invasive cancer [93, 137-139].

Some form of screening for colorectal cancer in persons aged 50 and over at average risk is recommended by all major organizations, but controversy lingers about the most cost-effective forms of screening. In a decision analysis full colonoscopy every ten years appeared preferable to biennial FOB and to sigmoidoscopy every five years [92].Whereas the benefit of screening is universally accepted, the best screening strategy remains controversial. In a recent decision analysis full colonoscopy every ten years appeared more cost effective than biennial examination of FOB and sigmoidoscopy every five years [92]. A re-evaluation of the data suggests that colonoscopy every five years would be even preferable.

In view of the fact that the incidence of colorectal cancer increases with age even after age 80 [2, 3] and that early detection may prevent the need of emergency surgery, whose mortality and morbidity increase with age [140], some form of screening for cancer of the large bowel appears indicated for any person with a life-expectancy of 3-5 years. The examination of choice varies with the patient preference and risks of complications. For patients unable or unwilling to have colonoscopy, examination of the stool should be performed every two years at the very minimum.

2.2.3 *Prostate Cancer*

The value of screening asymptomatic men for prostate cancer is still controversial despite the demonstration that serial PSA examinations do lead to early diagnosis of prostate cancer [141, 142] and that radical prostatectomy for early prostate cancer reduces the risk of cancer-related mortality [117]. The crux of the controversy is whether a reduction in cancer-related deaths at the price of serious treatment complications is worthwhile when a clear improvement of overall survival cannot be documented. Other areas of controversy include the age at which screening should be initiated and discontinued, if it should be performed at all; the optimal interval between assessments, and the PSA values at which prostate biopsy should be performed.

The evidence that serial PSA determinations reduce the risk of cancer-related deaths is still circumstantial and consists of:

- ➢ Two randomized and controlled studies [141, 142] showing a decline in cancer-related death thanks to screening. Both studies however cannot be considered conclusive. In one, conducted in Tyrol, all male population of one Alpine village underwent screening, while the male population of another; "control" village did not [141]. Clearly it cannot be assumed that the populations of the two villages had equivalent risk of prostate cancer. In the other study, the male population of Quebec City was randomized to screening vs no screening [142] but only a minority of eligible individuals eventually accepted randomization.
- The mortality from prostate cancer in the Olmstead County, USA has declined since introduction of PSA screening [143].
- The American Cancer Society instituted the prostate cancer awareness week in 1986. During this week, that is repeated every year, PSA

screening is promoted to the USA male population aged 50 and older. After five years, the incidence of advanced stage newly diagnosed prostate cancer had declined from 20% to less than 5%, suggesting that early detection is effective in preventing metastatic disease [144, 145].

- Determination of PSA on blood banked during the physician health study showed that the PSA concentration in the serum increased approximately 6 years prior to the clinical diagnosis of prostate cancer. After diagnosis, the median survival was approximately 8 years [146]. As the majority of these individuals had a life-expectancy in excess of 14 years it is legitimate assume that prostate cancer was the cause of death for the physicians who developed it, and that cure of prostate cancer might have saved their lives.

In the original screening studies PSA levels above four ng/ml were considered abnormal and an indication for biopsy [144, 147] it is now clear that this criterion for biopsy is inadequate. The predictive value positive for PSA values between 4 and 10 was only around 20%. At the same time, a number of studies have now shown that as many as 50% of prostate cancer may occur with PSA levels lower than 4 ng/dl [131, 148-150]. The specificity of the PSA determination may be improved by adopting age-adjusted normal standards, measurement of PSA density that is the ratio between the PSA value and the prostate volume, and of PSA velocity [148], that is the yearly rate of increase in PSA concentration, the ratio between free and total PSA, that is lower in patients with cancer than in those with benign prostatic hypertrophy and the simultaneous measurement of PSA and Kallikrein2 levels [151, 152] The sensitivity of the test may be improved by lowering the PSA levels at which the biopsy is performed, or performing a biopsy anytime the PSA velocity is higher than .75 ng/year), or having the biopsy directed by the ratio between free and bound PSA irrespective of the total PSA level. These different strategies are explored in ongoing studies.

To illustrate the uncertainty related to the optimal screening interval and its dependence on the accuracy of the test, two recent decision analysis provided both reasonable, but quite different conclusions. Etzioni et al compared annual screening using as PSA cut-off point age-adjusted values and biannual screening with cut-off value 4.0 ng/ml or more, and concluded that biannual screening reduced by 50% the false positive rate of the test, and maintained 93% of its effectiveness [153]. In this model screening was initiated at age 50 and continued at regular interval up to age 75. Ross et al calculated that biennial determination of PSA, with 2.6 ng/ml as the cut-point value at which biopsy should be preformed was the most cost effective strategy for men aged 45-75 [154].

While ongoing clinical trials are maturing, it is reasonable to conclude that screening asymptomatic men for prostate cancer with serial PSA determinations may reduce the cancer-related mortality for men aged 50-75. These subjects should be informed of potential benefits and risks of screening. It is reasonable to space the determination of PSA every two-three years after two yearly determinations have been normal, and free PSA should be included in the testing as it can provide additional information. Irrespective of the PSA values, a biopsy should be performed for PSA velocity of .75 ng or higher.

As average life expectancy of men lengthen, prostate cancer may progressively become a more important cause of death, and prostate cancer screening may prove beneficial even in older individuals.

2.2.4 *Lung Cancer*

Lung cancer is becoming more and more a disease of older individuals. Over the last twenty years the lung cancer-related mortality has declined around 30% for people aged 55 and younger and has increased 15% for those 75 and older [2, 3, 97, 98, 155, 156]. Currently the median age of lung cancer is 68 and approximately 40% of these neoplasms occur in people aged 70 and older. At least in part, these trends may be explained by the fact that as more people quit smoking, their risk of dying from cardiovascular diseases declines, they live longer and have more opportunity to develop lung cancer [97]. This possibility is confirmed by the fact that lung cancer in ex-smoker is becoming more common and lung cancer in the elderly appear less aggressive than in younger individuals [157, 158].

Four randomized controlled studies in asymptomatic smokers compared in the 70s yearly chest radiograph with chest radiographs and serial sputum cytology [6]. Though these studies are referred to as negative, they taught some important lessons:

- First, these studies demonstrated that sputum cytology does not improve the lung cancer-related mortality over chest radiography. No definitive statement can be made about the value of chest radiography, as even controls received this examination. In one study, the patients whose cancer had been diagnosed at screening had a five-year survival around 35%. This value is substantially higher than the 5% five-year survival of persons whose cancer was diagnosed when they had become symptomatic.
- The screened population was composed of smokers, whose survival might have been shortened by a number of comorbidities, including second malignancies. In this population it might have been particularly difficult to document any effect of lung cancer screening on survival. Nowadays the main focus of screening would be ex-smokers, persons

who have a more prolonged life expectancy, lower prevalence of comorbidity and likely a less aggressive lung cancer.

- More accurate imaging examinations as well as a number of molecular tests may have improved the sensitivity of the screening tests. A number of non-randomized studies showed that low energy spiral CT might improve the detection rate of early lung cancer [155, 159-162]. The main problem with this screening strategy is that at least 60% of the screened individuals have non-calcified nodule, only 2% of which turned out to be lung cancer. Clearly, it is not feasible from either a safety or a cost standpoint to biopsy all suspicious lesions and criteria of risk need to be formulated. An ongoing randomized clinical trial started in 2002 explores the value of spiral CT over regular chest radiography to reduce the lung cancer-related mortality of ex-smokers.

2.2.5 *Cervical Cancer*

The incidence of cervical cancer decreases and the mortality for metastatic cervical cancer has been increasing with age [2, 3]. The influence screening may have on this increasing mortality is unclear. According to a retrospective study, at least one Papanicolau examination between ages 60

and 70 reduced the mortality for cervical cancer among women who had not undergone regular screening before age 60 [163]. Thus, it appears reasonable to recommend serial Papanicolau screening for women aged 60 an older who had not undergone regular screening, especially those at increased risk of cervical cancer.

2.3 Age-Related Barriers to Cancer Prevention

Germane to the issue of cancer screening in the elderly is the recognition of age-related barriers to screening, which may be both patient and provider related. The ones include cultural barriers, lack of information and of social support [164, 165]; the others include lack of knowledge and lack of enthusiasm [164, 165]. Both the patient and provider related barrier is influenced by ageism, a proteiform prejudice that may color all aspects of life. Recurrent themes of ageism include the impression that aging means shortened life expectancy and limited tolerance of even simple medical procedures. The corollary of this attitude is that older individuals are better off left alone than submitted to any form of medical intervention. Ageism's is responsible of many unnecessary deaths and of unnecessary suffering [166], disabilities and deterioration of quality of life. Interventions that may overcome these barriers deserve to be outlined:

- Public and professional education illustrating the life expectancy of older individuals, the risk of cancer, and the benefit of early cancer treatment in terms of cure, preservation of function, and quality of life may go a long way in overcoming ageism.
- Focused interventions may be indicated for selected ethnic groups. For example, Fox et al have shown that concerns about their legal status and suspicious of the American medical system, in addition to poor understanding of English and illiteracy may prevent Hispanic women from seeking screening for breast and cervical cancer [165]. As these women generally utilize Hispanic practitioners, it is important to focus professional education on these practitioners as well.
- The recommendations of the primary care physician, and the degree of enthusiasm expressed by this practitioner may be the single most important determinant of cancer screening by older individuals. The involvement of these individuals is essential to promote cancer screening of the older population. This problem is compounded by the fact that more than 50% of individuals aged 65 and older lack a primary care provider, though they may be attending specialty clinics [166].

2.4 Conclusions

It is reasonable to implement screening for cancer of the breast and f the large bowel in persons with a life expectancy of 5 years and longer. No definite recommendation may be issued at present related to screening for prostate, lung and cervical cancer. Ongoing clinical trials may answer some of these questions.

REFERENCES

1. Cova D; Balducci L: Cancer chemotherapy in the elderly. In: Balducci L; Lyman GH; Ershler WB: Comprehensive geriatric oncology, Harwood Academic Publishers, in press, 2003
2. Berlin A: The conquest of cancer. Cancer Invest, 1995,13,540-550
3. Yancik R; Ries LAG: Aging and cancer in America: demographic and epidemiologic perspectives. Hematol/Oncol Clin, N America, 2000,14, 17-24
4. Yancik RM; Ries L: Cancer and age: magnitude of the problem. In: Balducci L; Lyman GH; Ershler WB: Comprehensive geriatric oncology. Harwood Academic Publishers, London, 1998, 95-104
5. Rcpetto L; Balducci L: A case for geriatric oncology. Lancet Oncology 2002, 3, 289-297s
6. Balducci L; Beghe' C: Prevention of cancer in the older person, Clin Ger Med 2002, 18, 505-528
7. Fried LP; Bandeen-Roche K; Kasper JD et al: Association of comorbidity with disability in older women: the women's health and aging study. J Clin Epidemiol, 1999, 52, 27-37

8. Barnabei R; Gambassi G; Lapana K et al: Management of pain in elderly patients with cancer. SAGE study group. Systematic assessment of geriatric drug use via epidemiology. JAMA, 1998, 17, 1877-1882
9. Balducci L; Extermann M: A practical approach to the older patient with cancer. Current problems in cancer, 2001, 25, 1-76
10. Diab SG; Elledge RM; Clark GM: Tumor characteristics and clinical outcome of elderly women with breast cancer. J Natl Cancer Inst, 2000, 92, 550-556
11. Repetto L; Granetto C; Venturino A et al: Prognostic evaluation of the older cancer patient. In: Balducci L; Lyman GH; Ershler WB: Comprehensive geriatric oncology, Harwood Academic Publishers, Amsterdam, 1998, 281-286
12. Sugimura T: Multistep carcinogenesis: a 1992 perspective. Science, 1992, 258, 603-607.
13. Anisimov V: Interactions of aging and carcinogenesis. Ref this book
14. Lippman SM; Spitz MR: Lung cancer chemoprevention: an integrated approach. J Clin Oncol, 2001, 19, suppl, 74s-82s.
15. Kinzler KV; Vogelstein B: Cancer-susceptibility genes. Gatekeepers and caretakers. Nature, 1997, 386, 761-763
16. Guengerich FP: Metabolic activation of carcinogens. Pharmacol Ther, 1992, 54, 16-71.
17. Oesch F; Doehmer J; Friedberg T et al: Control of ultimate mutagenic species by different enzymes. Progr Clin Biol Res 1990, 340B, 49-65.
18. Chung FL; Kelloff G; Steele V et al: Chemopreventive efficacy of arylalkyl isothiocianantes and N-actyl-cystein for lung tumorigenesis in Fisher rats. Cancer Res, 1996, 56, 772-778
19. Hecht SS: Chemoprevention by isothiocyanates. J Cell Biochem Suppl, 1995, 22, 195-209
20. Stoner GD; Mukhtar H: Polyphenols as cancer chemopreventive agents. J Cell Biochem Suppl, 1995, 22, 169-180
21. Morse MA; Elkind KI; Amin SG et al: Effects of alkyl chain length on the inhibition of NNK-induced lung neoplasia in A/J mice by arylalkyl isothiocyanates. Carcinogenesis, 1989, 10, 1757-1759
22. Brady JF; Ishikazi H; Fukuto JM et al: Inhibition of cytochrome P-450 2E1 by diallyl sulfide and its metabolites. Chem Res Toxicol, 1991, 4:642-647
23. Chen L; Lee M; Hong JY et al: Relationship between cytochrome p450E1 and acetone catabolism in rats as studied with diallyl sulfide as an inhibitor. Biochem Pharmacol, 1994, 48, 2199-2205
24. Rao CV; Tokomo K; Kelloff G et al: Inhibition of dietary oltipraz of experimental intestinal carcinogenesis induced by azoxymethane in male F344 rats. Carcinogenesis, 1991, 12, 1051-105.5
25. Hursting SD; Slaga TJ; Fisher SM et al: Mechanism-based cancer prevention approaches: targets, examples, and the use of transgenic mice. J Natl Cancer Inst, 1999, 91,215-225
26. Sancar A: Mechanism of DNA repair. Science, 1995, 266, 1954-1956
27. Fischer SM; DiGiovanni J: Mechanisms of tumor promotion: epigenetic changes in cell signaling. Cancer Bull, 1995, 47, 456-463
28. Furstenberger G; Marks F: Prostaglandin, epidermal hyperplasia, and skin tumor promotion. In: Horn KV; Marnett LJ: Prostaglandins, leukotrienes and cancer. Martinus-NiJoff, Boston, 1985, 22-37
29. Kong AN; Yu R; Hebbar V et al: Signal transduction events elicited by cancer prevention compounds. Mutat Res, 2001, 1, 231-241
30. Baron JA; Sandler RS: Nonsteroidal antiinflammatory drugs and cancer prevention. Ann Rev Med, 2000, 51, 511-523

31. Prescott SM; Fitzpatrick FA: Cyclooxygenase 2 and carcinogenesis. Biochem Biophys Acta, 2000, 1470, M69-78
32. Lippman SM; Brown PH: Tamoxifen prevention of breast cancer: an instance of the fingerpost (J Natl Cancer Inst, 1999,91, 1809-1819
33. Meyskens FL; Gerner EW: Development of difluoromethylornithine as a chemopreventive agent. Clin Cancer Res, 1999, 5, 945-951
34. Steele VE; Holmes CA; Hawk ET et al: Potential use of lipooxygenase inhibitors for cancer prevention. Expert Opin Investig Drugs. 2000, 9, 2121-2138
35. Fisher B; Costantino JP; Wickerham DL et al: Tamoxifen for prevention of breast cancer: report from the national Adjuvant breast and Bowel Project. J Natl cancer Inst, 1998, 90, 1371-1388
36. Agnusdei D; Liu-lerae S; Augendre-Ferrant B: Results of International Clinical Trials with Raloxifene. Ann Endocrin(paris), 1999, 60, 342-346
37. Ettinger B; Black D; Cummings S et al: Raloxifene reduces the risk of incident vertebral fractures: 24 months interim analysis. Osteoporos Int, 1998, 8 (suppl 3), 11
38. Yaffe K, Krueger K, Sarkar S, Grady D, Barrett-Connor E, Cox DA, Nickelsen T: Multiple outcomes of raloxifene evaluation investigators. N Engl J Med, 2001, April 19:344(16): 1207-1213
39. Jordan VC; Lababidi MK; Langhan-Fahey S: Suppression of mouse mammary tumorigenesis by long-term tamoxifen therapy. J Natl Cancer Inst, 1991; 83, 492-496
40. Minton SE: Chemoprevention of breast cancer in the older patient, Hematol Oncol Clin N America, 2000, 14, 113-130
41. Lieberman R; Nelson WG; Sakr WA et al: Executive summary of the National Cancer Institute workshop: highlights and recommendations. Urology, 2001 57 (suppl 1), 4-27
42. Lieberman R: Androgen deprivation therapy for prostate cancer chemoprevention: current status and future directions for agent developments. Urology, 2001, 58, (suppl 1), 83-90
43. Thompson IM; Goodman DJ; Tanger CM et al: The influence of finasteride on the development of prostate cancer. N Engl J Med, 2003, 349, 215-224
44. Hong WK; Endicott J; Itri LM et al: 13-cis-retinoic acid in the treatment of oral leukoplakia. N Engl J Med, 1986, 315, 1501-1505
45. Chambon B: The retinoid signaling pathway: molecular and genetic analysis. Semin Cell Biol, 1994,5, 115-125
46. Mangelsdorf DJ; Umesono K; Evans RM: The retinoid receptors. In: Sporn MB; Roberts AB; Goodman DS: The retinoids. Raven press, New York, 1994, 319-349
47. Boehm MF; Zhang L: Synthesis and structure-activity relationship of novel retinoid X receptor-selective retinoids J Med Chem, 1994,37,2930-2941
48. Oridate N; Lotan D; Xu XC et al: Differential induction of apoptosis by all-trans-retinoic acid and N-(4-hydroxiphenyl)retinamide in human head and neck squamous cell carcinoma cell lines. Clin Cancer Res, 1996, 2, 855-863
49. Steinbach G; Phillips RKS; Lynch PM: The effect of Celecoxib, a cyclooxygenase 2 inhibitor in familial adenomatous polyposis. N Engl J Med, 2000, 342, 1996-1952
50. Meyskens FL: Criteria for the implementation of large and multiagent clinical chemoprevention trials. J Cell Biochem Suppl 2000, 34, 115-120
51. Benner SE; Pajak TF; Lippman SM et al: Prevention of second primary tumors with isotretinoin in squamous cell carcinoma of the head and neck: long term follow up. J Natl Cancer Inst, 1994, 86, 140-141
52. Day R; Ganz PA; Costantino JP et al: Health-related quality of life and tamoxifen in breast cancer prevention: a report from the National Surgical Adjuvant Breast and Bowel Project P1 study. J Clin Oncol, 1999, 17, 2559-2569
53. Kerlikowske K; Salzman P; Phillips KA et al: Continuing screening mammography in women aged 70 to 79 years. JAMA, 1999, 282, 2156-2163

54. Vineis P; Veglia F: Selection and validation of biomarkers for chemoprevention: the contribution of epidemiology. IARC Sci Publ 2001, 154:57-68
55. Kensler TW; Davidson NE; Groopman JD et al: Biomarkers and surrogacy: relevance to chemoprevention. IARC Sci Publ, 2001, 154, 27-47
56. Follen M; Meyskens FL; Atkinson EN et al: Why most randomized phase II Cervical Cancer Chemoprevention Trials are uninformative. J Natl Cancer Inst, 2001, 93,1293-96
57. Mao L; El Naggar AK; Papadimitrakopoulou VM et al: phenotype and genotype in advanced premalignant head and neck lesions after chemopreventive therapy. J Natl Cancer Inst, 1998, 90, 1545-1551
58. Costantino JP; Gail MH; Pee D et al: Validation studies of model projecting the risk of invasive and total breast cancer incidence. J Natl Cancer Inst., 1999, 91:1541-1548
59. McCarthy EP; Burns RB; Freund KM et al: Mammography use, breast cancer stage at diagnosis, and survival among older women. J Am Ger Soc, 2000, 48, 1226-1233
60. McPherson CP; Swenson KK; Lee MW: The effects of mammographic detection and comorbidity on the survival of older women with breast cancer. J Am Ger Soc, 2002, 50, 1061-1068
61. Early Breast Cancer Trialists Collaborative Group: Tamoxifen for early breast cancer: an overview of the randomized trials. Lancet 351:1451-1467, 1998
62. Cummings SR; Duong T; Kenyon E et al: Serum Estradiol Level and risk of breast cancer during treatment with raloxifene JAMA, 2001, 287, 216-220
63. Fisher B; Dignam J; Wolmark N et al: Tamoxifen in treatment of intraductal breast cancer: National breast and bowel project B24 randomized controlled study. Lancet, 1999, 353, 1993-2000
64. Tan-Chiu E; Costantino J; Wang J et al: The effect of tamoxifen on benign breast disease. Findings from the national Surgical Adjuvant Breast and Bowel Project (NSABP) Breast cancer prevention trial. Breast Cancer Res Treat, 2001, 69, 3, 210
65. Veronesi U; Maisonneuve P; Costa A et al: Prevention of breast cancer with tamoxifen: preliminary findings from the Italian randomised trial among hysterectomysed women. Lancet, 1998, 352, 93-97
66. Powles T; Eles R; Ashley S et al: Interim analysis of the incidence of breast cancer in the Royal Marsden Hospital tamoxifen Randomised chemoprevention trial. Lancet, 1998, 352, 98-101
67. Gail MH; Costantino JP; Bryant J et al: Weighing the risks and benefits of tamoxifen treatment for preventing breast cancer. J Natl Cancer Inst, 1999, 91, 1829-1846
68. Paganini-Hill A, Clark LJ: Preliminary assessment of cognitive function in breast cancer patients. Breast Cancer Research Treat, 2000, Nov; 64(20: 165-176
69. Chlebowski RT; Ernst T; Chang L et al: Tamoxifen and estrogen effect on brain chemistry determined by MRI spectroscopy. ASCO Proc, 2001,20, 28a, abstr 108
70. Vogel VG; Costantino JP; Wickerham DL et al: The study of Tamoxifen and Raloxifen: preliminary enrollment data from a randomized breast cancer risk reduction trial. Breast Cancer Res Treatm, 2001, 69, 225 (abstr 135)
71. Messina MJ; Loprinzi CL: Soy for breast cancer survivors: a critical review of the literature. J Nutr, 2001, 13 (11 suppl), 3095s-3108s
72. Presenti E; Masferrer JL; Di Salle E: Effect of exemestane and celecoxib alone or in combination on DMBA induced mammary carcinoma in rats. Breast Cancer Res Treat, 2001, 69, 288 (abstr 445)
73. Baum M, on behalf of the ATAC Trialists' Group: The ATAC (Arimidex Tamoxifen Alone or in Combination) adjuvant breast cancer trial in post-menopausal women. Breast Cancer Res Treat, 2001, 69, 210, abstr 8
74. Boyle P: Severi G: epidemiology of prostate cancer chemoprevention. Eur Urol, 1999,75, 370-376

75. Stanford JL; Ostrander EA: Familial Prostate Cancer. Epidemiol Rev, 2001, 23, 19-23
76. Shaneyfelt T; Husein R; Bubley G et al: Hormonal predictors of prostate cancer: a meta-analysis. J Clin Oncol, 2000, 847-854
77. Moyad MA: Soy, disease prevention and prostate cancer. Semin Urol Oncol, 1999 17, 97-103
78. Giovannucci E: Tomatoes, tomato-based products, lycopene and cancer: review of the epidemiologic literature. J Natl Cancer Inst, 1999, 91, 317-331
79. Yoshizava K; Willett WC; Morris SJ et al: Study of prediagnostic selenium level in toenails and the risk of advanced prostate cancer. J Natl Cancer Inst, 1998, 90, 1219-1224
80. Nelson WG; Wilding G: Prostate cancer prevention agent development: criteria for candidate chemoprevention agents. Urology, 2001, 57, 56-63
81. Bostwick DG: Prostatic intra-epithelial neoplasia is a risk factor for cancer. Semin Urol Oncol, 1999, 17, 187-198
82. Bostwick DG; Montironi R; Sesterhenn IA: Diagnosis of prostatic intraepithelial neoplasia: Prostate work group consensus report. Scand J Urol Nephr Suppl, 2000, 205, 3-10
83. Balducci et al: prostate cancer: a model of cancer in the elderly. Arch Ger Gerontol, 1989
84. van der Kast TH; Labrie F; Tetu B: Prostatic intra-epithelial neoplasia and endocrine manipulation. Eur Urol, 35, 1999, 508-510
85. Lieberman R; Bermejo C; Akaza H et al: progress in prostate cancer chemoprevention: modulators of promotion and progression. Urology, 2001, 58, 835-842
86. Steiner MS; Raghov S; Neubauer BL: Selective estrogen receptor modulator for the chemoprevention of prostate cancer. Urology, 2001, 57, 68-72
87. Raghow S; Kuliyev E' Steakley M et al: Efficacious chemoprevention of primary prostate cancer by flutamide in an autochronos transgenic model. Cancer Res, 2000, 60, 4093-4097
88. Badawi AF; El-Sohemi A.: Non-steroidal anti-inflammatory drugs in chemoprevention of breast and prostate cancer. Med Hypotheses, 2001, 57, 167-168
89. Klein EA; Lippman SM; Thompson EM et al: The selenium and Vitamin E cancer prevention Trial. World J Urology, 2003, 21, 21-27
90. The Alpha-tocopherol, Beta carotene cancer prevention Study Group: the effect of vitamin E and beta carotene on the incidence of lung cancer and other cancers in male smokers. N Engl J med, 1994, 330, 1029-1035
91. Jamal A; Murray T; Samuels A et al: Cancer Statistics 2003. CA. A Cancer Journal for Clinician. , 2003, 53, 5-26
92. Frazier AL; Colditz GA; Fuchs CS: Cost-effectiveness of screening for colorectal cancer in the general population. JAMA, 2000, 284, 1954-1961
93. Winawer SJ; Zauber AG; Ho MN et al: Prevention of colorectal cancer by colonoscopic polypectomy. The National Polyp Study Workgroup. N Engl J Med, 1993, 329, 1977-1981
94. Mandel JS; Church Tr; Ederer F et al: Colorectal cancer mortality: effectiveness of biennial screening for fecal occult blood. J Natl Cancer Inst, 1999, 91, 434-437
95. Thun MJ; Namboodiri MM; Heath CW Jr et al: Aspirin use and reduced risk of fatal colon cancer. N Engl J Med, 1991, 325, 1593-1596
96. Mukerjee D; Nissen SE; Topol EJ: Risk of cardiovascular events associated with selective COX-2 inhibitors. JAMA, 2001, 286, 954-959
97. Halpern MT; Gillespie BW; Warner KE: Patterns of absolute risk of lung cancer mortality in former smokers. J Natl Cancer Inst, 1993,17, 457-464
98. Wingo PA; Cardinez CJ; Landis SH et al: Long term trends in cancer mortality in the United States. Cancer, 2003, 97, suppl 12; 3133-3275

99. Sinha R; Kulldorff M; Swanson CA et al: Dietary heterocyclic amines and the risk of lung cancer among Missouri women. Cancer res, 2000, 60, 3753-3756
100. Vineis P; Malats N; Lung M et al: Metabolic Polymorphism and susceptibility to cancer. Lyon, France, International Agency on Cancer Res, 1999
101. Ooi WL; Elston RC; Chen VW et al: Increased familial risk for lung cancer. J Natl Cancer Inst, 1986, 76, 217-222
102. Wei Q; Cheng L; Amos CI et al: Repair of tobacco-carcinogen induced DNA adducts and lung cancer risk. J Natl Cancer Inst, 2000, 92, 1764-1772
103. Wei Q; Cheng L; Hong WK et al: Reduced DNA repair capacity in lung cancer patients. Cancer Res, 1996, 56, 4103-4107
104. Wu XF; Hsu TC; Spitz MR: Mutagen sensitivity exhibits a dose-response relationship in case-control studies. Cancer Epidemiol Biomark Prev, 1996, 5, 577-578
105. Heimburger DC; Alexander B; Birch R et al: Improvement in bronchial squamous metaplasia in smokers treated with folate and Vitamin B12: report of a preliminary randomized double-blind intervention trial. JAMA, 1988, 259, 1525-1530
106. Arnold AM; Browman GP; Levine MN et al: The effect of the synthetic retinoid etretinate on sputum cytology: Results from a randomized trial. Br J Cancer, 1992, 65, 737-743
107. Lee JS; Lippman SM; Benner SE et al: A randomized placebo-controlled trial of isotretinoin in chemoprevention of bronchial squamous metaplasia. J Clin Oncol, 1994, 12, 937-945
108. Kurie JM; Lee JS; Khuri FR et al: N-(4-hydroxyphenyl)retinamide in the chemoprevention of squamous metaplasia of the bronchial epithelium. Clin Cancer res, 2000, 6, 2973-2979
109. McLarty JW; Holiday DB; Girard WM et al: Beta-carotene, vitamin A and lung cancer chemoprevention: results of an intermediary end-point study. Am J Clin Nutr, 1995, 62, 1431S-1438S
110. Omenn GS; Goodman GE; Thornquist MD et al: Effects of a combination of beta-carotene and vitamin A on lung cancer and cardiovascular disease. N Engl J Med, 1996, 334, 1150-1155
111. Pastorino U; Infante M; Maioli M et al: Adjuvant treatment of Stage I lung cancer with high-dose vitamin A. J Clin Oncol, 1993, 11, 1216-1222
112. Van Zandwijk N; Dalesio O; Pastorino U et al: EUROSCAN: a randomized trial of vitamin A and N-Acetylcysteine in patients with head and neck cancer or lung cancer. J Natl Cancer Inst, 2000, 92, 977-986
113. Lippman SM; Lee JJ; Karp dd et al: Randomized phase III intergroup trial of Isotretinoin to prevent second primary tumors in stage I non-small cell lung cancer. J Natl Cancer Inst, 2001, 93, 605-618
114. Wang X-D; Liu C; Bronson RT et al: Retinoid signaling and activator-protein 1 expression in ferrets given beta carotene and exposed to tobacco smoke. J Natl Cancer Inst, 1999, 91, 60-66
115. Papadimitrakapoulou VA; Hong WK; Lee JS et al: Low dose isotretinoin versus beta-carotene to prevent oral carcinogenesis: long-term follow-up. J Natl Cancer Inst, 1997, 89, 257-258
116. Chemoprevention Working Group: Prevention in the next millennium: Report of the Chemoprevention Working Group to the American Association for Cancer Research. Cancer Res, 1999, 59, 4743-4758
117. Holmberg L; Bill-Axelson A; Hegelsen F et al: A randomized trial comparing radical prostatectomy with watchful waiting in early prostate cancer. N Engl J Med, 2002, 347, 781-789

118. Steineck G; Helgesen F; Adolfsson J et al: Quality of life after radical prostatectomy or watchful waiting. N Engl J Med, 2002, 347, 790-796
119. Silverman MA; Zaidi U; Burnett S et al: Cancer screening in the elderly population. Hematol Oncol Clin, 2000, 14, 89-112
120. Walter LC; Covinsky KE: Cancer screening in elderly patients: a framework for individual decision-making. JAMA, 2001, 285, 2750-2756
121. Cohen HJ; Harris T; Pieper CF: Coagulation and activation of inflammatory pathways in the development of functional decline and mortality in the elderly. Am J Med, 2003, 114,180-187
122. Saliba D; Elliott M; Rubenstein LZ et al: The Vulnerable Elders Survey: a tool for identifying vulnerable older people in the community. J Am Ger Soc, 2001, 49, 1691-1699
123. Gill TM; Baker DI; Gottschalk M et al: A program to prevent functional decline in physically frail elderly persons who live at home. N Engl J Med, 2002, 347, 1068
124. Chen H; Haley W; Extermann M et al: treatment preference in the elderly cancer patients. AACR Proc, 2003, in press
125. Miller AB; Baines CJ; To T et al: Canadian national breast Screening Study 2: breast cancer detection and death rates among women aged 50-59 years. Can Med Ass J, 1992, 147, 1477-1488
126. Miller AB; To T; Baines CJ et al: Canadian National Breast Screening Study-2: 13-year results of a randomized trial in women aged 50-59 years. J Natl Cancer Inst, 2000, 92, 1490-1499
127. Nystrom L; Rutqvist LE; Wall S et al: Breast Cancer Screening with mammography: overview of the Swedish randomized trials. Lancet, 1993, 341, 973-978
128. Shapiro S: Periodic screening for breast cancer: The health insurance pilot project and its sequelae, 1963-1986. Baltimore MD. Johns Hopkins University Press, 1988
129. Wald N; Chamberlain J; Hackshaw A and EUSOMA Evaluation Committee: Report of the European Society for mastology breast screening evaluation committee. J Eur Soc mastology, 1993, 13,1-25
130. Kerlikowske K; Grady D; Rubin SM et al: Efficacy of screening mammography. A meta-analysis. JAMA, 1995, 273, 149-154
131. Gotzsche PC; Olsen O: Is screening for breast cancer with mammography justifiable? Lancet, 2000, 355, 129-133
132. Roberts C; Torgerson DJ: Baseline imbalance in randomized controlled trials. BMJ, 1999, 319, 185-191
133. de Koning HJ: Assessment of nationwide cancer-screening programs. Lancet, 2000, 355, 80-81
134. Van Dijck JAAM; Holland R; Verbeeck ALM et al: Efficacy of mammographic screening in the elderly: a case-referent study in the Nijmegen program in the Netherlands. J Natl cancer Inst, 1994, 86, 934-938
135. Randolph WM; Goodwin JS; Mahnken JD et al: Regular mammography use is associated with elimination of age-related disparities in size and stage of breast cancer at diagnosis. Ann Int Med, 2002, 137, 783-790
136. Mitra I: Breast screening: the case for physical examination without mammography. Lancet, 1994, 343, 342-344
137. Burt RW: Colon cancer Screening. Gastroenterology, 2000, 119, 837-853
138. Kronborg O; Fenger C; Olsen J et al: Randomised study of screening for colorectal cancer with fecal occult blood test. Lancet, 1996, 348, 1467-1471
139. Nelson DB; McQuaid KR; Bond JH et al: VA cooperative colonoscopy screening study group. Population based colonoscopy screening for colorectal cancer is feasible and safe: preliminary results from the VA colonoscopy screening trial. Gastrointest Endosc, 1999, 49, abstr 65

140. Kemeny MM; Bush-Devereaux E; Merriam LT et al: Cancer Surgery in the elderly. Hematol/Oncol Clin N America, 2000, 14, 169-192
141. Horninger W; Reisigl A; Rogatsch H et al: Prostate cancer screening in Tyrol, Austria, experience and results. Eur J Cancer, 2000, 36, 1322-1335
142. Labrie F; Candas B; Dupont A et al: Screening decreases prostate cancer death: first analysis of the Quebec randomized controlled trial. Prostate, 1999, 38, 83-91
143. Roberts RO; Bergstrahl EJ; Katusic SK et al: Decline in prostate cancer mortality from 1980 to 1997 and an increase in incidence trend in Olmsted County, Minnesota. J Urol, 1999, 16, 529-533
144. Mettlin C: Screening and early treatment of prostate cancer are accumulating strong evidence and support. Prostate, 2000, 43, 223-224
145. Mettlin C; Murphy GP; Babaian RJ et al: The results of a five-year early prostate cancer detection intervention. Investigators of the American cancer Society National prostate Cancer Detection Project. Cancer, 1996, 77,150-159
146. Gann PH; Hennekens PH; Stampfer MJ: A prospective evaluation of plasma prostate specific antigen for early detection of prostate cancer. JAMA, 1995, 273, 289-294
147. Oesterling JE; Jacobsen SJ; Chute CG et al: Serum prostate specific antigen in a community-based population of healthy men. Establishment of age-specific reference ranges. JAMA, 1993, 270, 860-864
148. Schroder FH; van der Crijisen-Koeter I; De Koning HJ et al: Prostate cancer detection at low prostate specific antigen. J Urol, 2000, 163, 806-812
149. Catalona WJ; Smith DS; Ornstein DK et al: Prostate cancer detection in men with serum PSA concentration up to 4.0 ng/ml and benign prostate examination. Enhancement of specificity with free PSA measurements. JAMA, 1997, 277, 1452-1455
150. Punglia RS; D'Amico AV; Catalona WJ et al: Effect of Verification Bias of Screening for Prostate Cancer by Measurements of Prostate Specific Antigen. New Engl J Med, 2003,349, 335-342
151. Catalona WJ; Partin AW; Slawin KM et al: Use of the percentage of free-prostate specific antigen to enhance differentiation of prostate cancer from benign prostatic disease: a prospective multicenter clinical trial. JAMA, 1998, 279, 1542-1547
152. Carsten S; Jung K; Lein M et al: Molecular forms of prostate-specific antigen and human kallikrein 2 as promising tools for early diagnosis of prostate cancer. Cancer Epidemiol, Biomark and prev, 2000, 9, 1133-1148
153. Etzioni R; Cha R; Cowen ME: Serial Prostate specific antigen screening for prostate cancer: a computer models evaluates competing strategies. J Urol, 1999, 162, 741-748
154. Ross K; Carter HB; Pearson JD et al: Comparative efficiency of prostate specific antigen screening strategies for prostate cancer detection. JAMA, 2000, 284, 1399-1405
155. Henschke C; McCauley DI; Yankelevitz DF et al: Early Lung Cancer Action Project: overall design and finding from baseline screening. Lancet, 1999, 354, 99-105
156. Gohagan JK; Porok PC; Hayes RB et al: The Prostate, Lung, Colorectal and Ovarian (PLCO) Screening Trial of the National Cancer Institute: history, organization, and status. Control Clin Trials, 21, 2000, suppl 6, 251s-272s
157. Holmes FF; Hearne E: Cancer stage to age relationship: implications for cancer screening in the elderly. J Am Ger Soc, 1981, 29, 55-61
158. Ershler WB; Longo DL: Aging and cancer: issues of basic and clinical sciences. J Natl Cancer Inst, 1997,89, 1489-1497
159. Sagawa M; Tsubono Y; Saito Y et al: A case-control study for evaluating the efficacy of mass screening program for lung cancer in the Miyagi prefecture. Japan Cancer, 2001, 93,588-594

160. Sono S; Li F; Yang ZG et al: Results of three year mass screening program for lung cancer using mobile, low-dose spiral computed tomography scanner. Br J Cancer, 2001,84, 25-32
161. Henschke CI; Naidich DP; Yankelevictz DF et al: Early Henschke CI; Naidich DP; Yankelevictz DF et al: Lung cancer action project: initial findings on repeat screening. Cancer, 2001, 92,153-159
162. Swenson SJ; Jett JR; Harman TE et al: Lung Cancer Screening with CT: Mayo Clinic Experience. Radiology, 2003,226,756-761
163. Celentano DD; Klassen AC: The impact of aging on screening for cervical cancer. In: Balducci L; Lyman GH; Ershler WB: Geriatric Oncology. JB Lippincott, 1992, 105-117
164. Fox SA; Roetzheim RG; Kington RS: Barriers to cancer prevention in the older person. Clinic Ger Med, 1997, 13, 79-96
165. Fox SA; Roetzheim RG; Kington RS: barriers to cancer prevention in the older person. In: Balducci L; Lyman GH; Ershler WB: Comprehensive geriatric Oncology. Harwood Academic Publishers, Amsterdam, 1998
166. Landi F; Onder G; Cesari M et al: Pain management in frail, community living elderly patients. Arch Intern Med, 2001, 161, 2721-2724

Chapter 11

DECISION ANALYSIS FOR CANCER PREVENTION AND CANCER TREATMENT IN THE ELDERLY

Martine Extermann

Program Leader, Senior Adult Oncology Program, H. Lee Moffitt Cancer Center and Research Institute, Tampa, Florida, Associate Professor of Oncology and Medicine, University of South Florida College of Medicine, Tampa, Florida.

Decision analysis can be an extremely useful tool in the approach to cancer in the elderly. Several factors contribute to this: the paucity of direct evidence from randomized trials, comorbidity, and wide variations in functionality and life expectancy. On an individual basis, the respective advantages of various treatment choices need to be estimated precisely enough to support the decision-making process. On a population level, political decisions need to be made, such as screening recommendations. We will address these various points below.

1. PAUCITY OF DIRECT DATA

Clinical trials tend to accrue younger and healthier patients than the average population of cancer patients [1,2]. This is due to design constraints, such as toxicity of treatment (e.g. high-dose Ara-C), or requirements for intact organ function (especially for early phase studies). It is unfortunately also due to a lesser propensity of physicians to offer trials to the elderly, despite a similar acceptance rate from the patient [3].

2. COMORBIDITY

Comorbid diseases can interact with cancer in several ways. They can first interfere with diagnosis, either by favoring incidental finding of early stage tumors, or by masking symptoms from a growing tumor. Certain diseases are associated with an increased incidence of cancer. This is the case for several autoimmune diseases. We describe some of them in a parallel chapter. However, more common diseases, such as diabetes, can increase the incidence of epithelial tumors, usually poorly sensitive to immune regulation, such as colon cancer. Comorbidity can also alter significantly a patient's life expectancy (Table 1) [4]. It can do it independently from the tumor, or altering the prognosis of the tumor itself [5-7]. Finally, comorbidities such as cardiovascular diseases, chronic diarrhea, etc., can force a different treatment choice than the standard treatment. Trials can rarely address comorbidity in detail. Therefore decision analysis models can be very helpful to integrate it in treatment decisions [8,4].

3. FUNCTIONALITY AND LIFE EXPECTANCY

Functional status (e.g. ECOG PS) has been repeatedly shown to alter the prognosis of cancer and its treatment [9]. However, in our experience, most elderly cancer patients do have a good performance status (0 or 1). Geriatric instruments, such as the Activities of Daily Living [10] and the Instrumental Activities of Daily Living [11], can provide additional insight into the functioning of older adults. About 60% of older cancer patients present some dependence in IADLs [12]. This is mostly a need for help rather than a full dependence. Nevertheless, geriatric studies have shown that even elderly with a low level of impairment in their function where at higher risk of developing dependence or death over the next 3 years [13]. This group of people is increasingly recognized as "vulnerable elderly", a state between a healthy and a frail elderly. Some studies did show that ADL and IADL add prognostic information when compared to ECOG PS in a multivariate model [14, 15].

4. COST-EFFECTIVENESS

The cost-effectiveness of many interventions is age-dependent. To state the obvious, life expectancy decreases as age advances. Competing causes of mortality will blunt the effect of cancer treatment on overall survival.

Table 1. Life expectancy according to comorbidity

Age	Life expectancy (Years: women)		
(Years)	Olympian	Average	Sick
65	20.0	18.5	9.7
70	15.8	14.8	8.6
75	12.1	11.5	7.3
80	8.8	8.4	5.9
85	6.1	5.9	4.5
Age		Men	
65	15.9	14.9	8.5
70	12.5	11.8	7.4
75	9.5	9.1	6.2
80	7.0	6.8	4.5
85	5.0	4.9	3.8

However, this decrease is highly heterogeneous, as shown in Table 1. Therefore the end point of interest may change: morbidity, independence, or quality of life for example. On the other hand, the incidence of most cancers increases with age. This would impact favorably the cost-effectiveness of screening and prevention strategies. Certain physiological changes of aging may also modify the yield of a test. For example fatty involution of the breast with age increases the sensitivity and specificity of mammography [16]. Cost-effectiveness analyses can help choose the best strategies in integrating modifiable factors more supply than clinical trials. Sensitivity analyses on cost-effectiveness models can also identify the main sources of costs for a strategy and help target them for reduction.

5. INDIVIDUAL DECISION TOOL VERSUS EPIDEMIOLOGICAL APPROACH

Two major approaches can be used in decision analysis for older cancer patients. The first one is epidemiological/public health. It looks at the general features of a disease in a population, its average prognosis, and defines a global approach to it. A good example is mammography screening in the elderly, or the establishment of guidelines.

The second approach is clinical decision-making. These models seek to integrate individual information with data from the literature to allow the clinician and his/her patient to make a decision. For example: should a 75 years old woman with a T1N1M0 breast cancer and moderate comorbidity receive adjuvant chemotherapy?

5.1. Some examples

5.1.1. *Individual decision tools*

5.1.1.a. Breast cancer

One of the problems a physician faces in the elderly is knowing when to give adjuvant systemic treatment, and which type. Whereas some good data are available on hormonal therapy, data on chemotherapy in women 70 and older are very sparse: 1180 women in the latest EBCTCG meta-analysis. A decision analysis model is a very good way to quantify the benefits from adjuvant treatment. It also allows for integration of various comorbidities, as long as some idea as to the prognosis of these comorbidities is available. We designed such a model [4]. A first interesting point is to note that comorbidity can outweigh age in predicting survival. A healthy 75 years old has a longer life expectancy than a 65 years old with a history of myocardial infarction (Table 1). A second point is to note that the impact of adjuvant treatment on relapse varies little with age. The impact on survival, however, begins to markedly diverge after the age of 75 (Figure 1). Another decision analysis model exists as a computer program: Adjuvant! [17]. It is designed for women of all ages. Unfortunately, it only allows to take into account a mild to moderate comorbidity.

5.1.1.b. Prostate cancer

A recently published model [18] addressed an important question: what should be the initial treatment of prostate cancer in elderly men? Radical prostatectomy, external beam radiation therapy, or watchful waiting? The

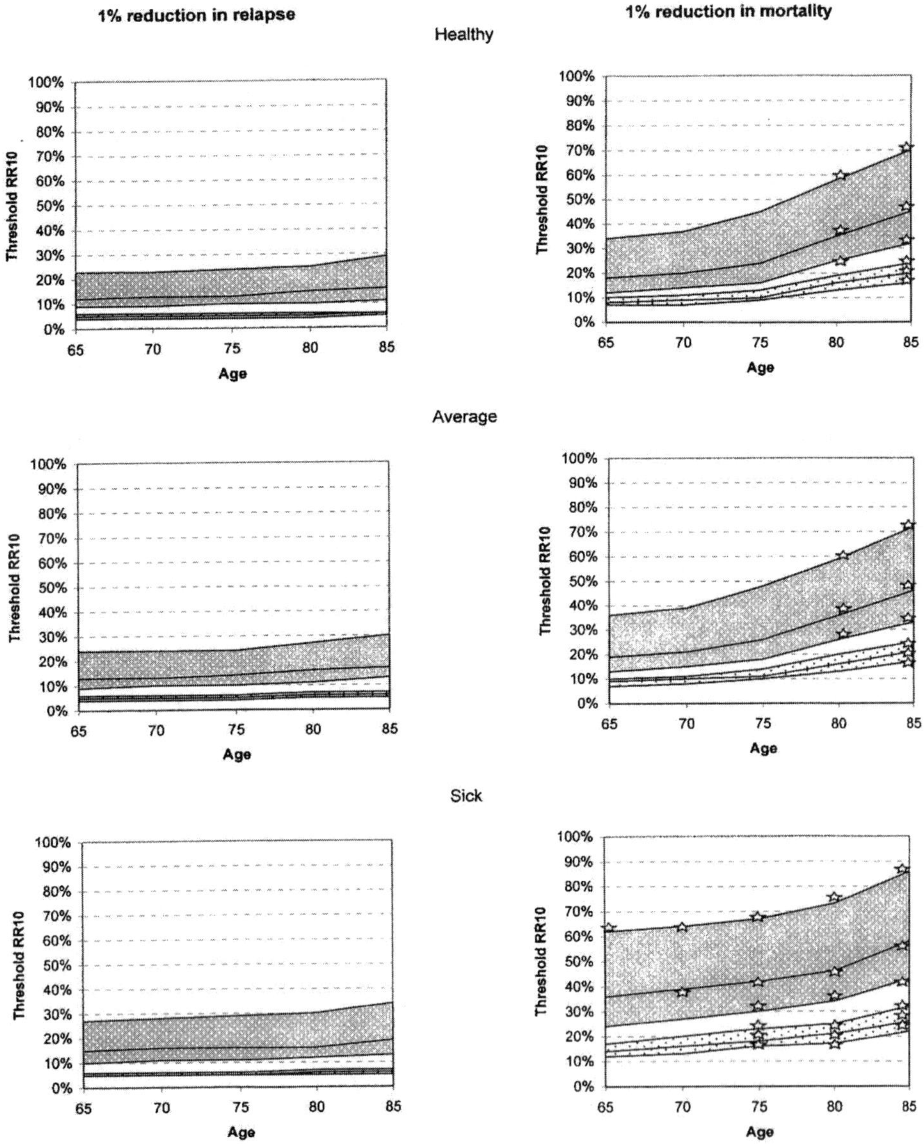

Figure 1.
Threshold RR10 for an absolute 1% reduction in relapse and mortality risks (ER+ tumors). On the left are the threshold RR10s for an absolute 1% reduction in relapse risk at 10 years. On the right are the threshold RR10s for an absolute 1% reduction in mortality risk at 10 years or, if, at 5 years. Graphs are organized from top to bottom with increasing level of comorbidity. Chemotherapy, gray area; tamoxifen, dotted area. The line in the middle of each band represents the baseline effectiveness of each treatment (50% for tamoxifen, 18% for chemotherapy). The bands represent the boundaries of the sensitivity analysis on that effectiveness (42% to 58% for tamoxifen, 10% to 26% for chemotherapy). (Reproduced with permission from Extermann 00.)

authors subclassified the cancers into three grades: Gleason 2-4, 5-7, 8-10. Their results are shown in Figure 2. They also analyzed the impact of comorbidity on the outcome. In men with Gleason 5-7 cancer, radical prostatectomy, but not radiation therapy resulted in higher quality adjusted life expectancy (QALE) for patients with mild comorbidity up to age 75, and men with moderate comorbidity up to age 65. For aggressive disease, potentially curative therapy improves QALE in men with even moderate comorbidity up to age 75.

5.1.2. *Population Approach*

5.1.2.a. Mammography screening

Two studies analyzed the impact of mammography screening of older women with an adjustment for comorbidity. The first study is a study by J. Mandelblatt and colleagues [19]. The comorbidities introduced in the model were hypertension and CHF. Screening mammography was providing savings in life expectancy up to age 85, whatever the comorbidity level. Under the baseline assumptions, the benefits were ranging from 2.17 days for healthy 65-69 years old women to 0.69 day for a healthy 85 years old, and 0.49 day for an 85 years old woman with CHF. Although these numbers may look small, the benefit for women actually having breast cancer were 617 days for an average health 65-69 years old, and 178 days for an 85 years old. For women with CHF, the benefits were 311 and 126 days respectively. When the model was adjusted for quality of life, the benefits were about 0.5 days lower on the whole population, thus canceling the benefit for the oldest and sickest women. Importantly, the model was very sensitive to the baseline risk of breast cancer. Therefore a suggested strategy to improve the effectiveness and cost-effectiveness of mammography screening would be to validate predictive risk models such as the Gail model [20] beyond the age of 70-75 years and target the higher risk women.

Another decision analysis study attempted an approach of this type [21]. The authors used bone density as a surrogate marker of estrogen levels and risk of breast cancer. They concluded that continuing mammography up to age 79 in women with the top 3 quartiles of bone mineral density would prevent 9.4 deaths/10,000, and add on average 2.1 days to life expectancy, at a marginal cost of $66,773. If mammography were used in all patients, it would prevent only 1.4 deaths/10,000, and add only 7.2 hours at a marginal cost-effectiveness of $117,689.

Recently the U.S. Preventive services task force conducted a systematic review of the cost-effectiveness of screening mammography after the age of 65 [19]. They concluded that extending a biennial screening mammography up to the age of 75-80 reduced mortality at reasonable

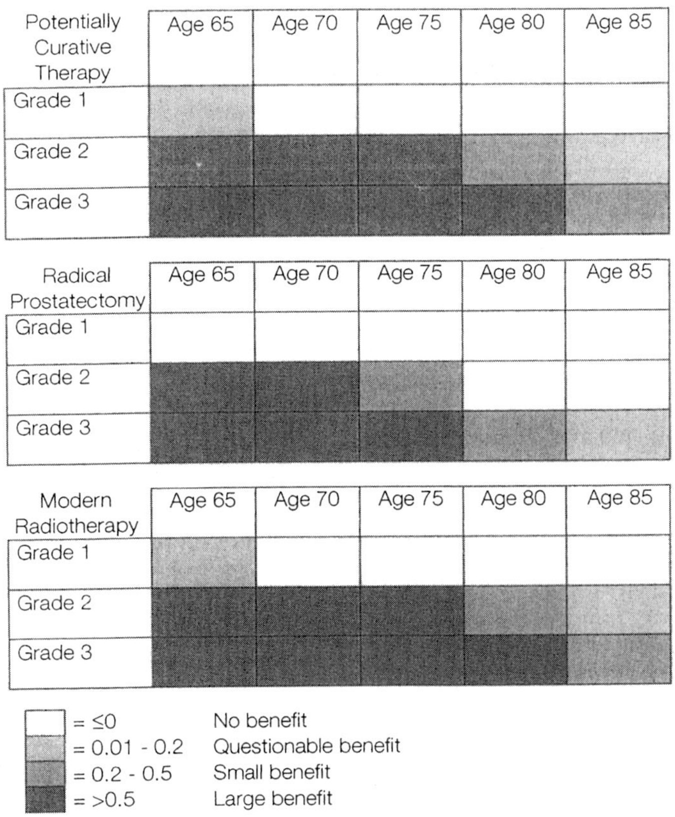

Figure 2.
QALY gained by prostate cancer patients with various treatment modalities for prostate cancer. (Reproduced with permission from Alibhai 03)

costs ($34,000 to $88,000, 2002 US dollars, per life year saved).

5.1.2.b. Colon Cancer Screening

Analyzing colon cancer screening poses a different challenge from breast cancer screening, and illustrates another possible use of decision analysis. Whereas in breast cancer, the screening strategies are quite defined and limited (i.e. mostly mammography), several options are available in colon cancer. Fecal occult blood test, digital rectal exam, sigmoidoscopy, colonoscopy, CT colonoscopy, barium enema, or any combinations thereof at variable frequencies are available. Decision analysis can help define a set of strategies that offer the best cost-effectiveness ratio and help eliminate strategies that are both less effective and more costly. A recent example is a study by Vijan et al [22]. The authors analyzed the effectiveness and cost-effectiveness of various strategies. A twice-lifetime colonoscopy at age 50 and 60 was the most effective screening strategy in terms of average gain in life expectancy and more cost-effective than flexible sigmoidoscopy combined with fecal occult blood test.

5.2. Can we integrate biological parameters?

Decision analysis models can provide ideal tools in the integration of biological markers of aging, frailty, or cancer aggressiveness. Once a model is designed, it is fairly easy to update it when new markers are discovered. Decision analysis models could also serve as screening tools when several markers or indexes are suggested, helping choose the best candidates for formal prospective testing.

6. CONCLUSIONS

Decision analysis models are a major asset for geriatric oncology. They are particularly adapted for the analysis of multiple variables that cannot be directly addressed by specific clinical trials. Technical developments such as PDAs can make these tools available at bedside for daily practice.

REFERENCES

1. Lewis JH, Kilgore ML, Goldman DP, Trimble EL, Kaplan R, Montello MJ, Housman MG, Escarce JJ. Participation of patients 65 years of age or older in cancer clinical trials. J Clin Oncol. 2003 Apr 1;21(7):1383-9

2. Hutchins LF, Unger JM, Crowley JJ, Coltman CA Jr, Albain KS. Underrepresentation of patients 65 years of age or older in cancer-treatment trials. N Engl J Med. 1999 Dec 30;341(27):2061-7

3. Kemeny MM, Peterson BL, Kornblith AB, Muss HB, Wheeler J, Levine E, Bartlett N, Fleming G, Cohen HJ. Barriers to clinical trial participation by older women with breast cancer. J Clin Oncol. 2003 Jun 15;21(12):2268-75

4. Extermann M., Balducci L, Lyman GH: What threshold for adjuvant therapy in older breast cancer patients? J Clin Oncol 18:1709-1717, 2000

5. Satariano WA, Ragland DR. The effect of comorbidity on 3-year survival of women with primary breast cancer. Ann Intern Med. 1994 Jan 15;120(2):104-10

6. Newschaffer CJ, Bush TL, Penberthy LE, Bellantoni M, Helzlsour K, Diener-West M. Does comorbid disease interact with cancer? An epidemiologic analysis of mortality in a cohort of elderly breast cancer patients. J Gerontol A Biol Sci Med Sci. 1998 Sep;53(5):M372-8

7. Meyerhardt JA, Catalano PJ, Haller DG, Mayer RJ, Macdonald JS, Benson AB 3rd, Fuchs CS. Impact of diabetes mellitus on outcomes in patients with colon cancer. J Clin Oncol. 2003 Feb 1;21(3):433-40

8. Mandelblatt JS, Wheat ME, Monane M, Moshief RD, Hollenberg JP, Tang J. Breast cancer screening for elderly women with and without comorbid conditions. A decision analysis model. Ann Intern Med. 1992 May 1;116(9):722-30

9. Frasci G, Lorusso V, Panza N, Comella P, Nicolella G, Bianco A, De Cataldis G, Iannelli A, Bilancia D, Belli M, Massidda B, Piantedosi F, Comella G, De Lena M. Gemcitabine plus vinorelbine versus vinorelbine alone in elderly patients with advanced non-small-cell lung cancer. J Clin Oncol. 2000 Jul;18(13):2529-36

10. Katz S, Ford AB, Moskowitz RW, Jackson BA, Jaffe MW: Studies of Illness in the Aged. The index of ADL: A standardized measure of biological and psychosocial function. JAMA 185:94-9, 1963

11. Lawton MP, Moss M, Fulcomer M, Kleban MH: A research and service oriented multilevel assessment instrument. J Gerontol 37:91-99, 1982

12. Extermann M, Overcash J, Lyman GH, Parr J, Balducci L: Comorbidity and functional status are independent in older cancer patients. Journal of Clinical Oncology 16:1582-7, 1998

13. Saliba D, Elliott M, Rubenstein LZ, Solomon DH, Young RT, Kamberg CJ, Roth C, MacLean CH, Shekelle PG, Sloss EM, Wenger NS. The Vulnerable Elders Survey: a tool for identifying vulnerable older people in the community. J Am Geriatr Soc. 2001 Dec;49(12):1691-9

14. Repetto L, Fratino L, Audisio RA, Venturino A, Gianni W, Vercelli M, Parodi S, Dal Lago D, Gioia F, Monfardini S, Aapro MS, Serraino D, Zagonel V. Comprehensive geriatric assessment adds information to Eastern Cooperative Oncology Group performance status in elderly cancer patients: an Italian Group for Geriatric Oncology Study. J Clin Oncol. 2002 Jan 15;20(2):494-502

15. Zagonel V, Fratino L, Piselli P, Milan I, La Copnca G, Serraino D, Monfardini S. The comprehensive geriatric assessment (CGA) predicts mortality among elderly cancer patients. Proc Am Soc Clin Oncol 21:365a, 2002

16. Carney PA, Miglioretti DL, Yankaskas BC, Kerlikowske K, Rosenberg R, Rutter CM, Geller BM, Abraham LA, Taplin SH, Dignan M, Cutter G, Ballard-Barbash R.Individual and combined effects of age, breast density, and hormone replacement therapy use on the accuracy of screening mammography. Ann Intern Med. 2003 Feb 4;138(3):168-75

17. Ravdin PM, Siminoff LA, Davis GJ, et al. Computer program to assist in making decisions about adjuvant therapy for women with early breast cancer. J Clin Oncol. 2001 19:980-91

18. Alibhai SM, Naglie G, Nam R, Trachtenberg J, Krahn MD. Do older men benefit from curative therapy of localized prostate cancer? J Clin Oncol. 2003 Sep 1;21(17):3318-27

19. Mandelblatt J, Saha S, Teutsch S, Hoerger T, Siu AL, Atkins D, Klein J, Helfand M; Cost Work Group of the U.S. Preventive Services Task Force. The cost-effectiveness of screening mammography beyond age 65 years: a systematic review for the U.S. Preventive Services Task Force. Ann Intern Med. 2003 Nov 18;139(10):835-42

20. Gail MH, Benichou J. Validation studies on a model for breast cancer risk.J Natl Cancer Inst. 1994 Apr 20;86(8):573-5. Erratum in: J Natl Cancer Inst 1994 ;86(10):803

21. Kerlikowske K, Salzmann P, Phillips KA, Cauley JA, Cummings SR. Continuing screening mammography in women aged 70 to 79 years: impact on life expectancy and cost-effectiveness. JAMA. 1999 Dec 8;282(22):2156-63

22. Vijan S, Hwang EW, Hofer TP, Hayward RA. Which colon cancer screening test? A comparison of costs, effectiveness, and compliance. Am J Med. 2001 Dec 1;111(8):593-601

Chapter 12

GUIDELINES FOR THE MANAGEMENT OF THE OLDER CANCER PATIENT

Lodovico Balducci

Lodovico Balducci, Program Leader, Senior Adult Oncology Program, H. Lee Moffitt Cancer Center and Research Institute, Tampa, Florida, Professor of Oncology and Medicine, University of South Florida College of Medicine, Tampa, Florida.

Age may influence the management of cancer in the older person in at least three areas: evaluation of the patient, increased risk of treatment complications, and changes in the biology of common tumors. The assessment of the patient involves, in addition to an estimate of life expectancy and risk of treatment complications, recognition of reversible conditions that may compromise the safety and efficacy of treatment, the patient's function and quality of life. These may include comorbidity, mild dementia, depression, anemia, and lack of adequate social support [1]. Age is also associated with increased risk of certain therapeutic complications, such as mielodepression, mucositis, neuro and cardiotoxicity following cytotoxic chemotherapy [2]. It is well recognized that the prognosis of different tumors may change with age. For example, acute myeloid leukemia and non – Hodgkin's lymphomas may become more resistant to chemotherapy, whereas the course of breast cancer may become more indolent.

The recognition that age may influence the management of cancer prompted a number of organizations to issue guidelines for the management of older individuals with cancer. The National Cancer Center Network (NCCN) and the European Organization for the Research and Treatment of Cancer (EORTC) have published a detailed set of guidelines addressing the issues of the elderly (Table 1) [3, 4]. In addition the American Society of Clinical Oncology (ASCO) has inserted age-related provisions in the

Table 1. Management Guidelines

NCCN Guidelines related to the management of older cancer patients

- All cancer patients aged 70 and older should undergo some form of geriatric assessment
- Colony-stimulating factors should be use to support prophylactically persons aged 65 and over receiving moderately toxic chemotherapy (CHOP, CA)
- Patient's hemoglobin should be kept at 12 gm/dl or higher with erythropoietin
- Doses of chemotherapy should be adjusted to the renal function of patients aged 65+
- Capecitabine should be used "in lieu " of intravenous fluorinated pyrimidines, when feasible
- Acute myelogenous leukemia in patients aged 70 + should be managed in a cancer center

EORTC Guidelines

- Prophylactic filgrastim in elderly patients with non-Hodgkin's lymphoma, small cell lung cancer, and urothelial tumors [4]

---

recommendations for the use of hemopoietic growth factors [5]. This chapter reviews the evidence that justifies existing guidelines [6] and highlight areas in which more information is wanted.

1. GUIDELINES: PRINCIPALS AND GOALS

The goals of guidelines for the diagnosis and management of diseases include [6]:

- A simple and uniform approach to the practice of medicine, comprehensive of relevant new information. To this end, the guidelines need two attributes: accessibility and plasticity.
- A framework of reference for quality assurance of medicine, nursing and health allied profession;
- Analysis of the levels of evidence that support current approach to disease. This is basilar to identify areas in which more information is necessary and urgent and to prioritize ongoing research. The level of evidence is classified according to the criteria of the United States Preventive Service Task Force [7, 8] (Table 2). At this point it is useful to underline that the goal of the guidelines is to promote the acquisition of new and better evidence in areas of uncertainty, not to discourage time-honored successful practices, such as appendectomy

for acute appendicitis, that have resulted in reduction of mortality and morbidity, even if they were developed before the definition of the rules of evidence.

Not unique of, but germane to, geriatric oncology is the definition of the adequate management end-points. The most desirable end-points of any diagnostic and treatment intervention are a reduction in mortality and a prolongation of survival. In the case of older individuals, with limited life expectancy, preservation of function and quality of life may be considered alternative end-point. In the following discussion, when appropriate, the effectiveness of an intervention will be assessed according to these end-points as well.

2. ASSESSMENT OF THE OLDER CANCER PATIENT

The NCCN recommends that individuals aged 70 and older undergo some forms of geriatric assessment [3], while the EORTC does not afford the issue. The potential benefits of the geriatric assessment include:

- Estimate of life-expectancy and tolerance of chemotherapy
- Recognition and management of conditions that may interfere with the treatment of cancer
- Adoption of a common language in the description of older patients, that may be used to interpret retrospective treatment analysis and to enroll patients in prospective clinical trials
- Preservation of function and reduction of hospitalization

The NCCN does not recommend a specific form of geriatric assessment. It recognizes that a comprehensive geriatric assessment (CGA) may not be feasible in a busy oncology practice and suggests that some form of screening be adopted to identify subjects in need of a more comprehensive evaluation. These recommendations take into account that a number of different instruments have been developed, including questionnaires, tests of physical performance and even laboratory tests, that may provide rapid and reliable information.

2.1 Evidence Supporting the Recommendation

2.1.1 Estimate of Life Expectancy and Treatment Tolerance

A number of cohort studies have demonstrated that functional deterioration, [9-13], cognitive decline [14-17], depression [18-22], comorbidity [24-26], and some geriatric syndromes, including falls [27], incontinence [28], delirium [29], failure to thrive [30], and neglect and abuse [31-33], are all associated with increased mortality (quality of evidence 2a). Though an interaction exists

Table 2. Levels of evidence

I.	Based on two or more randomized controlled clinical trials
IIa.	Based on one randomized clinical trial or on well done cohort studies
IIb.	Based on retrospective clinical studies
IIc.	Based on personal experience or anecdotic reports
IId.	Based on authoritative opinion
III.	No supportive evidence whatsoever

among functional and cognitive decline and comorbidity [34], a comprehensive index predicting the risk of mortality based on these different parameters is still wanted. The most practical application of the geriatric assessment to the prediction of life expectancy may involve the life-table methods, for long-term life expectancy (Table 3) [13]; whereas the formula of Walter et al may be used to predict short-term (one-year) mortality (Table 4) [9].

Patients who are dependent in ADLs, or who present one or more geriatric syndromes, or who have some serious forms of comorbidity fall in the lower quartile of life expectancy, those who are fully independent and with negligible comorbidity in the upper quartile, and those between these two situations in the intermediate quartiles.

2.1.2 Prediction of Chemotherapy-Related Toxicity

Two cohort studies of older cancer patients demonstrated that dependence in IADL was an independent risk factor for myelotoxicity in patients treated with moderately toxic chemotherapy [36, 37] (quality of evidence 2A). It is reasonable to recommend that both performance status and degree of functional dependence be assessed in older patients as they appear as independent variables [38].

2.1.3 Recognition of Conditions that May Interfere with Cancer Treatment and are Potentially Reversible

This claim is supported by three cohort studies (quality of evidence 2A). Of 200 patients treated in the Senior Adult Oncology Program (SAOP) at the H. Lee Moffitt Cancer Center in Tampa, who had undergone CGA at the time of the initial visit approximately 70% had severe comorbidity; 20% presented

Table 3. Life table assessment of life expectancy. Each age group is divided in quartiles of average life expectancy in years. The geriatric assessment suggests in which quartile is found each individual.

Men

Age	70	75	80	85	90
Upper quartile	18	14.2	10.8	7.9	4.3
Intermediate quartiles	12.4	9.3	6.7	4.7	2.3
Lower quartile	6.7	4.9	3.3	2.2	1

Women

Age	70	75	80	85	90
Upper quartile	21.3	17	10.8	7.9	4.3
Intermediate quartiles	15.7	11.9	6.7	3.2	2.3
Lower quartile	9.5	6.8	3.3	1.5	1

malnutrition, depression, and dementia 70% were dependent in ADL, 70% in IADL and 50% had polypharmacy [38]. The majority of these findings would have been missed without the CGA. Similar findings were recently reported by Repetto et al among Italian patients aged 65 and over [39], and by Ingram et al among Veterans aged 65 and over treated for cancer at the Durham VA Medical Center [40]. None of the studies reported the number of cases in which inadequate social support was detected. This benefit of the geriatric assessment emerged from a pilot study by Extermann et al involving 15 women aged 70 and older with early stage breast cancer. Almost 50% of these patients lacked an adequate caregiver able to support them during the administration of adjuvant treatment [41].

2.1.4 Preservation of Functional Independence and Quality of Life

A number of randomized controlled studies have demonstrated that a CGA leads to reduced hospitalization rate, and reduced rate of admission to assisted living facility in the general geriatric population (quality of evidence 1) [42-50]. It is controversial whether the performance of a CGA does lead also

Table 4. Prediction of one-year mortality following hospitalization, according to Walter [13].

A. Scores for each variable

Risk factor	Point
Male sex	1
Function: 1-4 ADL all ADL	 2 5
Comorbidity Congestive heart failure Solitary cancer Metastatic cancer Creatinine > 3 mg/dl	 2 3 8 2
Albumin 3.0-3.4 gm/dl < 3.0 gm/dl	 1 2

B. Total score and risk of one-year mortality

Total Score	1-year mortality
0-1	13%
2-3	20%
4-6	37%
>6	68%

to reduced mortality rate [42,51-54]. While no data specific for older persons with cancer are available, it is reasonable to infer that the CGA may be beneficial to all older individuals including those with cancer.

Table 5. Taxonomy of age (modified from Hamerman [34])

Type	Description	Rehabilitative needs
Primary	Fully independent Negligible Comorbidity	Health and Function Maintenance
Intermediate	• May be dependent in one or more IADL • < 3 comorbid conditions; intermediate comorbidity scores	May be rehabilitated to some extent
Secondary or frailty	Classical definition: one or more of the following: • ADL dependence • $\geq$ 1 geriatric syndrome • $\geq$ 3 comorbid conditions Alternate definition: at least three of the following: • unintentional weight loss $\geq$ 10% original body weight over one year; • self-reported exhaustion • decreased grip strength • slow movements • Difficulty in initiating movements	Prevention of further functional deterioration
Near death	Life-expectancy $\geq$ 3 months; no treatment available	No rehabilitation

2.1.5 Adoption of a Common Language in the Classification of Older Individuals Receiving Cancer Treatment or Entering Clinical Trials of Cancer Treatment

Clearly, the CGA assessment provides elements of common language, such as functional dependence, geriatric syndromes, polypharmacy, etc. These elements have not been integrated yet in a common and accepted language. Two types of approaches to the construction of such language are currently undertaken. One approach consists in subdividing older individuals into groups of different life expectancies and tolerance of treatment. Such taxonomy of aging was first proposed by Hamerman who recognized four states of aging [55] (Table 5). This classification reflects to some extent the cohort study by Rockwood et al, who demonstrated different life expectancies according to functional status and presence of one or more geriatric syndrome [28]. The main advantage of this approach is its simplicity. The main disadvantage is two fold: The definition of frailty is controversial [56, 57] and so is its reversibility. For some authors frailty represent an exhaustion of functional reserve [56], whereas for other authors it represent a critical reduction thereof that makes older individuals more vulnerable to stress [57-62]. Furthermore, even advanced stages of frailty may be reversible to some extent [63]. Second, the intermediate group of individuals is too vaguely defined and encompasses too large a gamut of conditions to be helpful in treatment-related decisions. Nevertheless, Hamerman's taxonomy has the merit to provide a frame of reference for a physiologic rather than chronologic classification of aging [55]. The other approach consists in the formulation of a comprehensive index of vulnerability capable to predict exactly the risk of death, functional decline, and therapeutic complications [58]. An example of this index is the so-called CRASH index (chemotherapy-related susceptibility high age adults) proposed by Extermann et al, which integrates both chemotherapy-related and patient-related elements. [64].

2.2 Evolution of the Geriatric Assessment

In its present forms, the geriatric assessment presents two problems: it is time-consuming and produces data that are in part subjective. Ongoing research efforts are aimed to make the geriatric assessment more user-friendly and more objective.

2.2.1 Screening Tests to Recognize Patients at Risk of Death and Functional Decline

Screening test to recognize patients who may benefit of a more "in depth" assessment include screening questionnaires, and tests of physical performance. To minimize the time investment of the geriatric assessment in a busy oncology practice, the NCCN has proposed that all patients be screened with the instrument of Lachs, a 14 item questionnaire with a sensitivity for CGA abnormalities of approximately 70% [3, 65] Other instruments, developed since the issuance of the guidelines may prove more appropriate. Examples of these instruments include the Vulnerable Elderly Survey 13 (VES 13), a 13 item questionnaire (Table 6) [58] capable to predict death and functional dependence, and a self-reported lengthy questionnaire including function, comorbidity, emotional and social resources whose feasibility was described by Ingram et al in more than 500 Veterans with cancer studied at the Durham VA Hospital [40]. These new findings illustrate

Table 6. Vulnerability

A. Vulnerability scale

Element of assessment	Score
Age • 75-84 • ≥ 85	 1 3
Self-reported health • Good or excellent • Fair or poor	 0 1
ADL/IADL. Needs helps in • Shopping • Money management • Light housework • Transferring • Bathing	 1 1 1 1 1
Activities. Needs help in •STOOPING, CROUCHING OR KNEELING •LIFTING OR CARRYING 10LBS •WRITING OF HANDLING SMALL OBJECTS •REACHING OR EXTENDING ARM ABOVE SHOULDER •WALKING 1/4 MILE •HEAVY HOUSEWORK	 1 1 1 1 1 1

B. Vulnerability scores, functional decline and survival

Score	Risk of functional decline or death
1-2 3+	11.8% 49.8%
1-3 4+	14.8% 54.9%

the evolution of the geriatric assessment and the new opportunity that may become available for a more efficient and meaningful testing.

A number of physical performance tests predict the risk of disability, functional decline and death [66-71]. Some of these tests may reasonably be used to identify older individuals in need of a complete CGA. Two tests of physical performance appear particularly promising: the "arm chair" test and the seven-item test [70, 71]. The armchair test consists of asking a person to get up from an armchair, walk ten feet and come back. The score includes: one point for using the arms of the chair to get up, one point for taking more than a second for completing the task, and one point for uncertain gait. The final score can vary from 0 to 3: the higher the score, the higher the risk of death and functional dependence. The seven-item performance test involves the performance of seven simple tasks and is scored according to the easiness by which each task is performed. Terret et al determined that this test was more sensitive than performance status in identifying abnormalities of the CGA in older patients with cancer [71].

2.2.2 *Laboratory Assessment of Aging*

A number of potential biochemical markers of aging have been described. Aging may be construed as the result of successive inflammatory episodes that lead to an accumulation of catabolic cytokines in the circulation. In addition to favor catabolism, these cytokines may activate the clotting cascade. The validity of this construct was proven by a recent study of Cohen et al [60]. These authors demonstrated that in home-dwelling individuals aged 70 and over, an increased concentration of Interleukin 6 or of D-Dimer in the circulation predicted an increment of 40-60% in risk of mortality or functional dependence in two years. When the concentration of both substances was increased, the increment in risk was 150%. For a long time, it has been known that the concentration of Interleukin 6 (IL-6) is increased in a number of aging-related conditions, from osteoporosis to Alzheimer dementia [59, 72, 73], and IL-6 has been considered a biomarker of aging. These laboratory findings suggest that measurement of circulating levels of IL-6 and possibly of other cytokines, whose concentration is associated with neurodegenerative disorders typical of aging should be included in future studies of geriatric assessment. The value of the laboratory in the clinical assessment of aging is unestablished.

2.2.3 *Conclusive Recommendations*

Some form of geriatric assessment is clearly beneficial to the management of older individuals with cancer. It appears reasonable to screen individuals aged 70+ with a short questionnaire of with some simple tests of physical performance and to execute a full assessment in individuals at risk. The value of laboratory tests and the most cost-effective screening test will be established in future studies.

2.3 Treatment-Related Recommendations

2.3.1 Dose-Adjustment According to the Glomerular Filtration Rate (GFR) in Persons Aged 65 and Older

This recommendation is based on the following findings:

- The GFR undergoes a decline in the majority of people aged 65 and older [74].
- The adjustment of the dose of methotrexate and cyclophosphamide to the GFR in women aged 65 and over with metastatic breast cancer reduced the toxicity but not the effectiveness of chemotherapy [75].
- This recommendation is fraught with a number of difficulties including the fact that the AUC of a drug is unpredictable to large extent and is at least in part dependent on pharmacogenomic [76]. The determination of the GFR is problematic: direct measurement with radioactive hippurate is not practical; and the 24-hour urine collection for the determination of the creatinine clearance is seldom accurate. The most popular measurement of the GFR include the use of formula accounting for the subject's age, sex, and serum creatinine, but this formula imply a similar decline in GFR and muscular mass in all subjects [77, 78]. Another difficulty involves the calculation of the excretion of active drug metabolites, such as idarubicinol and daunorubicinol, that account for most of the activity of the parent compound [79].
- It may be advisable to adjust the first dose of chemotherapy in individuals aged 65 and over, as long as the dose is escalated during the following cycles of chemotherapy if no toxicity is seen.

2.3.2 Use of Colony Stimulating Factors After Age 65, for Patients Receiving Moderately Toxic Chemotherapy (CHOP, CA)

This recommendation is based on multiple pieces of evidence:

- The risk of neutropenia and neutropenic infections increased after age 65 and older in the experience of three major cooperative groups: the South West Oncology Group (SWOG) [80], the Eastern Cooperative Oncology Group (ECOG) [81] and in the International Breast Cancer Study Group (IBCSG) [82] (level 2B evidence).
- In eight prospective studies of treatment of lymphoma with CHOP or CHOP like combination chemotherapy, in older patients the rate of grade iv neutropenia was consistently higher than 50%, the risk of neutropenic infections varied between 20-47% and the risk of infectious death between 5-15%, with one exception (Table 7) [83-90]. The lower patient age was 60, 65 or 70 in different studies. The

single exception to these findings was the study of Dijurdijn et al, where patients aged 65 and over were randomized to receive prophylactic G-CSF or no G-CSF. The study was well balanced in terms of age and comorbidity between the two groups of patients; however, patients randomized to G-CSF had more advanced local disease that may imply a worse prognosis [91]. Of special interest was the finding that during the first course of treatment the infection rate was much higher among the people not receiving G-CSF (32% vs 20%). The decline of infections in the following cycles may be explained by the fact that the immune defenses were restored among patients who obtained a remission of their disease, but also by the fact that most patients susceptible to infection had been eliminated from the study. The drop out rate due to infectious complications was twice as high among individuals who had not received G-CSF. Other reasons of concerns were the fact that the five year survival in both group of patients was lower than in other studies, and the infection rate was much lower both than the experience of other studies and than the North American practice experience [92]. For this reason, the NCCN has decided not to change its recommendations on account of this study.

- The demonstration by Dees et al in a small number of breast cancer patients that myelotoxicity from doxorubicin cyclophosphamide was cumulative for women aged 65 and older but not for those younger [93].
- The demonstration that filgrastim appear as active in individuals aged 70 and older as it is in younger individuals [83, 88, 91, 94-96].
- Economic considerations. Lyman et al showed that threshold risk of neutropenic infections beyond which neutropenia prophylaxis with filgrastim was cost-effective was around 20% [97], which is the case in all lymphoma studies involving individuals over 60. The threshold may even be lower for these individuals as the duration of their hospitalization is 25% longer than for the young ones [98].
- Alternative strategies to ameliorate the risk of infectious complications may not seem to work as well. Dose reduction has consistently resulted in poorer outcome [84-86, 88, 99, 100]. This finding was supported by the report of the German Lymphoma Study Group demonstrating that CHOP every two weeks in individuals aged 60-75 resulted in higher response rate and survival than standard three weekly CHOP [101]. The effectiveness of another strategy, the use of prophylactic oral antibiotics has not been proven in randomized controlled trials in the elderly [102].

In the case of acute myelogenous leukemia colony stimulating factors may improve the patient survival [103-105] and definitely reduce

Table 7. Myelodepression in elderly patients treated with a CHOP-like chemotherapy combination.

Author (s)	Patient #	Regimen	Age	Neutro-penia	Neutro-penic Fever	Treat-ment related Deaths
Zinzani (83)	161	VNCOP-B	60+	44%	32%	1.3%
Sonneveld (84)	148	CHOP CNOP	60+ 60+	NR NR	NR NR	14% 13%
Gomez (85)	249	CHOP	60+ 70+	24% 73%	8% 42%	0 20%
Tirelli (86)	119	VMP CHOP	70 + 70+	50% 48%	21% 21%	7% 5%
Bastion (87)	444	CVP CTVP	70+ 70+	9% 29%	7% 13%	12% 15%
Osby (88)						
O'Reilly (89)	63	POCE	65+	50%	20%	8%
Coiffier (90)	399	CHOP CHOP-Rituxan	60+	NR	12-20%	5%
Doorjidin (91)	374	CHOP	65+	-	32% (first course)	4%

- the duration of hospitalization for neutropenic infections (Level 1 evidence) [106].

Two major international organizations have recently issued similar recommendations. The American Society of Clinical Oncology recommended that individual aged 65 and older be treated with prophylactic filgrastim or pegrilgrastim when receiving moderately toxic chemotherapy [5]. The EORTC recommended that filgrastim be used prophylactically in patients aged 70 and older receiving adjuvant chemotherapy for breast cancer or treatment with CHOP and CHOP-like regimens for non-Hodgkin's lymphoma [4].

The prophylactic use of filgrastim or pegfilgrastim appears at present as the most prudent and cost-effective course of action for individuals aged 65-70 and over receiving moderately toxic chemotherapy regimens. In the case of large cell lymphoma and the adjuvant treatment of breast cancer this recommendation may appear even more advisable by he suggestion that dose dense treatment may improve the outcome of these patients [101]. Also in the case of lymphoma, the addition of Rituximab to the CHOP regimens, as supported be two large clinical trials [90], may enhance the risk of mielodepression.

A number of issues emerged from clinical trials may change this approach in the future and should be recognized and addressed. Perhaps the most important is the issue of cost. The basic assumption of the decision analysis of Lyman was that all episodes of neutropenic infections warranted hospital admission [97]. That policy has evolved in the USA. At present hospital admission is not warranted anymore in the absence of sepsis, liver or kidney disfunction, or pneumonia [107]. These patients may be treated as oral antibiotics as outpatients with a significant reduction of cost. Even for those who need intravenous antibiotics, the administration of these medications may occur in the outpatient setting. The study by Doordijin et al [91] suggested that the main benefit of filgrastim for older individuals treated with CHOP was a reduction in these minor infections and in the use of oral antibiotics. An analysis of all lymphoma trials in elderly individuals by Korourkis et al suggested that performance status rather than age was the main risk factor for neutropenic infections and the prophylactic use of growth factors may be limited to these individuals. Other issues of interest include the effects of growth factors on quality of life, survival, quality of life adjusted survival, and function [108].

2.3.3 Maintenance of Hemoglobin Levels ≥ 12 gm/dl with Erythropoietin

In cancer patients, the main basis of this recommendation was the increased risk of myelotoxicity associated with anemia during treatment with anthracyclines, alkaloids, épipodophyllotoxines, and camptothecins (level 2b evidence) [36, 109-113], and the increased risk of functional dependence [114-117] which is of special concerns to older individuals, more vulnerable to this complication.

This recommendation is also supported by other findings, including:

- Anemia as an independent risk factor for mortality in elderly patients [115,118-120] reported in three retrospective [118-120] and one cohort study [115].
- Anemia as a risk factor for decreased response and survival among patients receiving radiation therapy for cancer of the cervix and of the head and neck [121, 122].
- The demonstration that the highest incremental improvement in fatigue is seen when hemoglobin levels raise from 11 to 13 gm/dl [123, 124]. To this it should be added that among elderly patients the prevalence of functional independence increases in parallel with

hemoglobin levels, even within ranges of hemoglobin levels that are considered normal [115, 116, 121].

- The association of chronic anemia with coronary death, congestive heart failure and memory disorders [125-128].

2.3.4 Substitution of Intravenous Fluorinated Pyrimidines with Capecitabine

This recommendation stems from the increased incidence of mucosal toxicity from fluorinated pyriminine in older individuals, well documented in two retrospective studies (level of evidence 2c). In favor of capecitabine are:

- Two randomized controlled studies comparing capecitabine to intravenous fluorouracil in cancer of large bowel, reporting a substantial reduction in the risk of mucositis [129]. This finding could be expected, as capecitabine is a prodrug activated mainly in the liver and in the neoplastic tissue: consequently, the exposure of normal tissues to the active principle is minimized [129].
- The oral formulation allows a major flexibility in dosage

At present there is not enough evidence to extend this recommendation to other oral preparation of fluorinated pyrimidines. It should be remembered that the dose of capecitabine should be adjusted to the glomerular filtration rate that is commonly reduced in older individuals.

2.3.5 Management of Individual Tumors

The NCCN recommended that the management of individual tumors in the elderly is best trusted to the committees charged with the formulation of clinical guidelines for the management of these neoplasms. In this session we will outline age-related issues that deserve special attention and possible approaches.

2.3.5a. Acute Myelogenous Leukemia. The incidence of Acute Myelogenous Leukemia increases with age. The prognosis of AML in older individuals is poorer than in younger individuals for a number of reasons including higher prevalence of multidrug resistance, unfavorable cytogenetic changes and hypoplastic marrow [130]. In addition, poor patient conditions may make these individuals more vulnerable to treatment complications. Common sense dictates that if AML in a person aged 60 and over is treated with standard chemotherapy, this should be done preferentially in a cancer center, where supportive care with blood product and antibiotics is easily available and where a dedicated staff may provide all attention these patients need and deserve. In addition to reversal of MDR, issues to be defined include less toxic forms of induction, including monoclonal antibodies and new medications, value of supportive treatment with growth factor in patients with hypoplastic disease or myelodysplasia.

2.3.5b. Non-Hodgkin's Lymphomas.

The incidence of these conditions increases with age, and age of 60 and higher is generally considered a poor prognostic factor [131]. For large cell lymphoma there is general agreement that maintenance of the dose intensity of chemotherapy should be maintained and that filgrastim or pegfilgrastim be used to minimize myelosuppression and allow administration of chemotherapy in time. There is also general agreement the combination of rituximab and chemotherapy with CHOP is superior to CHOP alone [90]. Issues to be defined include the value of dose dense chemotherapy [101], the management of individuals with cardiovascular diseases preventing the use of an anthracycline, and the value of weekly chemotherapy over a shorter period of time [89].

For low grade lymphoma the main issue is when treatment should be initiated, and what is the most effective initial treatment, whether low dose single agent chemotherapy, combination chemotherapy, monoclonal antibodies or a combination of these compounds. Also the role of radioimmunochemotherapy should be defined.

2.3.5c. Breast Cancer. The main area of controversy is the use of adjuvant chemotherapy in women over 70, and in particular the balance of benefits and risks: A number of decision analyses may assist the practitioner in this decision [132, 133]. It appears reasonable to recommend that the use of chemotherapy be guided by an individual estimate of risk and benefit rather than by the patient chronologic age. Other issues include long-term complications of adjuvant aromatase inhibitors, and the use of single agent or combination chemotherapy in metastatic disease.

2.3.5d. Non-Small Cell Lung Cancer. The incidence of this disease among older individuals is progressively increasing [133]. The issues of concern include benefits and risk of simultaneous versus sequential radiation and chemotherapy in older individuals with locally advanced disease [134], the benefits of combination vs single agent chemotherapy in metastatic disease, and the need of a platinum compound in older individuals [135-137].

2.3.5e. Cancer of the Large Bowel. A recent meta-analysis clearly showed similar benefits of adjuvant chemotherapy for stage III disease in patients below 50 and in those over 70 [138]. Issue of interest concern the use of oral preparation and especially capecitabine in lieu of fluorinated pyrimidines and the benefits of combination chemotherapy both in the adjuvant and the metastatic setting.

3. CONCLUSIONS

The review allows the following conclusions:

1. Some form of geriatric assessment appear beneficial for older cancer patients; this assessment may allow to estimate life-expectancy and tolerance of treatment, to reveal reversible conditions that may influence the treatment, and to provide a common language to classify older individuals in clinical practice and clinical trials. The geriatric assessment is also the background of any decision analysis related to the study and the management of older patients, capable to accommodate new insights in the biology of cancer and aging and to address problems related to the management of specific diseases.
2. Some age related changes may affect the pharmacology of antineoplastic agents in the majority of older individuals and justify some general guidelines for the administration of chemotherapy that include:
   - Adjustment of the doses of the first chemotherapy to the glomerular filtration rate in individuals aged 65 and older. If no toxicity is observed, the following doses should be increased to prevent under-treatment
   - Prophylactic use of filgrastim or pegfilgrastim in patients aged 65 and older receiving chemotherapy of moderate dose intensity, comparable to CHOP
   - Maintenance of the hemoglobin of patients receiving chemotherapy at 12 gm/dl or higher
   - Aggressive management of mucositis with timely fluid resuscitation
   - Prevention of mucositis by substituting capecitabine for intravenous fluorinated pyrimidine

Specific guidelines for the management of individual diseases may be necessary as illustrated. The geriatric assessment may provide the framework of reference to estimate benefits and risks.

REFERENCES

1. Balducci L; Beghe' C: The application of geriatric principles to the management of the older cancer patient. Crit Rev Oncol Hematol, 2000, 35, 147-154

2. Cova D; Balducci L: Cancer chemotherapy in the older person. In Balducci L; Lyman GH; Ershler WB: Comprehensive Geriatric Oncology 2003, in press

3. Balducci L, Yates G: General guidelines for the management of older patients with cancer. Oncology, NCCN Proceedings, November 2000, 221-7

4. Repetto L; Biganzoli L; Kohene CH et al: EORTC cancer in the elderly task force guidelines for the use of colony-stimulating factors in elderly patients with cancer. Eur J Canc, 2003, 39, 2264-2272

5. Ozer H; Artmitage JO; Bennett CL; Crawford J; Demetri GD et al: 2004 update of recommendations for the use of hematopoietic colony-stimulating factors: evidence-based, clinical practice guidelines. J Clin Oncol, 2004, in press

6. Siddall R: Managers and medicine: weight of evidence. Health Service J, 2002, 112, 34-36

7. Harris RP; Helfan M; Woolf SH et al: Current methods of the US Preventive Service Task Force: a review of the process. Am J Prev Med, 2001, 20 (3 suppl), 21-35

8. Balducci L: The geriatric cancer patient: equal benefit from equal treatment. Cancer Control: Journal of the Moffitt Cancer Center, March/April, 8:Suppl 2:1-25, 2001

9. Reuben DB; Rubenstein LV; Hirsch SH et al: Value of functional status as predictor of mortality. Am J Med, 1992, 93, 663-669

10.Inouye SK; Peduzzi PN; Robison JT et al: Importance of functional measures in predicting mortality among older hospitalized patients. JAMA, 1998, 1187-1193

11.Siu AL; Moshita L; Blaustein J: Comprehensive geriatric assessment in a day hospital. J Am Ger Soc, 1994, 42, 1094-1099

12.Ramos LR; Simoes EJ; Albert MS: Dependence in activities of daily living and cognitive impairment strongly predicted mortality in older urban residents in Brazil. J Am Ger Soc, 2001, 49, 1168-1175

13.Walter LC; Brand RJ; Counsell RS et al: Development and validation of a prognostic index for 1 year mortality in older adults after hospitalization JAMA 2001, 285,2987-2993

14.Stump TE; Callahan CM; Hendrie HC: Cognitive impairment and mortality in Older Primary care patients. J Am Ger Soc, 2001, 49, 934-940

15.Nakanishi N; Tatara K; Ikeda K et al: Relation between intellectual dysfunction and mortality in community-residing older people. J Amer Ger Soc, 1998, 46, 583-589

16.Eagles JM; Beattie JAG; Restall DB et al: Relationship between cognitive impairment and early death in the elderly. Br Med J, 1990, 300, 239-240

17.Bruce ML; Hoff RA; Jacobs SC et al: The effect of cognitive impairment on 9-year mortality in a community sample. J Gerontol, 1995, 50B;P289- 296

18.Kivela S-L; Pahkala K: Depressive disorder as predictor of physical disability in old age. J Am Geriatr Soc, 2001, 290-296

19.Blazer DG; Hybels CF; Pieper CF: The association of depression and mortality in elderly persons: a case for multiple independent pathways. J Gerontol Med Sci, 2001, 56A, M505-509

20.Covinsky KE; Kahana E; Chin MH et al: De ressive Symptoms and three-year mortality in older hospitalized medical patients. Ann Int Med, 1999, 130, 563-569

21.Bruce ML; Leaf PJ; Rozal GP et al: Psychiatric Status and nine year mortalitydata in the new haven Epidemiologic catchment Area Study. Am J Psych, 1994, 151, 716-721

22.Lyness JM; Ling DA; Cox C et al: The importance of subsyndromal depression in older primary care patients. Prevalence and associated functional disability. J Am Ger Soc, 1999, 47, 647-652

23.Lyness JM; Noel TK; Cox C et al: Screening for depression in elderly primary care patients: a comparison of the center for Epidemiologic Studies Depression Scale and the Geriatric Depression Scale. Arch Intern Med, 1997, 157, 449-454

24.Satariano WA & Ragland DR: The effect of comorbidity on 3-year survival of women with primary breast cancer. Ann Int Med, 1994, 120, 104-110
25.Piccirillo JF; Feinstein AR: Clinical symptoms and comorbidity: significance for the prognostic classification of cancer. Cancer, 1996, 77, 834-842
26.Yancik R; Ganz PA; Varricchio CG et al: Perspectives on comorbidity and cancer in the older patient: approach to expand the knowledge base. J Clin Oncol, 2001, 19, 1147-1151
27.Tinetti ME; Williams CS: The effects of falls and fall injuries in functioning in community dwelling older persons. J Gerontol, 1998, 53A M112-119
28.Rockwood K; Stadnyk K; Macknigt C et al: A brief instrument to classify frailty in elderly people. Lancet, 1999,353, 205-206
29.Bucht G; Gustafson Y; Sandberg O: Epidemiology of delirium. Dement Ger Cogn Disord, 1999, 10, 315-318
30.Verdery RB: Failure to thrive in old age: follow-up on a workshop. J Gerontol Biol Scie Med.1997, 52, M333-336
31.Pavlik VN; Hyman DJ; Festa NA: Quantifying the problem of abuse and neglect in adults: analysis of a statewide database. J Am Ger Soc, 2001, 49, 45-48
32.Lachs MS; Williams C; O'Brien S et al: Risk factors for reported elder abuse and neglect: a nine-year observational cohort study. Gerontologist, 1997, 37, 469-474
33.Dyer CB; Pavlick VN; Murphy KP et al: The high prevalence of depression and dementia in elder abuse or neglect. J Am Ger Soc, 2000, 48, 205-208.
34.Njegovan V; Hing MM; Mitch SL et al: The hierarchy of functional loss associated with cognitive decline I older persons. J Gerontol A Biol Sci Med Sci, 2001, 56, M638-643
35.Walter LC; Covinsky KE: Cancer screening in elderly patients: a framework for individual decision making. JAMA, 2001, 285, 2750-2756
36.Extermann M; Chen A; Cantor AB et al: Predictors of toxicity from chemotherapy in older patients. Proc Am Soc Clin Oncol, 2000, 19, 617a
37.Zagonel V; Fratino L; Piselli P et al: The comprehensive Geriatric Assessment predicts mortqality among elderly cancer patients. Proc Am Soc Clin Oncol, 2002,, 21, 365 a, abstr 1458
38.Extermann M; Overcash J; Lyman GH et al: Comorbidity and functional status are independent in older cancer patients. J Clin Oncol, 1998, 16, 1582-1587
39.Repetto L; Fratino L; Audisio RA et al: Comprehensive geriatric assessment adds information to the Eastern Cooperative Group Performance status in elderly cancer patients. An Italian Group for Geriatric Oncology Study. J Clin Oncol, 2002, 20, 494-502
40.Ingram SS; Seo PH; Martell RE et al: Comprehensive assessment of the elderly cancer patient: the feasibility of self-report methodology. J Clin Oncol, 2002, 20, 770-775
41.Extermann M; Chen H; Cantor AB; Corcoran MB; Meyer J; Grendys E; Cavanaugh D; Antonek S; Camarata A; Haley WE; Balducci L: Predictors of tolerance to chemotherapy in older cancer patients: a prospective pilot study. European Journal of Cancer, 38, 1466-1473, 2002
42.Cohen HJ; Feussner JR; Weinberger M et al: A controlled trial of inpatient and outpatient geriatric assessment. N Engl J Med, 2002, 346,905-912
43.Reuben DB; Franck J; Hirsch S et al: A randomized clinical trial of outpatient geriatric assessment (CGA), coupled with an intervention, to increase adherence to recommendations. J Am Ger Soc, 1999, 47, 269-276.
44.Bula CJ; Berod AC; Stuck AE et al: Effectiveness of preventive in-home geriatric assessment in well functioning, community dwelling older people: secondary analysis of a randomized trial. J Am Ger Soc, 1999, 47, 389-395
45.Tulloch AJ; Moore V: A randomized controlled trial of geriatric screening and surveillance in general practice. J R Coll Gen Pract, 1979, 29, 733-742
46.Landi F; Onder G; Russo A et al: A new model for integrated home care in the elderly: impact on hospital use. J Clin Epidemiol, 2001, 54, 968-970

47.Bernabei R; Venturiero V; Tarsitani P et al: The comprehensive geriatric assessment: when, where, how. Crit Rev Hematol Oncol, 2000, 33,45-56
48.Boult C; Boult LB; Morishit L et al: A randomized clinical trial of outpatient geriatric evaluation and management. J Am Ger Soc, 2001, 49, 351-359
49.Inouye SK; Bogardus ST; Charpentier PA et al: A multicomponent intervention to prevent delirium in hospitalized older patients. N Engl J Med, 1999, 340:669-674
50.Tinetti ME; McAvay G; Claus G et al: A multifactorial intervention to reduce the risk of falling among elderly people living in the community. N Engl J Med, 1994, 331, 821-827
51.McCorkle R; Strumpf NE; Nuamah IF et al: A specialized home care intervention improves survival among old post-surgical cancer patients. J Am Ger Soc, 2000, 48, 1707-1713
52.Burns R; Nichols LO; Martindale-Adams J et al: Interdisciplinary geriatric primary care evaluation and management. Two-year outcomes. J Am Ger Soc, 2000, 48, 8-13
53.Stuck AE; Siu AL; Wieland GD et al: Comprehensive geriatric assessment: meta-analysis of controlled trials. Lancet, 1993, 342, 1032-1036
54.Stuck AE; Egger M; Beck JC et al: A controlled trial of geriatric evaluation. N Engl J Med, 2002,347, 371-373
55.Hamerman D: Toward an understanding of frailty. Ann Intern Med, 1999, 130, 945-950
56.Balducci L and Stanta G: Cancer in the frail patient: a coming epidemic. Hematol Oncol Clin N America, 2000, 14, 235-250
57.Fried LP; Tangen CM; Walston J et al: Frailty in older adults: evidence for a phenotype. J Gerontol Med Sci, 2001, 56A, M146-M156
58.Saliba D; Elliott M; Rubenstein LZ et al: The vulnerable elders survey: a tool for identifying vulnerable older people in the community. J Am Ger Soc, 2001, 49, 1691-1699
59.Ferrucci L; Harris TB; Guralnik JM et al: Serum Il-6 level and the development of disability in older persons. J Am Ger Soc, 1999, 47, 639-646
60.Cohen HJ; Pieper CF; Harris T: Markers of inflammation and coagulation predict decline in function and mortality in community-dwelling elderly. J Am Ger Soc, 2001, 49, S1, A3
61.Martin F: Frailty and somatopause. Growth Hormone IGF Res, 1999, 9, 3
62.Binder EF; Schechtman KB; Ehsani AA et al: Effects of exercise training on frailty in community dwelling older adults: results of a randomized controlled trial. J Am Ger Soc, 2002, 50, 1921-1928
63.Hamerman D; Berman JV; Albers GW et al: Emerging evidence of inflammation in conditions frequently affecting older adults: reports of a symposium. J Am Ger Soc, 1999, 47, 1016-1025
64.Extermann M; Bonetti M; Sledge GW; O'Dwyer PJ; Bonomi P; Benson AB III: MAX2: A convenient index to estimate the average per patient risk of chemotherapy toxicity (in submission)
65.Lachs MS; Feinstein AR; Cooney LM et al: A simple procedure for general screening for functional disability in elderly patients. Ann Intern Med, 1990, 112, 699-706
66.McDermott M; Greenland P; Ferrrucci L et al: Lower extremity performance is associated with daily life physical activity in individuals with and without peripheral arterial disease. J Am Ger Soc, 2002, 50, 247-255
67.Pavol MJ; Owings TM; Foley KT et al: Influence opf lower extremities strength of healthy older adults on the outcome of induced trip. J Am Ger Soc, 2001, 50, 256-262
68.Daltroy LH; Larson MG; Eaton HM et al: Discrepancies between self-reported and observed physical function in the elderly: the influence of response shift and other factors. Soc Sci Med, 1999, 48, 1549-1561
69.Merrill SS; Seeman TE; Kasl SV et al: Gender differences in the comparison of self-reported disability performance measures. J Gerontol Biol Sci Med Sci, 1997, 52, 19-26
70.Gill TM; Baker D; Gottshalk M et al: A program to prevent functional decline in physically frail, elderly persons who live at home. N Engl Jrnl Med, 2002, 347, 1068-1074

71. Terret C: Management and geriatric assessment of cancer in the elderly. Expert Rev Anticancer Ther, 2004, 4, 669-675
72.Ershler WB; Keller ETR: Age-associated increased interleukin-6 gene expression, late life disease and frailty. Ann Rev Med, 2000, 51, 245-270
73.Wilson CJ; Cohen HJ; Pieper CF: Cross-linked fibrin degradation products (D-dimer) , plasma cytokines, and cognitive decline in community dwelling elderly persons. J Am Ger Soc, 2003, 51, 1374-1381
74.Duthie E: in Balducci L; Lyman GH; Ershler WB: Comprehensive Geriatric Oncology, 2003, in press
75.Gelman RS; Taylor SG: Cyclophosphamide, methotrexate and 5-fluorouracil chemotherapy in women more than 65-year-old with advanced breast cancer. The elimination of age trends in toxicity by using doses based on creatinine clearance. J Clin Oncol, 1984, 2, 1406-1414
76.Gurney H: Dose calculations of anticancer drugs: a review of the current practice and introduction of an alternative. J Clin Onc, 1996, Vol. 14:2590-2611
77.Waller DG; Fleming JS; Ramsay B et al: The accuracy of creatinine clearance with and without urine collection as a measure of glomerular filtration rate. Postgrad Med J, 1991, 67, 42-46
78.Levey AS; Bosch JP; Lewis JB et al: A more accurate method to estimate glomerular filtration rate from serum creatinine: a new prediction equation. Ann Intern Med, 1999, 130, 461-470
79.Kintzel PE; Dorr RT: Anticancer Drug Renal Toxicity and elimination: dosing guidelines for altered renal function. Cancer Treat Rev, 1995,21,33-64
80.Kim YJ; Rubenstein EB; Rolston KV et al: Colony-stimulating factors (CSFs) may reduce complications and death in solid tumor patients with fever and neutropenia. Proc ASCO, 2000, 19, 612a, abstr 2411
81.Begg CB; Carbone P: Clinical trials and drug toxicity in the elderly. The experience of the Eastern Cooperative Oncology Group. Cancer, 1983, 52, 1986-1992
82.Crivellari D; Bonetti M; Castiglione-Gertsch M et al: Burdens and benefits of adjuvant cyclophosphamide, methotrexate and fluorouracil and Tamoxifen for elderly patients with breast cancer: The International Breast Cancer Study Group Trial vii. J Clin Oncol, 2000, 18, 7, 1412-1422
83.Zinzani PG; Storti S; Zaccaria A et al: Elderly aggressive histology non-Hodgkin's lymphoma: first line VNCOP-B regimen: experience on 350 patients. Blood, 1999, 94, 33-38
84.Sonneveld P; de Ridder M; van der Lelie H et al: Comparison of doxorubicin and mitoxantrone in the treatment of elderly patients with advanced diffuse non-Hodgkin's lymphoma using CHOP vs CNOP chemotherapy. J Clin Oncol 13:2530-2539, 1995
85.Tirelli U; Errante D; Van Glabbeke M et al: CHOP is the standard regimen in patients ≥ 70 years of age with intermediate and high grade non-Hodgkin's lymphoma: results of a randomized study of the European Organization for the Research and Treatment of Cancer Lymphoma Cooperative Study. J Clin Oncol, 1998,16,27-34
86.Bastion Y; Blay J-Y; Divine M et al: Elderly patients with aggressive non-Hodgkin's lymphoma: Disease presentation, response to treatment and survival. A Groupe d'Etude des Lymphomes de l'Adulte Study on 453 patients older than 69 years. J Clin Oncol 15: 2945-2953, 1997
87.Gomez H; Mas L; Casanova L et al: Elderly patients with aggressive non-Hodgkin's lymphoma treated with CHOP chemotherapy plus granulocyte-macrophage colony-stimulating factor: identification of two age subgroups with differing hematologic toxicity. J Clin Oncol 16:2352-2358, 1998
88.Osby E; Hagberg H; Kvaloy S et al: CHOP is superior to CNOP in elderly patients with aggressive lymphoma while outcome is unaffected by filgrastim treatment: results of a Nordic Lymphoma Group randomized trial. Blood, 2003, 101, 3840-3848

89.O'Reilly SE; Connors JM; Howdle S et al: In search of an optimal regimen for elderly patients with advanced-stage diffuse large-cell lymphoma: results of a phase II study of P/DOCE chemotherapy. J Clin Oncol 2250-2257, 1993

90.Coeffier B; Lepage E; Briere J; Herbrecht R; Tilly H; Bouabdallah R; Morel P; Van Den Neste, E; Salles G; Gaulard P; Reyes F; Lederlin P; Gisselbrecht C: CHOP chemotherapy plus rituximab compared with CHOP alone in elderly patients with diffuse large-B-cell lymphoma. N Engl J Med, Jan 24; 346(4): 235-42, 2002

91.Doorduijn JK; van derr Holt B; van der Hem KG et al: Randomized trials of granulocyte-colony stimulating factor (G-CSF) added to CHOP in elderly patients with aggressive non-Hodgkin's lymphoma. J Clin Oncol, 2003, 21, 2041-2050

92.Morrison VA; Picozzi V; Scotti S et al: The impact of age on delivered dose-intensity and hospitalizations for febrile neutropenia in patients with intermediate-grade non-Hodgkin's lymphoma receiving initial CHOP chemotherapy: a risk factor analysis. Clin Lymphoma, 2001, 2, 47-56

93.Dees EC, O'Reilly S, Goodman SN, Sartorius S, Levin MA, Jones RJ, Donehower RC; Fetting JH: A prospective pharmacologic evaluation of age-related toxicity and adjuvant chemotherapy in women with breast cancer. Cancer Invest, 2000, 18(6): 521-9

94.Bertini M; Freilone R; Vitolo U et al: The treatment of elderly patients with aggressive non-Hodgkin's lymphomas: Feasiblity and efficacy of an intensive multidrug regimen. Leukemia Lymphoma 22:483-493, 1996

95.Price TH; Chatta GS; Dale DC: Effect of recombinant granulocyte colony-stimulating factor on neutrophil kinetics in normal young and elderly humans. Blood, 1996, 88,335-340

96.Zagonel V; Babare R; Merola MC et al: Cost-benefit of granulocyte colony-stimulating factor administration in older patients with non-Hodgkin's lymphoma treated with combination chemotherapy. Ann Oncol, 1994, 5, suppl 2 127-132

97.Lyman GH; Kuderer N: In: Balducci L; Lyman GH; Ershler WB: Comprehensive Geriatric Oncology, 2003, in press

98.Chrischilles E; Delgado DI; Stolshek BS et al: Impact of age and colony stimulating factor use in hospital length of stay for febrile neutropenia in CHOP treated non-Hodgkin's lymphoma patients. Cancer Control, 2002, 9, 203-211

99.Meyer RM; Browman GP; Samosh ML et al: Randomized phase II comparison of standard CHOP with weekly CHOP in elderly patients with non-Hodgkin's lymphoma. J Clin Oncol, 1995, 13, 2386-2393

100.Dixon DO, Neilan B, Jones SE, Lipschitz DA, Miller TP, Grozea PN, Wilson HE: Effect of age on therapuetic outcome in advanced diffuse hisiocytic lymphoma: the Southwest Oncology Group experience. Clin Oncol, 1986, Vol. 4, 295-305

101.Wunderlich A; Kloess M; Reiser M et al: Practicability and acute haematological toxicity of 2- and 3-weekly CHOP and CHOEP chemotherapy for aggressive non-Hodgkin's lymphoma: results from the NHL-B trial of the German High Grade Non-Hodgkin's Lymphoma Study Group. Ann Oncol, 2003, 14, 881-893

102.Kerr KG: The prophylaxis of bacterial infections in neutropenic patients. J. Antimicrob Chemother, 1999 Nov; 44(5): 587-91

103.Rowe JM; Andersen JW; Mazza JJ et al: Randomized placebo-controlled phase III study of granulocyte-macrophage colony stimulating factor in adult patients > 55-70 years with acute myelogenous leukemia: a study of the Eastern Cooperative Oncology Group (E1490). Blood, 1995, 86, 457-462

104.Witz F; Sadoun A; Perrin MC: A placebo-controlled study of recombinant human granulocyte macrophage colony-stimulating factor administered during an induction treatment for "de novo" acute myelogenous leukemia in older patients. Blood, 1998, 15, 2722-2730

105.Dombret H; Chastang C; Fenaux P et al: A controlled study of recombinant human granulocyte colony-stimulating factor in elderly patients after treatment for acute myelogenous leukemia. N Engl J Med, 1995, 332, 1678-1683

106.Balducci L; Hardy CL; Lyman GH: Hemopoietic growth factors and age. Curr Opinion Hematol, 2001, Vol. 8, No. 3, 170-87
107.Hartman LC; Tschetter LK; Haberman TM et al: Granulocyte colony-stimulating factor in severe chemotherapy induced febrile neutropenia. N Engl J Med, 1997,336, 1776-1780
108.Kouroukis CT; Browman GP; Esmail R et al: Chemotherapy for older patients with newly diagnosed, advanced stage, aggressive histology non-Hodgkin lymphoma: a systematic review. Ann Intern Med, 2002, 136, 144-152
109.Pierelli L; Perillo A; Greggi S et al: Erythropoietin addition to granulocyte-colony stimulating factor abrogates life-threatening neutropenia and increases peripheral blood progenitor-cell mobilization after epirubicin, paclitaxel and cisplatin in combination chemotherapy. J Clin Oncol, 1999, 17, 1288-1296
110.Ratain MJ; Schilsky RL; Choi KE et al: Adaptive control of etoposide administration: impact of interpatient pharmacodynamic variability. Clin Pharmacol Ther, 1989, 45, 226-233
111.Silber JH; Friedman M; Di Paola RS et al: First-cycle blood counts and subsequent neutropenia, dose reduction or delay in early stage breast cancer therapy. J Clin Oncol, 1998, 16, 2392-2400
112.Schijvers D; Highley M; DeBruyn E et al. Role of red blood cell in pharmakinetics of chemotherapeutic agents. Anticancer Drugs, 1999, 10, 147-53
113.Klein CE; Gupta E; Reid JM et al: Population pharmacokinetic model for irinotecan and two of its metabolites: SN-38 and SN-38 glucuronide. Clin Pharmacol Ther, 2002,72,638-647
114.Balducci L; Hardy CH: Anemia in the older cancer patient. In: Balducci L; Lyman GH; Ershler WB: Comprehensive Geriatric Oncology, 2003, in press
115.Chaves PH; Volpato S; Fried L: Challenging the world health organization criteria for anemia in the older woman. J Am Ger Soc, 2001, 49, S3, A10
116.Nissenson AR; Goodnough LT; Dubois RW et al: Anemia: not just an innocent bystander. Arch Intern Med, 2003,163, 1400-1404
117.Ferrucci JAGS, in press
118.Kikuchi M; Inagaki T; Shinagawa N: Five-year survival of older people with anemia: variation with hemoglobin concentration. J Am Ger Soc, 2001, 49, 1226-1228
119.Izaks GJ; Westendorp RGJ; Knook DL. The definition of anemia in older persons. JAMA. 1999; 281(18): 1714–7
120.Anía BJ, Suman VJ, Fairbanks VF, et al. Incidence of anemia in older people: an epidemiologic study in a well defined population. J Am Geriatr Soc, 1997, Jul: 45(7):825-31
121.Lee WR; Berkey B; Marcial V et al: Anemia is associated with decreased survival and increased locoregional failure in patients with locally advanced head and neck cancer: a secondary analysis of RTOG 85-27. Int J Rad Oncol Biol Phys, 1998,42, 1069-1075
122.Dunst J; Kuhnt T; Strauss HG et al: Anemia in cervical cancer: impact on survival, patterns of relapse, and association with hypoxia and angiogenesis. Int J Rad Oncol Biol Phys, 2003, 56,778-787
123.Gabrilove JL; Einhorn LH; Livingston RB et al: Once-weekly dosing of epoetin alfa is similar to three-times weekly dosing in increasing hemoglobin and quality of life. Proc Am Soc Clin Oncol 1999; 18:574a
124.Cleeland CS; Demetri GD; Glaspy J et al: Identifying hemoglobin levels for optimal quality of life. Results of an incremental analysis. Proc Am Soc Clin Oncol 1999; 18:574A (abstract 2215)
125.Liao S; Ferrell BA: fatigue in an older population. J Am Ger Soc, 2000, 48, 426-430Metivier F, Marchais SJ, Guerin AP, Pannier B, London GM. Pathophysiology of anaemia: focus on the heart and blood vessels. Nephrol Dial Transplant 2000; 15(3):14–8
126.Metivier F; Marchais SJ; Guerin A; Pannier B, London GM: Pathophysiology of anaemia: focus on the heart and blood vessels. Nephrol Dial Transplant, 2000:15(3): 14-8
127.WU WC; Rathore SS; Wang Y et al: Blood transfusions in elderly patients with acute myocardial infarction, N Engl Jrnl Med, 2001, 345, 1230-1236

128.Pickett JL; Theberge DC; Brown WS; Schweitzer SU; Nissenson AR:. Normalizing hematocrit in dialysis patients improves brain function. Am J Kidney Dis 1999; 33(6): 1122–30

129.Carreca I; Balducci L: Oral chemotherapy in the older cancer patient. Am J Cancer, 2002, in press

130.Buchner T: Acute leukemia in the elderly. In: Balducci L; Lyman GH; Ershler WB: Comprehensive Geriatric Oncology, 2003, in press

131.The International Non-Hodgkin's Lymphoma Prognostic Factors Project: a predictive model for aggressive non-Hodgkin's lymphoma. N Engl J Med, 1993,329,987-994

132.Extermann M; Balducci L; Lyman G: What threshold for adjuvant tamoxifen in older breast cancer patients? A decision analysis. Eur Jrnl Can 34(suppl 1):S40, 1998

133.Baum M; Ravdin PM: Decision making in early breast cancer: guidelines and decision tools. Eur J Cancer, 2002, April; 38(6):745-9

134.Balducci L; Beghe C: Prevention of cancer in the older person. Clinics in Geriatric Medicine, 18, 505-28, 2002

135.Langer C; Scott C; Byhardt R et al: Effect of advanced age on outcome of Radiation Therapy Oncology Group Studies of locally advanced NSCLC. Lung Cancer 2000, 29, (suppl 1), 104

136.Gridelli C; Perrone F; Gallo C et al: Chemotherapy for elderly patients with advanced non-small-cell lung cancer in the elderly study (MILES) phase III randomized trial. J Natl Cancer Inst, 2003, 95, 341-343

137.Frasci G; Lorusso V; Panza N et al: Gemcitabine plus vinorelbine versus vinorelbine alone in elderly patients with advanced non small cell lung cancer. J Clin Oncol, 2000, 18, 2529-2536

138.Sargent DJ; Goldberg RM; Jacobson SD et al: A pooled analysis of adjuvant chemotherapy for resected colon cancer in elderly patients. N Engl J Med, 2001, 345, 1091-1097

INDEX